Basic Sciences for
Obstetrics and Gynaecology

Basic Sciences for Obstetrics and Gynaecology

Core Materials for MRCOG Part 1

Edited by

Austin Ugwumadu

Consultant Obstetrician and Gynaecologist,
St George's Healthcare NHS Trust
and Senior Lecturer,
St George's, University of London, London

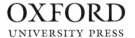

OXFORD

UNIVERSITY PRESS

OXFORD
UNIVERSITY PRESS

Great Clarendon Street, Oxford, OX2 6DP,
United Kingdom

Oxford University Press is a department of the University of Oxford.
It furthers the University's objective of excellence in research, scholarship,
and education by publishing worldwide. Oxford is a registered trade mark of
Oxford University Press in the UK and in certain other countries

© Oxford University Press 2014

The moral rights of the author has been asserted

First Edition published in 2014

Impression: 1

British Library Cataloguing in Publication Data
Data available

Library of Congress Cataloguing in Publication Data
Data available

ISBN 978-0-19-953508-8

Printed in Great Britain by Ashford Colour Press Ltd, Gosport, Hampshire

Contents

Contributors

Behdad Afzali
Clinical Lecturer in Renal Medicine
MRC Centre for Transplantation
Guy's Hospital
London
UK

Arisudhan Anantharachagan
Specialist Registrar in Obstetrics & Gynaecology
St. George's Hospital
London
UK

Tom Bolton
Ion Channels & Cell Signalling Centre
Professor of Pharmacology
Basic Medical Sciences
St George's University of London
UK

Aodhán Breathnach
Consultant Medical Microbiologist
Department of Medical Microbiology
St George's Healthcare NHS trust
London
UK

Dupe Elebute
Consultant Haematologist
King's College Hospital
London
UK

Harold Ellis CBE FRCS
Emeritus Professor of Surgery
University of London
UK

Refik Gökmen
Clinical Lecturer in Renal Medicine
MRC Centre for Transplantation
Guy's Hospital
London
UK

Roger Horton
Emeritus Professor of Neuropharmacology
St George's, University of London
UK

David Makanjuola
Consultant Nephrologist, South West Thames Renal
Transplant Network
St Helier and St George's Hospitals
London
UK

Isaac Manyonda
Consultant & Reader in Obstetrics and Gynaecology
St George's Hospital NHS Trust
London
UK

Tony Michael
Head of Graduate School (Deputy Dean of Education)
and Reader in Reproductive Science
Division of Biomedical Sciences
St George's University of London
UK

Ippokratis Sarris
Senior Registrar in Obstetrics and Gynaecology
London Deanery
UK

Austin Ugwumadu
Consultant Obstetrician and Gynaecologist
St George's Healthcare NHS Trust and
Senior Lecturer
St George's, University of London
UK

Saffron Whitehead
Emeritus Professor of Endocrine Physiology
Basic Medical Sciences
St George's, University of London
UK

Abbreviations

5HIAA	5-hydroxyindoleacetic acid	**CCF**	congestive cardiac failure
5HT	5-hydroxytryptamine	**CD**	cluster of differentiation
α-**KG**	α-ketoglutarate	**CEA**	carcino-embryonic antigen
α-**KGDH**	α-ketoglutarate dehydrogenase	**CF**	cystic fibrosis
π_c	capillary oncotic pressure	**CI**	confidence interval
π_{IF}	interstitial osmotic pressure	**CJD**	Creutzfeldt–Jakob disease
AC	alternating current	**CMV**	cytomegalovirus
ACE	angiotensin-converting enzyme	**CNS**	central nervous system
ACEI	ACE inhibitors	**CO**	cardiac output
Ach	acetylcholine	**CoA**	coenzyme A
ACTH	adrenocorticotropic hormone	**CoASH**	coenzyme A (reduced)
ADH	antidiuretic hormone	**COMT**	catecholamine-O-methyltransferase
ADP	adenosine diphosphate	**COX**	cyclo-oxygenase
AFP	α-feto protein	**CPS**	carbamoyl phosphate synthase
AGN	acute glomerulonephritis	**CPT**	carnitine palmitoyl transferase
AIDS	acquired immune deficiency syndrome	**CrCl**	creatinine clearance
ALT	alanine transaminase	**CRH**	corticotrophin-releasing hormone
AMP	adenosine monophosphate	**CSF**	cerebrospinal fluid
ANA	antinuclear antibodies	**CTP**	cytidine triphosphate
ANP	atrial natriuretic peptide	**DA**	dopamine
ANS	autonomic nervous system	**DAD**	diffuse alveolar damage
APC	antigen-presenting cell	**dATP**	deoxy-adenosine triphosphate
APTT	activated partial thromboplastin time	**DBP**	diastolic blood pressure
AR	absolute risks	**DC**	direct current
ARB	angiotensin II receptor blocker	**DCT**	distal convoluted tubule
ARDS	adult respiratory distress syndrome	**dCTP**	deoxy-cytidine triphosphate
ARND	alcohol-related neurodevelopmental disorder	**dGTP**	deoxy-guanosine triphosphate
AS	ankylosing spondylitis	**DHEA**	dehydroepiandrosterone
ASD	atrial septal defect	**DHOA**	dihydroorotic acid
AST	aspartate transaminase	**DHT**	dihydrotestosterone
AT	angiotensin	**DIC**	disseminated intravascular coagulopathy
ATN	acute tubular necrosis	**DIT**	di-iodotyrosine
ATP	adenosine triphosphate	**DNA**	deoxyribonucleic acid
AV	atrioventricular	**DOPA**	dihydroxyphenylalanine
BAPP	β-amyloid precursor protein	**dsDNA**	double-stranded DNA
BBB	blood-brain barrier	**dTMP**	deoxy-thymidine monophosphate
BM	bone marrow	**DTs**	*delirium tremens*
BMR	basal metabolic rate	**dTTP**	deoxy-thymidine triphosphate
BP	blood pressure	**DVT**	deep vein thrombosis
bpm	beats per minute	**EBV**	Epstein-Barr virus
BTK	biltong tyrosine kinase	**EC**	endocardial cushion
CAH	congenital adrenal hyperplasia	**EDRF**	endothelial-derived relaxation factor
cAMP	cyclic adenosine monophosphate	**EpO**	erythropoietin
CBG	cortisol-binding globulin	**EPSE**	extrapyramidal side effects

ER	endoplasmic reticulum
ERPF	effective renal plasma flow
ERV	expiratory reserve volume
ESBL	extended-spectrum beta-lactamase
ESR	erythrocyte sedimentation rate
ETEC	enterotoxigenic E. coli
FAD	flavin adenine dinucleotide (oxidized)
FADH$_2$	flavin adenine dinucleotide (reduced)
FBC	full blood count
FDP	fibrin degradation product
FFP	fresh frozen plasma
FMN	flavin mononucleotide
FO	fossa ovalis
FRC	functional residual capacity
FSH	follicle-stimulating hormone
G6PD	glucose-6-phosphate dehydrogenase
GABA	γ-aminobutyric acid
GAP	glyceraldehyde-3-phosphate
GAPDH	glyceraldehyde-3-phosphate dehydrogenase
GFR	glomerular filtration rate
GH	growth hormone
GHRH	growth hormone-releasing hormone
GLUT	glucose transport (protein)
GMP	guanosine monophosphate
GnRH	gonadotropin-releasing hormone
Gp	glycoprotein
GPCR	G-protein coupled receptor
GTP	guanosine triphosphate
HAV	hepatitis A virus
Hb	haemoglobin
HbA	adult haemoglobin
HbF	fetal haemoglobin
HBcAg	hepatitis B core antigen
HBeAg	hepatitis B e-antigen
HbO$_2$	oxyhaemoglobin
HBsAg	hepatitis B surface antigen
HBV	hepatitis B virus
HCG	human chorionic gonadotrophin
HDN	haemolytic disease of the newborn
HEV	hepatitis E virus
HIB	haemophilus influenzae type B (vaccine)
HIV	human immunodeficiency virus
HLA	human leukocyte antigen
HMGCoA	3-hydroxy-3-methylglutaryl-CoA
HMP	hexose monophosphate
HNPCC	hereditary non-polyposis colorectal cancer
hPL	human placental lactogen
HPV	human papillomavirus
HR	heart rate
HRT	hormone replacement therapy
HSC	haematopoietic stem cell
HSD	hydroxysteroid dehydrogenase
hsp	heat shock protein
HSP	Henoch-Schoenlein purpura
HSV	herpes simplex virus
HTLV	human T cell leukaemia virus
HUS	haemolytic uraemic syndrome
IC	inspiratory capacity

ICAM	intercellular adhesion molecule
ICDH	isocitrate dehydrogenase
IF	intrinsic factor
IFN	interferon
IGF	insulin-like growth factor
IGFBP	insulin-like growth factor binding protein
IL	interleukin
IMP	inosine monophosphate
INR	international normalized ratio
IQR	interquartile range
IRV	inspiratory reserve volume
ITP	immune thrombocytopenic purpura
IUD	intra-uterine death
IV	intravenous
JGA	juxtaglomerular apparatus
KGDH	ketoglutarate dehydrogenase
LA	left atrium
LA	local anaesthetic
LASER	light amplification by stimulated emission of radiation
LDH	lactate dehydrogenase
L-DOPA	dihydroxyphenylalanine
LFA	lymphocyte function-associated antigen
LH	luteinizing hormone
LMWH	low-molecular weight heparin
LSD	lysergic acid diethylamide
MAC	membrane attack complex
MAC	minimum alveolar concentration
MAO	monoamine oxidase
MAOI	monoamine oxidase inhibitor
MAP	mean arterial pressure
MCH	mean corpuscular haemoglobin
MCHC	mean corpuscular haemoglobin concentration
MCV	mean corpuscular volume
MDH	malate dehydrogenase
MENS	multiple endocrine neoplasia syndrome
MHC	major histocompatibility complex
MIT	mono-iodotyrosine
MMR	measles, mumps, and rubella (vaccine)
MPT	mitochondrial permeability transition
MR	metabolic rate
MRI	magnetic resonance imaging
mRNA	messenger ribonucleic acid
MRSA	methicillin-resistant S. aureus
NA	noradrenaline
NAD$^+$	nicotinamide adenine dinucleotide (oxidized)
NADH	nicotinamide adenine dinucleotide (reduced)
NADP	nicotinamide adenine dinucleotide phosphate (oxidized)
NADPH	nicotinamide adenine dinucleotide phosphate (reduced)
NDPK	nucleotide diphosphokinase
NEFA	non-esterified fatty acid
NIH	negative in health
NIS	sodium iodide symporter
NK	natural killer (cell)
NO	nitric oxide
NOS	nitric oxide synthase

NPV	negative predictive value
NSAID	non-steroidal anti-inflammatory drug
NTHI	non-typeable *H. influenzae*
nvCJD	new variant CJD
OP	ostium primum
OR	odds ratio
OS	ostium secundum
PA	pernicious anaemia
PAH	*p*-aminohippurate
Pc	capillary hydrostatic pressure
PCO$_2$	partial pressure of carbon dioxide
PCR	polymerase chain reaction
PCT	proximal convoluted tubule
PDGF	platelet-derived growth factor
PDH	pyruvate dehydrogenase
PE	pulmonary embolism
PEP	phosphoenolpyruvate
PEPCK	phosphoenolpyruvate carboxykinase
PFK	phosphofructokinase
PFO	patent foramen ovale
PGE	prostaglandin E
PGI$_2$	prostacyclin (or prostaglandin I$_2$)
PI	protease inhibitor
PID	positive in disease
P$_{IF}$	interstitial hydrostatic pressure
PKD	polycystic kidney disease
PKU	phenylketonuria
PO$_2$	partial pressure of oxygen
PPV	positive predictive value
PRF	prolactin-releasing factor
PRL	prolactin
PRPP	5-phosphoribosyl-1-pyrophosphate
PSA	prostate specific antigen
PT	prothrombin time
PTH	parathyroid hormone
PTT	partial thromboplastin time
RA	right atrium
RAAS	renin-angiotensin-aldosterone system
RAS	renin-angiotensin system
RBC	red blood cell
RCT	randomized controlled trial
RDS	respiratory distress syndrome
RF	radio frequency
RNA	ribonucleic acid
RR	relative risks
RSV	respiratory syncytial virus
RV	residual volume
SA	sinoatrial
SAA	serum amyloid A
SBP	systolic blood pressure
SCID	severe combined immunodeficiency (syndrome)
SCN	suprachiasmatic nucleus
SDH	succinate dehydrogenase
SEM	standard error of the mean
SG	specific gravity
SHBG	sex hormone-binding globulin
SLE	systemic lupus erythematosus
SNRI	serotonin-noradrenaline reuptake inhibitor
SP	septum primum
SS	septum secundum
SSPE	subacute sclerosing pan-encephalitis
SSRI	selective serotonin reuptake inhibitor
SV	stroke volume
SVR	systemic vascular resistance
T$_3$	tri-iodothyronine
T$_4$	thyroxine
TB	tuberculosis
TBG	thyroid-binding globulin
T$_C$	cytotoxic T cells
TCA	tricarboxylic acid
TCA	tricyclic antidepressant
TcR	T-cell receptor
TG	triglyceride
T$_H$	helper T cells
THC	tetrahydrocannibinol
THF	tetrahydrofolate
TIBC	total iron binding capacity
TK	tyrosine kinase
TLC	total lung capacity
TNF	tumour necrosis factor
TPO	thyroid peroxidise
TPR	total peripheral resistance
TRH	thyrotropin-releasing hormone
TSH	thyroid-stimulating hormone
TT	thrombin time
TTP	thymidine triphosphate
TTP	thrombotic thrombocytopenic purpura
TV	tidal volume
TXA$_2$	thromboxane A$_2$
UDP	uridine diphosphate
U-LGL	uterine large granular lymphocyte
VC	vital capacity
VCAM	vascular cell adhesion molecule
VDRL	Venereal Disease Reference Laboratory (test)
VLDL	very low density lipoprotein
VoD	volume of distribution
VP	vasopressin
VSD	ventricular septal defect
vWD	von Willebrand disease
vWF	von Willebrand factor
VZV	varicella-zoster virus
WASP	Wiskott-Aldrich syndrome protein
WBC	white blood cells

CHAPTER 1

General Embryology

Embryogenesis

Embryogenesis is the process by which the embryo is formed and it consists of three main phases, namely:

- fertilization
- gastrulation
- organogenesis.

  - Fertilization is the fusion of sperm and ovum to produce a zygote (see Figure 1.1). It occurs in the ampula of the fallopian tube approximately 12 hours after ovulation.

  - Following fertilization the second meiotic division of the ovum is completed, leading to the production of a haploid ovum and the second polar body.

  - Prior to nuclear fusion of the haploid gametes, the genetic material in each of the chromosomes is copied to make 23 chromosomes with 2n copies of the DNA.

  - Following the fusion of the haploid chromosomes with 2n copies of DNA, the spindles appear with the maternal and paternal 2n copies of the chromosomes arranged alongside and ready to separate. Each n copy of maternal and paternal chromosomes goes to the opposite pole to reconstitute the 46 chromosomes again. At the same time the cell membrane divides into two to make two cells, each with a diploid chromosome complement.

  - The first mitotic division of the zygote is achieved at 30 hours post-fertilization.

  - Gastrulation is the phase in early embryonic development when the three germ layers—ectoderm, mesoderm, and endoderm—are formed. It occurs in the third week of intra-uterine life. Each germ cell layer gives rise to specific organs in the developing embryo (see Figures 1.2 and 1.3). Gastrulation is followed by organogenesis.

  - The mesoderm is composed of the paraxial, intermediate, and lateral plate mesoderms (see Figure 1.3).

  - The paraxial mesoderms give rise to the somites—rounded elevations of paraxial mesoderm that appear on either side of the neural tube under the surface ectoderm on the dorsal aspect of the embryo from the base of the skull to the tail region (see Figure 1.3D). The first pair appears on day 20 of intra-uterine life and they develop at a rate of three pairs per day to a maximum number of 42–44 pairs.

  - Neurulation is the formation of the nervous system and begins when the notochord induces the ectoderm germ layer to form the neural plate, which subsequently forms the neural tube (see Figure 1.4).

  - The neural plate may be seen by day 18 of intra-uterine life while the neural tube is seen by day 22 of intra-uterine life.

  - The neural tube later differentiates into the spinal cord and the brain. The openings of the neural tube at the cranial and caudal ends are called the cranial and caudal neuropores respectively.

  - The cranial neuropore closes at day 24 while the caudal neuropore closes by day 26 of intra-uterine life. Failure of these closures leads to anencephaly and spina bifida respectively.

Chronology of the development of the embryo

The development of the embryo can be characterized chronologically by the 23 Carnegie stages based on the work by Streeter (1942) and O'Rahilly and Müller (1987), covering the first 60 days of embryonic development (see Figure 1.5).

The cardiovascular system is one of the first systems to develop. Initial components appear as angiogenic clusters in the extra-embryonic mesoderm, which line the yolk sac. The primitive heart begins to beat from about day 21 of intra-uterine life.

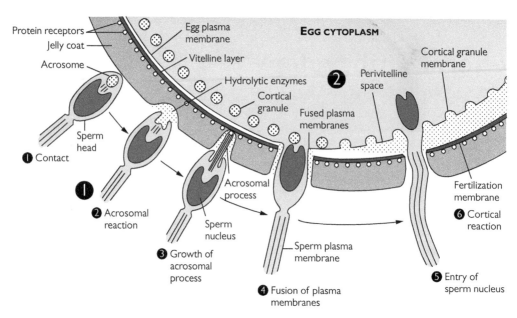

Figure 1.1 Steps of the process of fertilization of an ovum by sperm.
Reprinted from Macmillan Publishers Ltd: *Nature*, Naokazu Inoue *et al.*, 'The immunoglobulin superfamily protein Izumo is required for sperm to fuse with eggs', 434, pp. 234–238, Copyright 2005, with permission.

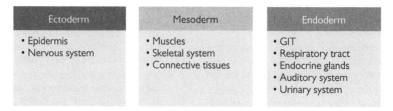

Figure 1.2 Germ cell layers and their derivatives.

The cardiovascular system consists of three main parts:

• the heart
• the arterial system
• the venous system.

■ The formation of the heart comprises of six steps, beginning with the specification of the cardiac precursor cells. These cells arise from the splanchnic mesoderm called the cardiogenic mesoderm, which can differentiate into the endocardium and myocardium.

■ The second stage of this process is the migration and merger of the cardiac precursor cells. The angiogenic cells migrate anteriorly towards the midline where they merge to form a pair of heart tubes. The heart tubes consist of the truncus arteriosus, bulbus cordis, a single ventricle and atrium, the sinus venosus, and an atrioventricular canal (Figure 1.6).

■ The heart tubes eventually fuse due to embryogenic folding to form a single heart tube. This is the third stage, also known as the 'fusion stage' of the primordial heart tubes. The single heart tube is the earliest structure similar to the mature fetal heart.

■ The fourth stage is the heart looping stage. The single heart tube eventually elongates in the pericardial cavity and by day 23 of intra-uterine life outgrows the volume of the pericardial cavity. This results in the bending or looping of the heart tube. The mechanism of this looping is poorly understood.

■ The fifth stage is the formation of the heart chambers.

■ The final stage is the formation of the valves (from the endocardial cushions) and septae.

A

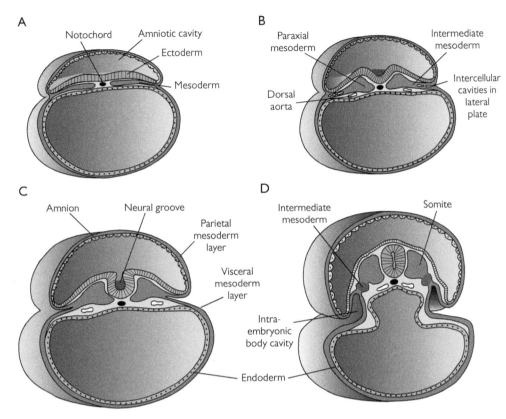

Figure 1.3 Gastrulation.

Reproduced from Thomas W. Sadler, *Langman's Medical Embryology*, 11th edition, Wolters Kluwer. Copyright 2009, with permission. http://www.lww.com.

The atrial septum is formed in five stages and begins at about the fourth week of intra-uterine life.

1. Formation of the septum primum: This septum develops from the roof of the atrium anteriorly and grows towards the endocardial cushions. The septum is crescent-shaped and thus does not completely separate the two atrial chambers (Figure 1.7a). This resultant gap is known as the ostium primum.

2. Closure of the ostium primum: As the septum primum develops, the ostium primum narrows and eventually closes.

3. Formation of the ostium secundum: This ostium forms on the septum primum as the ostium primum closes. It maintains the connection between the left and right atria.

4. Formation of the septum secundum: This septum forms to the right of the septum primum (Figure 1.7c). It originates from the posterior wall of the atria and grows over the septum primum leaving a small opening known as the foramen ovale (Figure 1.7d). The foramen ovale is continuous with the ostium secundum.

5. Regression of the septum primum: Eventually the septum primum becomes the flap that covers the foramen ovale on its left side and is known as the valve of

foramen ovale. After birth the foramen ovale becomes the fossa ovalis.

The ventricular septum is composed of two components:

1. A muscular part: This develops from the floor of the ventricle and grows towards the endocardial cushions, but stops short of these and leaves a gap.

2. A membranous part: This is formed by the endocardial cushion and the aortopulmonary septum. It accommodates the atrioventricular conducting bundle.

- The cardiac outflow tract develops from the truncus arteriosus and bulbus cordis (Figure 1.8A–H). The truncus arteriosus forms the ascending aorta and pulmonary trunk, whilst the bulbus cordis together with the primitive ventricle form the ventricles of the heart.

- The venous drainage of the heart consists of two sinuses, namely sinus venosum and sinus venarum.

- The arterial system comprises of a paired primitive aorta and the aortic arches (Figure 1.9). The primitive aorta is also known as the dorsal aorta and originates from the aortic sac. It is continuous with the umbilical artery posteriorly and the aortic arches anteriorly. They merge eventually to form the descending aorta (Figure 1.9).

3

The aortic arches are a series of six paired embryological vascular structures located in the pharynx (Figure 1.9). Although all of the arches do not exist at the same time, for convenience they will be considered together, and they give rise to the structures shown in Figure 1.10.

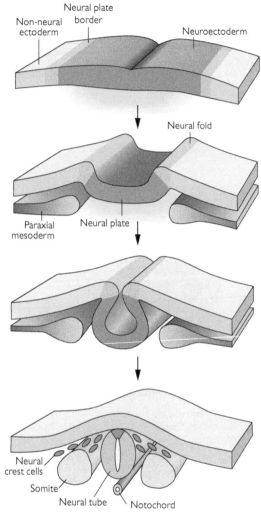

Figure 1.4 The process of neurulation.
Reprinted from Macmillan Publishers Ltd: *Nature Reviews Neuroscience*, L. S. Gammill and M. Bronner-Fraser, 'Neural crest specification: migrating into genomics', **4**, 10, pp. 795–805, Copyright 2003, with permission.

Respiratory system

The respiratory system lies relatively dormant in the fetus until birth. It consists of:

- lung buds and trachea
- respiratory accessories including visceral pleura, cartilage, smooth muscles, and blood vessels, all arising from the splanchnopleuric mesoderm
- larynx: the laryngeal epithelium arises from the endoderm while its cartilage and muscles arise from the pharyngeal arches.

- The respiratory epithelial components develop from the ventral wall of the endodermal lining of the foregut as a diverticulum, which grows into the surrounding splanchnopleuric mesoderm.
- The respiratory diverticulum eventually separates from the foregut by the development of bilateral longitudinal ridges. These ridges, which are also known as the tracheo-oesophageal folds, fuse together to form the tracheo-oesophageal septum, giving rise to the trachea and lung buds.

- The lung buds divide many times to form the bronchial tree in a process known as branching morphogenesis.
- The right lung bud divides into three secondary lung buds while the left lung bud divides into two secondary lung buds. The bronchial tree division is not complete until after birth.

Fetal lung maturation has four stages known as the glandular, canalicular, saccular, and alveolar periods. The glandular period occurs between 6 to 16 weeks of intra-uterine life. During this period most of the lung components are formed, except for the alveoli. Hence, gaseous exchange is not possible at the end of this period. The alveoli tend to develop in the canalicular period that occurs between 16 to 24 weeks of intra-uterine life. The saccular period is between 24 weeks of intra-uterine life to birth. It is during this period that the blood-air barrier is established and specialized cells of the respiratory epithelium appear. The blood-air barrier is also known as the alveolar-capillary barrier. There are two types of lung cells:

- Type 1 pneumocytes that line the alveoli
- Type 2 pneumocytes that appear at 24 weeks of intra-uterine life and are responsible for surfactant production.
  - The lung epithelium is initially cuboidal, but progressively thins with fetal maturation. Thus, respiration and gas exchange are possible only when this epithelium

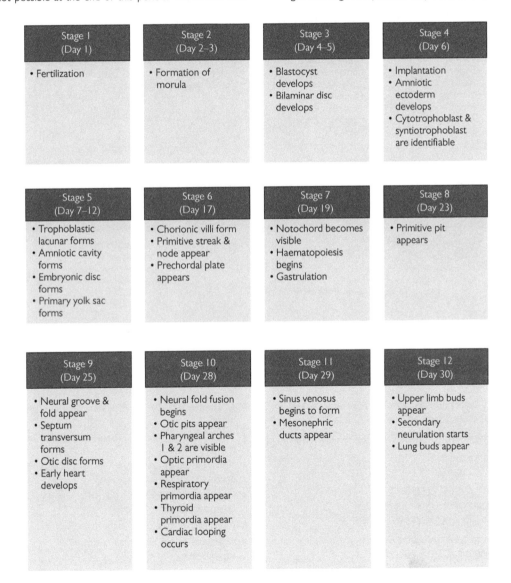

Figure 1.5 Carnegie stages.

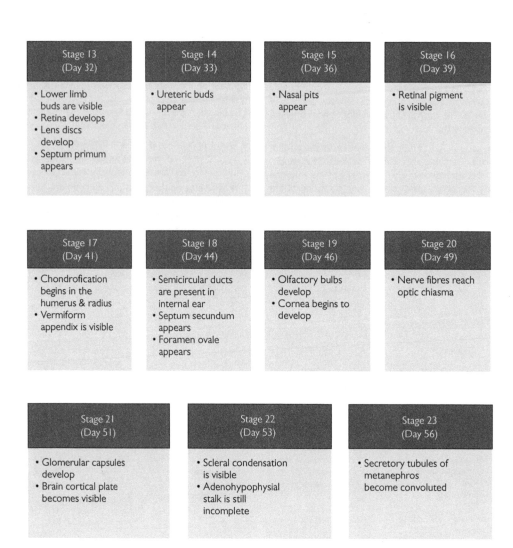

Figure 1.5 (cont.)

thins sufficiently to form a squamous epithelium. This process begins at 26 weeks of fetal life.

The diaphragm is composed of five components (Figure 1.11):

- septum transversum
- the body wall
- mesentery of the oesophagus
- pleuroperitoneal membrane
- third, fourth, and fifth cervical somites.

Structures that pass through the diaphragm and their transmitting channels:

- Caval opening (T8)—inferior vena cava and right phrenic nerve
- Oesophageal hiatus (T10)—oesophagus and vagal trunk
- Aortic hiatus (T12)—aorta, azygous vein, and thoracic duct
- Foramen of Morgagni (Larrey's triangle)—superior epigastric vessels
- Apertures of right crus—right splanchnic nerve
- Apertures of left crus—left splanchnic nerve and hemi-azygous vein.

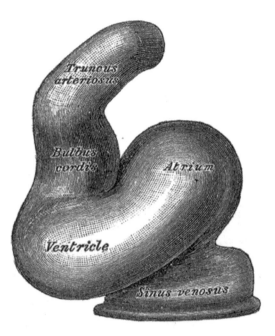

Figure 1.6 The heart tube.
This figure was published in Gray, *Anatomy of the Human Body*, Twentieth edition, throughly revised and re-edited by Warren H. Lewis, plate 462, Elsevier. Copyright the editors, 1918.

Gastrointestinal system

The gastrointestinal system is formed from the endodermal layer and comprises of:

- foregut
- midgut
- hindgut.

  ▪ The foregut begins at the mouth and ends at the entrance of the bile duct into the duodenum. It includes the oesophagus, stomach, duodenum, pancreas, and liver.

  ▪ During early fetal development the entire gut tube is suspended by the dorsal mesentery. Its essence is to facilitate the delivery of vessels and nerves from the dorsal aorta and the autonomic nervous system to developing body cavity structures. The residual adult mesentery is the double layer of peritoneum that suspends the jejunum and ileum from the posterior abdominal wall.

  ▪ The dorsal mesentery extends from the lower oesophagus to the cloaca but is lost over the duodenum, ascending colon, and descending colon, probably as a result of subsequent gut rotation.

  ▪ The ventral mesentery is smaller than the dorsal mesentery. It arises from the septum transversum and covers the stomach, terminal oesophagus, and initial portion of duodenum. The liver develops within the ventral mesentery while the spleen arises from the dorsal mesogastrium. The pancreas develops from the endodermal lining of the duodenum starting as two pancreatic buds, the dorsal and ventral buds, which begin to arise from week 4 of intra-uterine life. The dorsal bud lies within the dorsal mesentery and is the larger of the two buds, while the ventral bud lies within the ventral mesentery.

  ▪ The hepatic diverticulum arises above the pancreatic duct from the ventral wall of the duodenum. By week 10 of intra-uterine life the liver starts producing red blood cells. Prior to this the red blood cells contain a nucleus and are produced by the mesoblast.

  ▪ The midgut begins from the opening of the bile duct and ends about two-thirds of the way along the transverse colon. Its vascular supply arises from the superior mesenteric artery.

  ▪ Through fetal development the midgut rapidly elongates and outgrows the small volume of the peritoneal cavity. This leads to the herniation of the midgut via the umbilical cord at around 6 weeks of intra-uterine life (Figure 1.12a–f). As the midgut herniates out of the peritoneal cavity it rotates 90° anticlockwise along

Transection through embryonic atrial septum

En-face view of embryonic atrial septum from right atrium

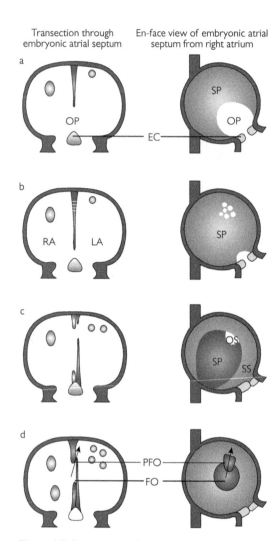

Figure 1.7 Development of the atrial septum *in utero*.
a. The septum primum grows from the roof of the atria.
b. Fenestrations develop within the septum primum. **c.** The septum secundum develops by an infolding of the atrial walls. The ostium secundum acts as a conduit for right-to-left shunting of oxygenated blood. **d.** At the anterosuperior edge of the fossa ovalis, the primum and secundum septa remain unfused, which constitutes a PFO. Arrow denotes blood flowing through the PFO from the embryonic right atrium to the left atrium. Abbreviations: EC, endocardial cushion; FO, fossa ovalis; LA, left atrium; OP, ostium primum; OS, ostium secundum; PFO, patent foramen ovale; SP, septum primum; RA, right atrium; SS, septum secundum.
Reprinted from Macmillan Publishers Ltd: *Nature Reviews Cardiology*, P. A. Calvert et al., 'Patent foramen ovale: anatomy, outcomes, and closure, **8**, 3, pp. 148–160, Copyright 2011, with permission.

its long axis. This process is known as physiological herniation. The herniation is reduced at 10 weeks of intra-uterine life when the volume of the peritoneal cavity is bigger than the length of the midgut. As the herniated midgut reduces into the peritoneal cavity it rotates a further 180° anticlockwise on its mesentery. These rotational movements explain the final positions of intra-abdominal organs in adult life.

■ The hindgut runs from the distal third of the transverse colon to the upper half of the anal canal. It derives its arterial supply from the inferior mesenteric artery. Initially the hindgut opens into the primitive cloaca, the precursor to the bladder (urogenital sinus), and the rectum (hindgut).

■ The primitive cloaca is connected to the umbilicus by the allantois, the endodermal evagination of the developing hindgut (Figure 1.13). The allantois is a sac-like structure webbed with blood vessels. It is primarily involved in nutrition and excretion, collection of liquid waste from the embryo, and the exchange of gases in the embryos of birds, reptiles, and some mammals.

■ In human embryos the allantois is comparatively small and involved with early blood formation and with the formation of the urinary bladder.

■ The allantois is initially continuous with the bladder, but as the bladder enlarges with further development and division of the urogenital sinus and the hindgut by the urorectal septum, the allantois constricts and becomes a thick, fibrous cord called the urachus, represented in the adult as the median umbilical ligament. This remnant structure lies in the space of Retzius, between the transversalis fascia anteriorly and the peritoneum posteriorly.

■ The blood vessels of the allantois become the umbilical arteries and vein (Figure 1.13). The cloacal membrane breaks down at week 7 of intra-uterine life.

■ The anal canal is derived from two embryological tissues demarcated by the pectinate line. The upper part of the anal canal is derived from endoderm while the lower part is derived from ectoderm. Thus, the upper two-thirds are lined with columnar epithelium and derive their blood supply from the superior rectal artery (which is a branch of the inferior mesenteric artery). The lower third, however, is lined with stratified squamous epithelium and derives its blood supply from the inferior rectal artery (which is a branch of the internal pudendal artery). The lumen of the anal canal is initially occluded at 7 weeks of intra-uterine life and recanalized at 9 weeks.

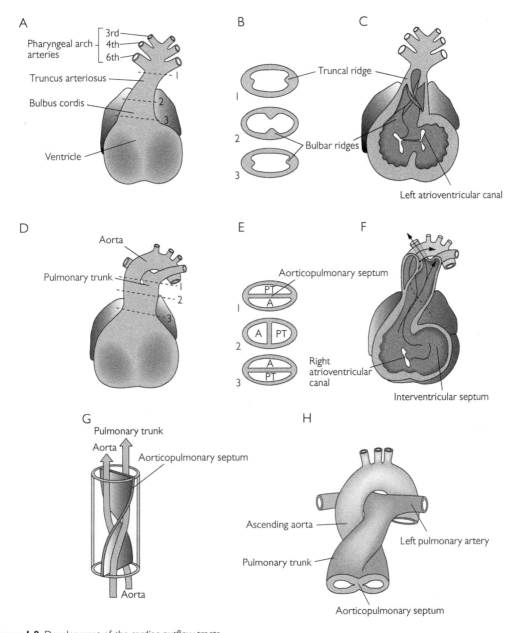

Figure 1.8 Development of the cardiac outflow tracts.
This figure was published in *Before we are Born* Seventh edition, K.L. Moore and T.V.N. Persaud, Copyright Elsevier 2008.

Urinary system

The initial structures that develop in the urogenital system have an excretory function. The two essential components necessary for the development of an excretory system are a capillary bed and the glomeruli.

The development of a kidney proceeds through three main phases:

- pronephros: appears by day 22 of intra-uterine life
- mesonephros
- metanephros: appears by fifth week of intra-uterine life.
  - Pronephros is a rudimentary organ that appears at the end of the third week of intra-uterine life. It is transient and is replaced by the mesonephros.

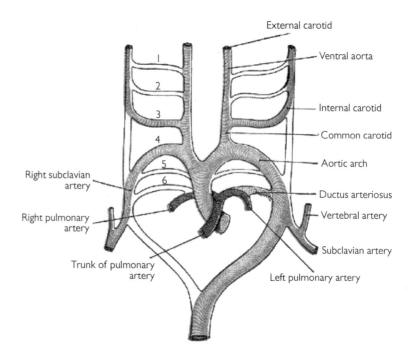

Figure 1.9 Aortic arches.
This figure was published in Gray, *Anatomy of the Human Body*, Twentieth edition, throughly revised and re-edited by Warren H. Lewis, plate 473, Elsevier. Copyright the editors, 1918.

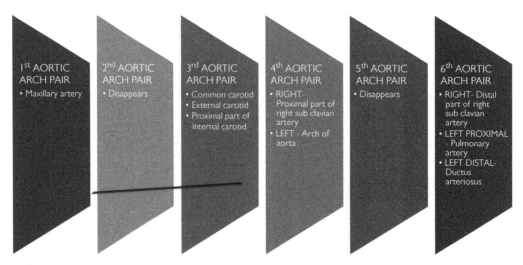

1st AORTIC ARCH PAIR	2nd AORTIC ARCH PAIR	3rd AORTIC ARCH PAIR	4th AORTIC ARCH PAIR	5th AORTIC ARCH PAIR	6th AORTIC ARCH PAIR
• Maxillary artery	• Disappears	• Common carotid • External carotid • Proximal part of internal carotid	• RIGHT- Proximal part of right sub clavian artery • LEFT - Arch of aorta	• Disappears	• RIGHT- Distal part of right sub clavian artery • LEFT PROXIMAL - Pulmonary artery • LEFT DISTAL- Ductus arteriosus

Figure 1.10 Aortic arches and their derivatives.

- The mesonephros develops in the lower thoracic and lumbar region. The cavities that appear in the mesonephros become the Bowman's capsule and join laterally to form the mesonephric duct (Figure 1.14). These ducts drain into the urogenital sinus and form the bladder trigone.

- In the male the mesonephric ducts also give rise to the ductus deferens and the efferent ductules of the testes. In the female they produce the Gardner's ducts.
- The metanephros eventually becomes the definitive adult kidney. It consists of the ureteric bud and the metanephric blastema.

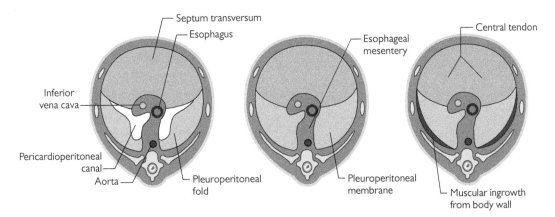

Figure 1.11 The diaphragm.
This figure was published in *Elsevier's Integrated Anatomy and Embryology*, B.I. Bogart and V. Ort, Copyright Elsevier 2007.

- The ureteric bud is an outgrowth of the mesonephric duct and begins to develop from week 5 of intra-uterine life. It eventually grows into the metanephric duct, which then forms the:
  1. definitive ureter
  2. renal pelvis
  3. calyces
  4. collecting ducts.

- The metanephric blastema is the condensation of nephrogenic cord tissue around the ureteric bud and forms the nephrons. Formation of the nephrons continues until 32 weeks of intra-uterine life. The nephrons are functional from as early as 10 weeks of intra-uterine life.

- The bladder arises from the urogenital sinus after the division of the cloaca.

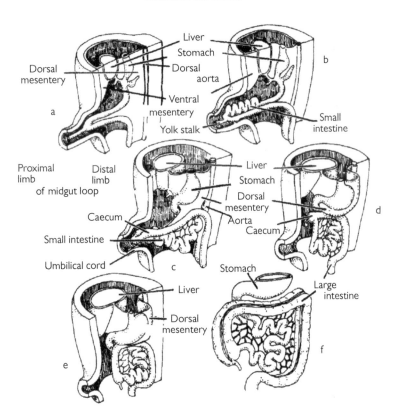

Figure 1.12 Midgut rotation.
This figure was published in *The Developing Human*, Keith L. Moore, 2nd edition. Copyright Elsevier 1977.

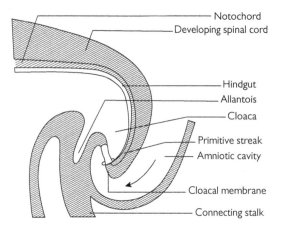

Notochord
Developing spinal cord

Hindgut
Allantois
Cloaca
Primitive streak
Amniotic cavity

Cloacal membrane
Connecting stalk

Figure 1.13 Hindgut.
This figure was publised in *The Developing Human*,
Keith L. Moore, 2nd edition. Copyright Elsevier 1977.

- The urogenital sinus also forms the Bartholin's glands and Skene's glands, which are analogous to the male prostate. It has three portions:
  1. vesico-ureteric: forms the bladder
  2. pelvic: forms the prostate
  3. phallic.
- The urogenital sinus is initially continuous with the allantois. After birth the allantois degenerates to become the urachus, forming the median umbilical ligament.

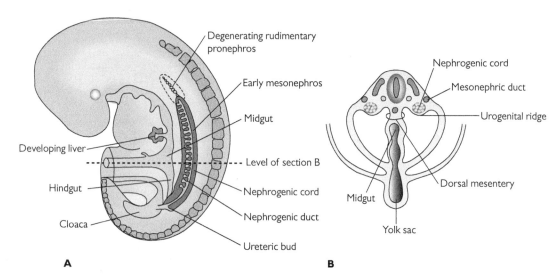

Degenerating rudimentary pronephros

Early mesonephros

Midgut

Developing liver

Level of section B

Hindgut

Nephrogenic cord

Nephrogenic duct

Cloaca

Ureteric bud

Nephrogenic cord

Mesonephric duct

Urogenital ridge

Dorsal mesentery

Midgut

Yolk sac

A   B

Figure 1.14 Development of the urinary system. **A.** Lateral view of a five-week embryo showing the extent of the mesonephros and the primordium of the metanephros or permanent kidney. **B.** Transverse section of the embryo showing the nephrogenic cords from which the mesonephric tubules develop. **C-F.** Transverse sections showing successive stages in the development of a mesonephric tubule between the fifth and eleventh weeks. Note that the mesenchymal cell cluster in the nephrogenic cord develops a lumen, thereby forming a mesonephric vesicle. The vesicle soon becomes an S-shaped mesonephric tubule and extends laterally to join the pronephric duct, now renamed the mesonephric duct. The expanded medial end of the mesonephric tubule is invaginated by blood vessels to form a glomerular capsule (Bowman's capsule). The cluster of capillaries projecting into this capsule is known as a glomerulus. This figure is adapted from a figure published in *The Developing Human. Clinically Oriented Embryology* Sixth edition, KL Moore and TVN Persaud, Copyright Elsevier 1998.

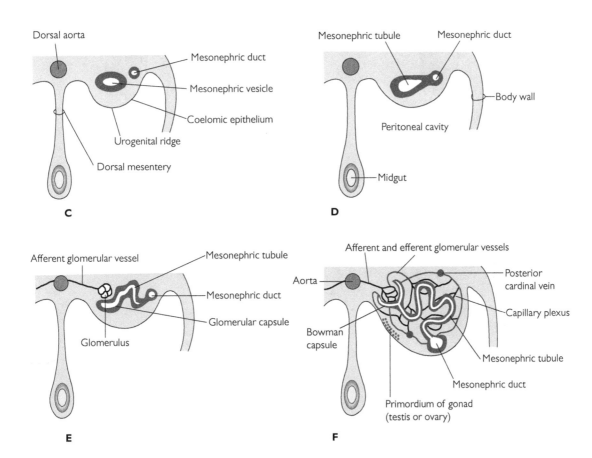

Figure 1.14 (cont.)

Reproductive system

The major organs of the reproductive system include the external and internal genitalia. The development of the reproductive system is closely related to the development of the urinary system. The development of the female internal genitalia occurs in the absence of testosterone and anti-Mullerian hormone. At first, two pairs of genital ducts arise. These are the mesonephric and paramesonephric ducts.

- The mesonephric ducts (commonly known as the Wolffian ducts) persist in the male and regress in the female due to the effect of circulating testosterone, which begins in the male fetus by 8 weeks of intra-uterine life. They connect to the urogenital sinus and lose their urinary function once the metanephros is formed (Figure 1.15). The mesonephric duct is responsible for the formation of the:
  - ductus deferens
  - epididymis
  - seminal vesicles
  - prostatic utricle
  - trigone of the bladder.

- The paramesonephric ducts are also known as the Mullerian ducts. Unlike the mesonephric ducts, they persist in the female and regress in the male. Regression of these ducts is due to the secretion of anti-Mullerian hormone in the male fetus. The ducts lie lateral to the mesonephric ducts and form the:
  - fallopian tubes
  - broad ligament
  - uterovaginal canal.

- The uterovaginal canal gives rise to the uterus, cervix, and upper half of the vagina. It eventually fuses with the sinovaginal bulb, which is the swelling on the urogenital sinus that forms the lower half of the vagina and the vaginal plate.

A

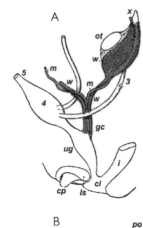

B

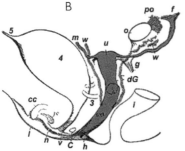

C

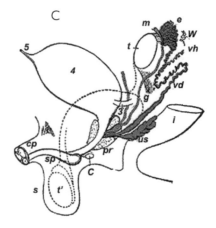

Figure 1.15 Wolffian duct degenerates in females and develops in males. This figure was published in Gray, *Anatomy of the Human Body*, Twentieth edition, throughly revised and re-edited by Warren H. Lewis, plate 1110, Elsevier. Copyright the editors, 1918.

A—Primitive urogenital organs in the embryo prior to sexual distinction	B—Female sexual organs	C—Male sexual organs
• 3. Ureter • 4. Urinary bladder • 5. Urachus • cl. Cloaca • cp. Elevation that becomes clitoris or penis • i. Lower part of the intestine • ls. Fold of integument from which the labia majora or scrotum are formed • m, m. Right and left Müllerian ducts uniting together and running with the Wolffian ducts in gc, the genital cord • ot. The genital ridge from which either the ovary or testis is formed • ug. Sinus urogenitalis • W. Left Wolffian body • w, w. Right and left Wolffian ducts	• C. Greater vestibular gland, and immediately above it the urethra • cc. Corpus cavernosum clitoridis • dG. Remains of the left Wolffian duct, such as give rise to the duct of Gärtner, represented by dotted lines; that of the right side is marked w • f. The abdominal opening of the left uterine tube • g. Round ligament, corresponding to gubernaculum • h. Situation of the hymen • i. Lower part of the intestine • l. Labium major • n. Labium minus • o. The left ovary • po. Epoophoron • sc. Corpus cavernosum urethrae • u. Uterus; the uterine tube of the right side is marked m • v. Vulva • va. Vagina • W. Scattered remains of Wolffian tubes near it (paroöphoron of Waldeyer)	• C. Bulbo-urethral gland of one side • cp. Corpora cavernosa penis cut short • e. Caput epididymis • g. The gubernaculum • i. Lower part of the intestine • m. Müllerian duct, the upper part of which remains as the hydatid of Morgagni; the lower part, represented by a dotted line descending to the prostatic utricle, constitutes the occasionally existing cornu and tube of the uterus masculinus • pr. The prostate • s. Scrotum • sp. Corpus cavernosum urethrae • t. Testis in the place of its original formation • t', together with the dotted lines above, indicates the direction in which the testis and epididymis descend from the abdomen into the scrotum • vd. Ductus deferens • vh. Ductus aberrans • vs. The vesicula seminalis • W. Scattered remains of the Wolffian body, constituting the organ of Giraldès, or the paradidymis of Waldeyer

- The external genitalia are undifferentiated until 9 weeks of intra-uterine life. The default development is towards the female phenotype in the absence of dihydrotestosterone (DHT). At about 5 weeks of intra-uterine life a cloacal fold forms on either side of the cloacal membrane. This fold forms the labia minora in females and the penile urethra in males. The fusion of the cloacal folds anteriorly gives rise to the genital tubercle. The genital tubercle elongates to form the clitoris in the female fetus and gives rise to the penis in the male fetus. Lateral to the cloacal folds are the genital swellings that form the labia majora or scrotum in the female or male fetus respectively.
- The development of the gonads starts in the form of a common primordium in the genital ridges adjacent to the developing kidney at around 4 weeks of intra-uterine life (Figure 1.16). At around 6 weeks of intra-uterine life, sex cords develop within the forming gonads. Later in intra-uterine life they differentiate into the male (testis) and female (ovary) sex organs. The differentiation into the testes is determined by the presence of the SRY gene on the Y chromosome.

- The ovary is formed by the gonadal ridge and mesonephros. It consists of a medulla and a surface germinal epithelium and contains the ova. The ova originate from the primordial germ cells that migrate from the endoderm of the yolk sac via the hindgut to the genital ridge (Figure 1.16).
- The testes comprise of two primary cells: Sertoli and Leydig cells. The Sertoli cells secrete the anti-Mullerian hormone while the Leydig cells produce testosterone. These hormonal secretions begin as early as 8 weeks of intra-uterine life.
- The testes are guided in their descent towards the labio-scrotal swelling by the gubernaculum during fetal maturation. This descent comprises of two phases. The first phase is an independent phase that occurs until the testes reach the deep inguinal ring at about 7 months of intra-uterine life. The second phase is hormone dependent and occurs from 7 to 9 months of intra-uterine life. The gubernaculum in female fetuses becomes the ovarian and round ligaments.

Placenta and fetal membranes

The choriodecidual interface is a functional fetomaternal organ and has two parts:

- chorion frondosum (the fetal part)
- decidua basalis (the maternal part).
  - The placenta begins its development from implantation and is derived from the trophoblast of the blastocyst. Trophoblastic differentiation gives rise to the cytotrophoblast and syntiotrophoblast.
  - The functional component of the placenta is the chorionic villi. The chorionic villi increase the surface area available for gaseous and substrate exchange with the maternal blood. It is the chorionic villi that are responsible for uterine decidual invasion. With time, the primary chorionic villi develop into the secondary and tertiary chorionic villi with the inclusion of mesoderm and blood vessels.
    1. Primary: Contains only trophoblast (Figure 1.17).
    2. Secondary: Contains trophoblast and mesoderm (Figure 1.18).
    3. Tertiary: Contains trophoblast, mesoderm, and blood vessels (Figures 1.18 and 1.19).
  - Fibrinoid deposition occurs in the placenta from as early as 4 months of gestation. Accumulation of the fibrin occurs in three regions of the placenta:

    1. subchorial Langhan's layer within the chorion plate
    2. Rohr's layer beneath the stem villi within the basal plate
    3. Nitabutch's layer in the decidua basalis within the basal plate (this is the layer from which the placenta detaches at birth).
  - 'Fetal membranes' is the term applied to structures derived from the blastocyte that do not contribute to the embryo. They are made up of the amnion, chorion, yolk sac, and allantois. The amnion has no blood vessels, lymphatics, or nerves and consists of five layers:
    1. cuboidal epithelium
    2. basement membrane
    3. compact layer
    4. fibroblast layer
    5. spongy layer (remnant of extra-embryonic coelom).
  - The chorion is composed of four layers:
    1. cellular layer
    2. reticular layer
    3. basement membrane
    4. trophoblast.

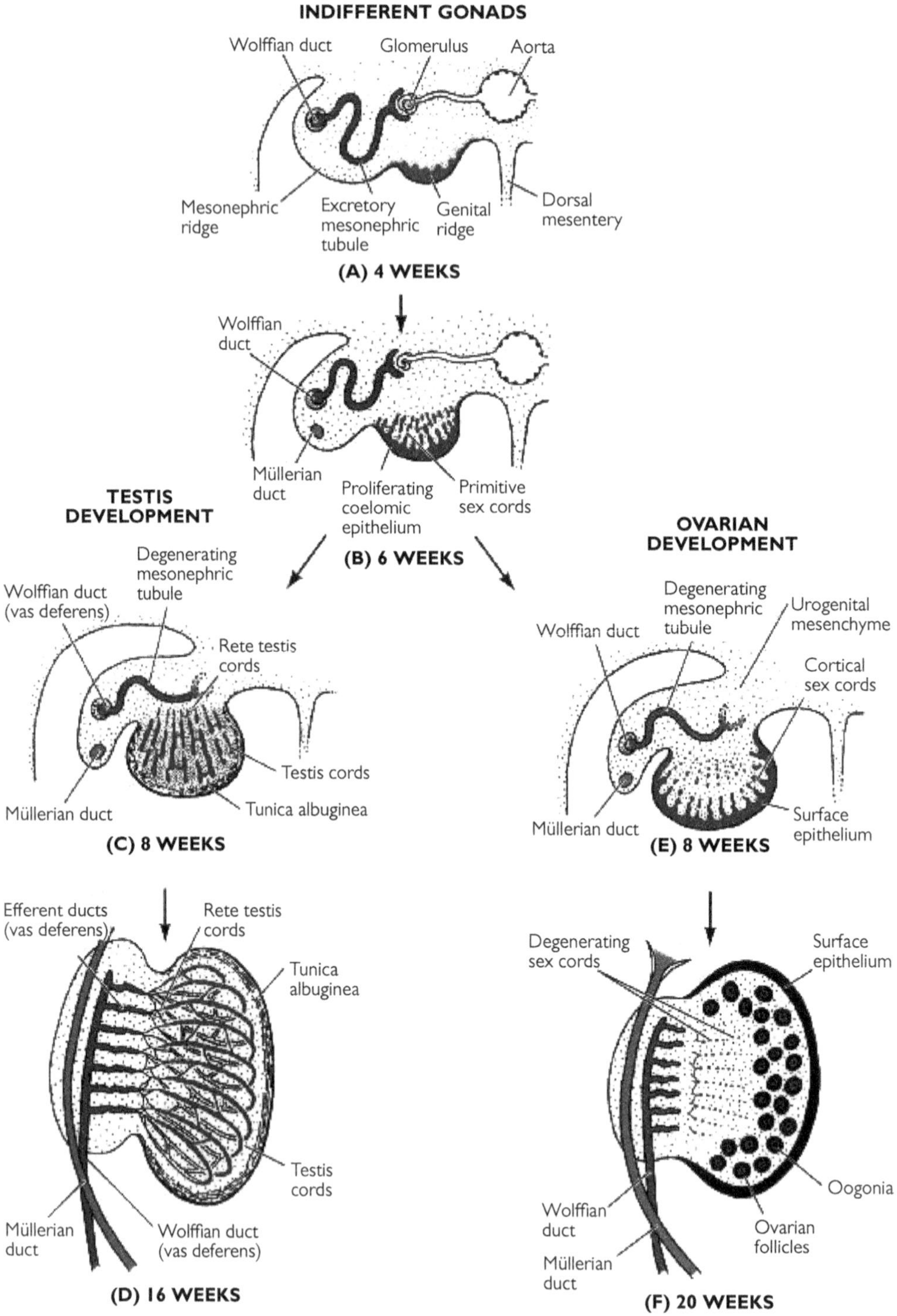

INDIFFERENT GONADS

Wolffian duct   Glomerulus   Aorta

Mesonephric ridge   Excretory mesonephric tubule   Genital ridge   Dorsal mesentery

(A) 4 WEEKS

Wolffian duct

Müllerian duct   Proliferating coelomic epithelium   Primitive sex cords

(B) 6 WEEKS

TESTIS DEVELOPMENT

Degenerating mesonephric tubule

Wolffian duct (vas deferens)

Rete testis cords

Müllerian duct

Testis cords

Tunica albuginea

(C) 8 WEEKS

Efferent ducts (vas deferens)   Rete testis cords

Tunica albuginea

Müllerian duct   Wolffian duct (vas deferens)

Testis cords

(D) 16 WEEKS

OVARIAN DEVELOPMENT

Degenerating mesonephric tubule   Urogenital mesenchyme

Wolffian duct

Cortical sex cords

Müllerian duct

Surface epithelium

(E) 8 WEEKS

Degenerating sex cords   Surface epithelium

Oogonia

Wolffian duct   Ovarian follicles

Müllerian duct

(F) 20 WEEKS

Figure 1.16 Differentiation of the human gonad in transverse section.
Reproduced from SF Gilbert, *Developmental Biology*, 6th edition, Sinauer, with permission. Copyright 2000.

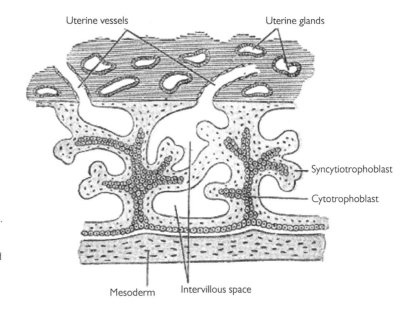

Figure 1.17 Primary chorionic villi.
This figure was published in Gray,
Anatomy of the Human Body,
Twentieth edition, throughly revised
and re-edited by Warren H. Lewis,
plate 36, Elsevier. Copyright the
editors, 1918.

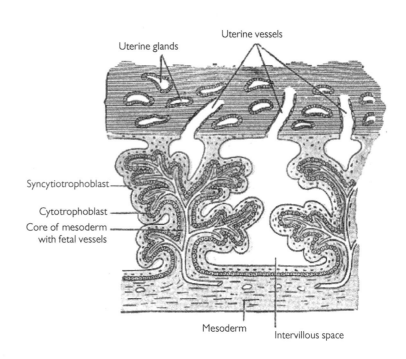

Figure 1.18 Secondary chorionic
villi.
This figure was published in Gray,
Anatomy of the Human Body,
Twentieth edition, throughly revised
and re-edited by Warren H. Lewis,
plate 37, Elsevier. Copyright the
editors, 1918.

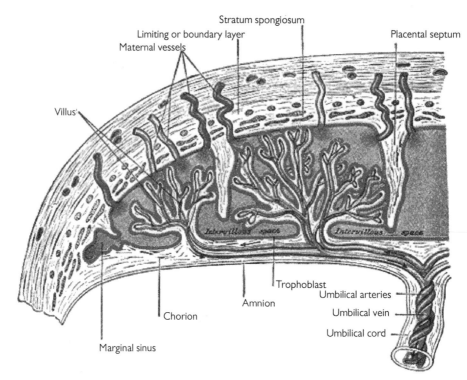

Figure 1.19 Placental circulation and its layers.
This figure was published in Gray, *Anatomy of the Human Body*, Twentieth edition, throughly revised and re-edited by Warren H. Lewis, plate 39, Elsevier. Copyright the editors, 1918.

References

O'Rahilly, R. & Muller, F. Developmental stages in human embryo development. *Carnegie Institution of Washington* 1987; Publ. 63

Streeter, G. L. Developmental horizons in human embryos. Description of age group XI, 13 to 20 somites, and age group XII, 21 to 29 somites. *Carnegie Institution of Washington* 1942; Publ. 541: *Contrib. Embryol.*, **30**, 211–245.

CHAPTER 2

Anatomy

The anterior abdominal wall

There is no deep fascia over the trunk; it would render deep breathing or abdominal distension impossible. The muscles of the anterior abdominal wall have several functions:

- They flex the trunk.
- They are accessory muscles of respiration in forcible expiration and coughing.
- They are used in defecation, micturition, and parturition.
- They protect the abdominal viscera against trauma.

The anterior abdominal wall muscles include the rectus abdominis and the three lateral muscles (Figure 2.1).

Rectus abdominis

- This arises from the pubic crest and inserts into the fifth to seventh costal cartilages.
- It occupies about two-thirds of the anterior abdominal wall. Its outlines can easily be defined in subjects of normal build by the midline linea alba and the linea semilunaris along its curved lateral border when the abdominal muscles are tensed.
- It is contained within the fibrous rectus sheath, formed in the main by a split in the aponeurosis of the internal oblique muscle.
- Posteriorly this is reinforced by the aponeurosis of the transversus abdominis and anteriorly by the external oblique.
- Below a level roughly halfway between the umbilicus and the pubic crest, demarcated by the rather ill-defined arcuate line of Douglas, the aponeuroses all pass in front of the rectus. This gap enables the inferior epigastric vessels, which arise from the external iliacs, to pass upwards into the posterior sheath (Figure 2.2).
- Above the costal margin the posterior sheath is also absent; the uppermost part of the rectus abdominis lies directly against, and attached to, the fifth to seventh costal cartilages. Here the anterior sheath is made up entirely of the aponeurosis of the external oblique.
- The anterior sheath is closely adherent to the rectus muscle, while the posterior part of the sheath is only loosely attached by connective tissue. This enables local anaesthetic solution to pass freely up and down this space in an abdominal wall field block.

The lateral muscles

- These fill the space between the lumbar muscles and rectus abdominis and between the costal margin and the iliac crest.
- Their medial aponeurotic expansions constitute the rectus sheath.
- Above the level of the iliac crest, the fibres of the *external oblique* muscle pass downwards and medially, those of the *internal oblique* pass upwards and forwards, and those of the *transverses abdominis* run transversely. Below this line, these muscles become aponeurotic and their fibres pass downwards and medially in the formation of the inguinal canal.
- The *inguinal ligament*, passing from the anterior superior iliac spine to the pubic tubercle, represents the rolled lower border of the external oblique aponeurosis.

Blood supply

The anterior abdominal wall has a rich blood supply from the lower intercostals and subcostal vessels. In addition, the posterior sheath contains the inferior epigastric vessels, which anastomose with the smaller superior epigastric artery and vein, the terminal branches of the internal thoracic vessels. This arterial anastomosis is an important communication between the subclavian artery above and the external iliac artery below, for example in occlusion of the lower aorta (Leriche syndrome) and in coarctation of the aorta. Of more immediate concern is that these vessels may be lacerated at insertion of the lateral trocar at laparoscopy.

Nerve supply

The anterior abdominal wall is innervated by the anterior primary rami of T7 to L1. The cutaneous segmental

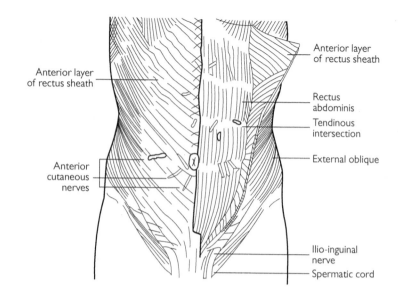

Figure 2.1 The anterior abdominal wall.
Reproduced from Harold Ellis, *Clinical Anatomy*, figure 43, Copyright Wiley, 2002, with permission.

supply is easily mapped out on the patient—T7 supplies the xiphoid region, T10 the level of the umbilicus, and L1 the groin. L1 divides on the posterior abdominal wall to form the iliohypogastric and ilioinguinal nerves. The former runs deep to the external oblique just above the inguinal canal to supply the suprapubic skin, while the latter traverses the inguinal canal in front of the round ligament. It emerges either through the external inguinal ring or through the adjacent aponeurosis to supply the skin of the anterior part of the labium majus together with the skin of the adjacent upper thigh.

Abdominal incisions

- *The midline incision:* This is made through the linea alba. Above the umbilicus this is wide, but below this level it becomes narrow and the surgeon may experience some difficulty in finding the exact line of cleavage between the two recti. Being made up of fibrous tissue, it provides an almost bloodless line along which the abdominal wall can be rapidly opened. Deep to the sheath is a variable amount of extraperitoneal fascis, depending on the build of the patient, and then the peritoneum. In a lower

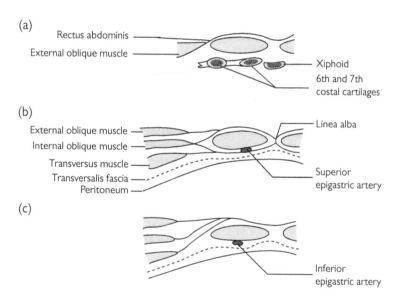

Figure 2.2 The layers of the rectus sheath.
Reproduced from Harold Ellis, *Clinical Anatomy*, figure 44, Copyright Wiley, 2002, with permission.

midline incision, the peritoneum should be opened at the upper end of the wound to ensure that bladder injury is avoided.

- *The Pfannensteil incision:* A curving interspinous skin crease incision is made about 5 cm above the pubis just inferior to the margin of the pubic hair line. The anterior rectus sheath is divided to its full extent at this level on each side and dissected off the adherent underlying rectus muscle almost to the umbilicus above and to the pubis below. The recti are then retracted laterally, exposing the peritoneum covered by a variable amount of extraperitoneal fascia. As with the lower midline incision, the peritoneum is opened at the superior end of the incision to ensure that the bladder (which should first invariably be emptied by a catheter) is not wounded.

The pelvic skeleton

The pelvic skeleton is made up of the innominate bones (Figure 2.3) on either side, the sacrum, and the coccyx. They are bound to each other by powerful and dense ligaments. The pelvis is involved in:

- walking (through its part in the formation of the hip joint and in its side-to-side swinging action in ambulation)
- supporting the weight of the body
- providing attachment for powerful muscles
- protection of the pelvic viscera.

Its marrow is an important area of haematopoiesis.

To the obstetrician, its particular interest is in its function as the bony birth canal. It is this aspect that will be mainly considered here.

The os innominatum

This is made up of three separate bones—the ilium, the ischium, and the pubic. In the fetus and child these are separate and connected to each other by cartilage. This is replaced by bone when growth ceases.

The *ilium* (Figure 2.3) bears an iliac crest, which is easily palpated through its course. It runs between the anterior and posterior superior iliac spines, below which are the corresponding inferior spines. The inner aspect bears a large auricular (ear-shaped) surface, which forms the synovial sacroiliac joint with the corresponding auricular surface on the lateral aspect of the sacrum. The iliopectineal line runs forwards from the apex of the auricular surface and clearly demarcates the true from the false pelvis.

The *pubis* (Figure 2.3) is made up of a body and a superior and inferior pubic ramus.

The *ischium* (Figure 2.3) has a vertically situated body that bears the ischial spine on its posterior aspect. This defines an upper (greater) and lower (lesser) sciatic notch. The interior pole of the bone bears the ischial tuberosity. This is easily palpated through the buttock when the hip is flexed and it is this on which you sit. From the tuberosity projects the ischial ramus, which passes forwards to join the inferior pubic ramus.

The *obturator foramen* is the opening, which is bounded by the body and rami of the pubis and the body and ramus of the ischium.

On the outer aspect, the three bones fuse together at the acetabulum. This forms the deep socket for the femoral head, for which it bears a large, smooth, crescentic articular surface.

The pelvis tilts forwards in the erect posture so that the plane of its inlet is at an angle, of 60 degrees to the horizontal. To place the articulated pelvis in the position it adopts in standing, position it against a wall so that the anterior superior iliac spine and the top of the body of the pubis touch it.

21

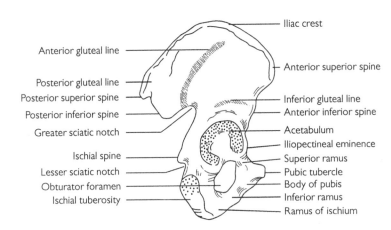

Labels (clockwise from top):
Iliac crest
Anterior superior spine
Inferior gluteal line
Anterior inferior spine
Acetabulum
Iliopectineal eminence
Superior ramus
Pubic tubercle
Body of pubis
Inferior ramus
Ramus of ischium
Ischial tuberosity
Obturator foramen
Lesser sciatic notch
Ischial spine
Greater sciatic notch
Posterior inferior spine
Posterior superior spine
Posterior gluteal line
Anterior gluteal line

Figure 2.3 The innominate bone. Reproduced from Harold Ellis, *Clinical Anatomy: Applied Anatomy for Students and Junior Doctors*, figure 92, Copyright Wiley, 2010, with permission.

The sacrum

- The sacrum is made up of five fused vertebrae and is roughly a triangle (Figure 2.4).
- The anterior border of its upper part forms the sacral promontory at the lumbosacral junction.
- It demarcates the entrance to the pelvic cavity posteriorly and is easily felt as a landmark at laparotomy.
- The anterior aspect of the sacrum presents a central mass and a line for four anterior sacral foramina on either side, which transmit the upper four sacral nerve roots. Lateral to these foramina on each side is the lateral mass.
- The superior aspect of the lateral mass on each side forms the ala (wing) of the sacrum.
- The central mass of the sacrum is rectangular. The triangular shape of the bone is due to the rapid shrinkage in size of the lateral masses from the top down.
- Posteriorly lies the sacral canal, which continues the vertebral canal downwards. The sacral canal is bounded by short pedicles, strong laminae, and small sacral spinous processes. Perforating through from the canal are the four posterior sacral foramina, which transmit the posterior primary rami of the upper four sacral nerves.
- Inferiorly, the canal terminates at the sacral hiatus, which faces posteriorly and transmits the fifth sacral nerve. The lower extremity of the hiatus bears a sacral cornu on either side, which can be easily palpated with the finger immediately above the natal cleft. This is a sure guide to the canal when performing a sacral block.

- On its lateral aspect, the sacrum bears the auricular facet for articulation with the corresponding surface of the ilium to form the synovial sacro-iliac joint. The fifth lumbar vertebra may occasionally fuse partly or wholly with the sacrum ('sacralization of L5'). The first segment of the sacrum may be partly or completely separate from the rest of the bone ('lumbarization of S1'). The posterior arch of the sacrum is often partially, and sometimes completely, bifid.
- The dural sheath terminates distally at the level of the second piece of the sacrum. This level corresponds to the level of the sacral dimple on either side. Below this level, the sacral canal is filled with the loose connective tissue of the extradural space, the lower filaments of the cauda equine, and the filum terminale. The extradural space can be entered through the sacral hiatus to perform an extradural anaesthetic block (Figure 2.4).

The coccyx

The coccyx (Figure 2.4) is made up of three to five diminutive vertebrae and articulates with the lower end of the sacrum. Occasionally the first segment is separate and in other specimens the coccyx will be found fused with the sacrum. It represents, of course, the tail of more primitive mammals.

Joints and ligaments of the pelvis

The *symphysis pubis* is the cartilaginous joint between the body of the pubis on either side. It is strengthened by fibrous ligaments, especially above and below (Figure 2.5).

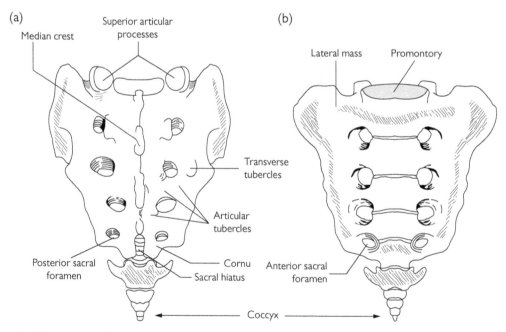

Figure 2.4 The sacrum and the coccyx.
Reproduced from Harold Ellis, *Clinical Anatomy*, figure 93, p. 126, Copyright Wiley, 2002, with permission.

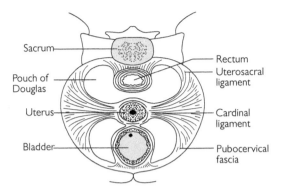

Sacrum

Pouch of Douglas

Uterus

Bladder

Rectum

Uterosacral ligament

Cardinal ligament

Pubocervical fascia

Figure 2.5 The pelvic ligaments seen from above. Reproduced from Harold Ellis, *Clinical Anatomy*, figure 107, p. 146, Copyright Wiley, 2002, with permission.

The *sacroiliac joint* on each side is a synovial joint between the auricular surface of the sacrum and that of the ilium. The sacrum hangs like a wedge between these two joints and is supported by the *posterior sacroiliac ligament* on each side. Since these support the whole weight of the body, it is not surprising that they are the most powerful ligaments in the body.

In addition, there are the *sacrotuberous* and the *sacrospinous ligaments*, which define two exits from the pelvis:

1. The *greater sciatic foramen*—between the greater sciatic notch and the sacrospinous ligament.
2. The *lesser sciatic foramen*—between the lesser sciatic notch and the sacrospinous and sacrotuberous ligaments.

Sex differences

There are a large number of differences between the typical male and female pelvic bones (Figure 2.6). These are associated principally with two features. First, the male pelvis tends to be larger, heavier, and with better-defined muscle markings. Second, the pelvis is wider and shallower in the female, correlated with its role as a bony part of the birth canal.

The numerous sex differences are summarized in Table 2.1, but the ones that are obvious when looking at an X-ray of the pelvis are:

1. The pelvic inlet is heart-shaped in the male and comparatively larger and oval in the female. The inlet is enlarged in the female by the fact that the ala of the sacrum on either side is as wide as the transverse width of the body of the sacrum. In the male, each ala is only about half the width of the body.
2. A very constant difference is that the angle between the inferior pubic rami is narrow in the male and wide in the female—thus, of course, widening the bony pelvic outlet. In the male it corresponds to the angle formed between the index and the middle finger, whereas in the female it corresponds to the angle formed between the outstretched thumb and index finger.
3. The soft tissue shadow of the penis and scrotum can be seen in the male, or else the lead screen used to shield the testes from irradiation.

Obstetrical pelvic measurements

These measurements are summarized in Table 2.2 and Figure 2.7.

- *The transverse diameter of the outlet* of the pelvis is assessed clinically by measuring the distance between the ischial tuberosities in a plane passing across the anal orifice.
- The *anteroposterior diameter of the outlet* is measured from the inferior aspect of the pubic symphysis to the coccyx.
- The most useful measurement is the *diagonal conjugate*, which is the distance between the lower margin of the pubic symphysis to the promontory of the sacrum. This normally measures 12.5 cm. From a practical point of view it is not possible, in the normal pelvis, to reach the sacral promontory on vaginal examination—if it is possible, the pelvis is seriously contracted.

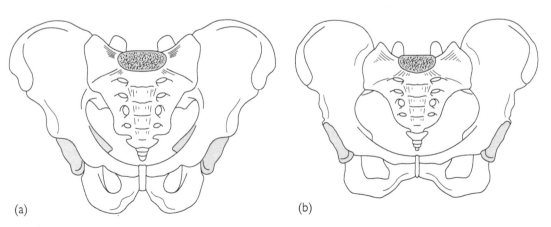

(a)   (b)

Figure 2.6 The male (a) and the female (b) pelvis. Reproduced from Harold Ellis, *Clinical Anatomy*, figure 94, p. 126, Copyright Wiley, 2002, with permission.

Table 2.1 Comparison of male and female pelvis

	Male	Female
General structure	Heavy and thick	Light and thin
Joint surfaces	Large	Small
Muscle attachments	Well marked	Rather indistinct
False pelvis	Deep	Shallow
Pelvic inlet	Heart-shaped	Oval
Pelvic canal	'Long segment of a short cone', i.e. long and tapered	'Short segment of a long cone', i.e. short with almost parallel sides
Pelvic outlet	Comparatively small	Comparatively large
First piece of sacrum	The superior surface of the body occupies nearly half the width of the sacrum	Oval superior surface of the body occupies about one-third the width of the sacrum
Sacrum	Long, narrow, with smooth concavity	Short, wide, flat, curving forward in lower part
Sacroiliac articular facet (auricular surface)	Extends well down the third piece of the sacrum	Extends down only to the upper border of the third piece
Subpubic angle (between inferior pubic rami)	'The angle between the middle and index finger'	'The angle between the thumb and index finger'
Inferior pubic ramus	Presents a strong everted surface for attachment of the crus of the penis	This marking is not present
Acetabulum	Large	Small
Ischial tuberosities	Inturned	Everted
Obturator foramen	Round	Oval

- Another useful and simple clinical guide is the *sub-arch*; the examiner's clenched fist should rest easily between the ischial tuberosities.

- These measurements of the bony pelvis are narrowed by the pelvis muscles, the rectum, the bladder, and the thickness of the uterine wall.

The muscles and fasciae of the pelvic floor

The canal of the bony and ligamentous pelvis is closed by a diaphragm of muscles and fasciae, which are pierced by the rectum, vagina, and urethra to reach the exterior. The muscles are divided into:

- the *pelvic diaphragm*, formed by levator ani and coccygeus
- a superficial group of muscles of the anterior (urogenital) and posterior (anal) perineum.

Note that the pelvic diaphragm forms the floor of the pelvis and the roof of the perineum.

Table 2.2 Obstetrical pelvic measurements

	Transverse	Oblique	Anteroposterior
Inlet	12.5 cm	11.5 cm	10 cm
Mid pelvis	11.5 cm	11.5 cm	11.5 cm
Outlet	10 cm	11.5 cm	12.5 cm

Levator ani

- This is a broad, thin muscle (Figure 2.8).
- It arises from the posterior aspect of the body of the pubis, from the ischial spine, and from the dense fascia covering obturator internus between these two attachments.
- The fibres pass medially and downwards to meet the muscle of the opposite side in a raphe.
- The anterior fibres pass backwards to loop around the posterior aspect of the vagina to meet in the fibrous perineal body.
- The middle fibres pass backwards and downwards around the posterior aspect of the terminal part of the rectum to the fibrous anococcygeal body and blend with the anal sphincter muscles.
- The posterior fibres pass to attach to the coccyx and to a midline raphe between the coccyx and the anococcygeal body.

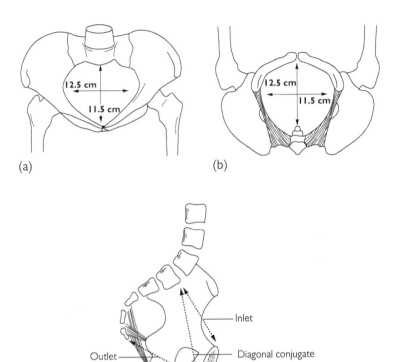

(a)

(b)

(c)

Inlet

Outlet

Diagonal conjugate

Figure 2.7 Obstetrical pelvic measurements.
Reproduced from Harold Ellis, *Clinical Anatomy*, figure 95, Copyright Wiley, 2002, with permission.

- Levator ani provides muscular support to the pelvic viscera, especially when intra-abdominal pressure is raised in micturition, defecation, and parturition.
- Its innermost fibres, often termed the *puborectalis*, form a sling around the anorectal junction. This maintains

the sharp angulation between the rectum and the anal canal, which can be appreciated on rectal examination and on sigmoidoscopy (Figure 2.8).
- Levator ani is supplied by the pudendal nerve.

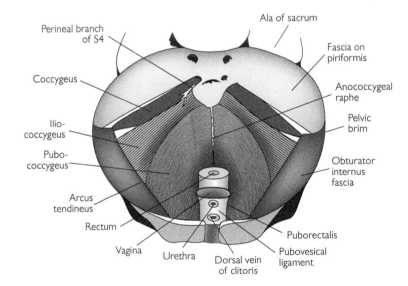

Perineal branch of S4

Coccygeus

Ilio-coccygeus

Pubo-coccygeus

Arcus tendineus

Rectum

Vagina

Urethra

Dorsal vein of clitoris

Pubovesical ligament

Puborectalis

Obturator internus fascia

Pelvic brim

Anococcygeal raphe

Fascia on piriformis

Ala of sacrum

Figure 2.8 Female pelvic floor from above. The pubococcygeus part of levator ani lies internal to the iliococcygeus part.
This figure was published in *Last's Anatomy* Ninth edition, R.M.H. McMinn, figure 5.53, p. 375, Copyright Elsevier 1994.

Coccygeus

- This is an insignificant and non-functional muscle in humans.
- It corresponds almost exactly to the sacrospinous ligament, which it overlies, passing from the side of the lower sacrum and the coccyx to the ischial spine.
- This ligament is regarded as a degenerate part of the coccygeus in humans.
- The muscle is well developed and the ligament often missing in animals with a well developed tail.

The anterior (urogenital) perineum

An imaginary line passing between the ischial tuberosities lies just in front of the anal orifice. Between this line and the inferior ischiopubic ramus on each side lies the urogenital part of the perineum (Figure 2.9). Attached to the sides of this triangle is a strong fascial sheath, the *perineal membrane*, which is pierced by the urethra, encased in its external urethral sphincter of voluntary muscles, and by the vagina. Enclosing the deep aspect of the external sphincter is a fascial sheath on the deep aspect of the levator ani, so that the sphincter is contained within a fascial space termed the *deep perineal pouch*, which also contains transversely running fibres of the *deep transverse perineal muscles*. Superficial to

the perineal membrane is the *superficial perineal pouch*. The contents of this pouch include:

- ischiocavernosus muscle
- bulbospongiosus muscle
- superficial transverse perineal muscle
- crura of the clitoris (crura of the penis in the male)
- vestibular bulbs (bulb of the penis in the male)
- the greater vestibular glands (Bartholin's).

The posterior (anal) perineum

This triangle lies between the ischial tuberosity on each side of the coccyx (Figures 2.9 and 2.10). It is roofed by levator ani, and contains the anal canal with its encircling sphincters and with the ischioanal fossa on either side.

The *ischioanal fossa* is of surgical importance because of the frequency with which it may become infected and because the pudendal nerve and vessels lie in its lateral wall. Its boundaries are:

- Medially—the fascia over the inferior aspect of the levator ani and the external anal sphincter.
- Laterally—the fascia over obturator internus on the inner side wall of the pelvis. Contained within a tunnel (the

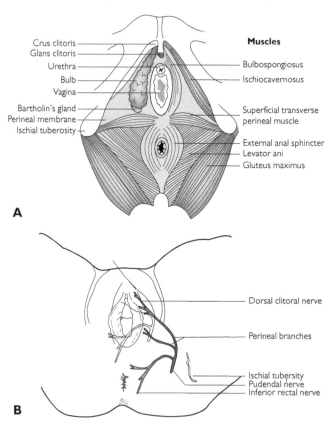

Figure 2.9 Structures in the anterior (urogenital) and the posterior (anal) perineum, and their relationships.
Reproduced from Harold Ellis, *Clinical Anatomy: Applied Anatomy for Students and Junior Doctors*, figure 99, p. 143, Copyright Wiley, 2010, with permission.

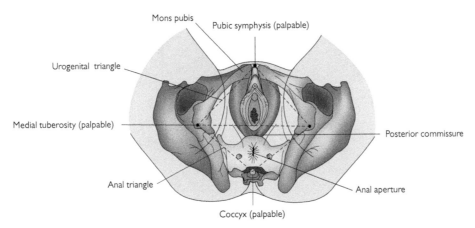

Mons pubis
Pubic symphysis (palpable)
Urogenital triangle
Medial tuberosity (palpable)
Posterior commissure
Anal triangle
Anal aperture
Coccyx (palpable)

Figure 2.10 The imaginary line between the ischial tuberosities in front of the anal orifice forms the bases of the anterior (urogenital) and the posterior (anal) triangles.
This figure was published in *Grays Anatomy for Students*, Richard Drake, Nque Vogl, Adam Mitchell, Figure 5.73a, p. 443, Copyright Elsevier, 2005.

pudendal or Alcock's canal) in the fascia covering this muscle are the pudendal nerve (S2, 3, and 4) and the internal pudendal artery and vein. These give off the inferior rectal vessels and nerve, supplying the external anal sphincter and perianal skin, and then pass forward to supply the perineal tissues.

- Anteriorly—the urogenital perineum.
- Posteriorly—the sacrotuberous ligament, covered behind by gluteus maximus.
- Floor—skin and subcutaneous fat.
- Contents—fat.

The pelvic fascia

The pelvic fascia is the connective tissue that covers the pelvic walls and the viscera lying within the pelvic cavity. It is divided into the parietal and the endopelvic fascia. The *parietal fascia* covers the walls and the floor of the pelvic cavity. It is thickened over obturator internus, where it gives attachment to levator ani. The spinal nerves lie outside this fascia, while the pelvic vessels lie internal to it. The *endopelvic fascia* is the extraperitoneal connective tissue that covers the uterus (the parametrium), vagina, bladder, and rectum. Three condensations of the connective tissue sling the pelvic organs from the walls of the pelvis (Figure 2.5).

1. The *cardinal ligaments* (also known as the transverse cervical or Mackenrodt's ligaments) pass laterally on each side from the cervix and upper vagina to the side wall of the pelvis. They are made up of fibrous connective tissue with some involuntary muscle and are pierced in their upper part by the ureter on each side.
2. The *pubocervical fascia* extends forward on either side of the bladder from the lateral part of the cardinal ligament on each side of the pubis, acting as a sling for the bladder.
3. The *uterosacral ligaments* pass backwards on either side from the posterolateral aspect of the cervix at the level of its isthmus, and from the lateral fornix of the vagina in

the lateral boundary of the pouch of Douglas. They attach to the periosteum in front of the sacroiliac joint and lateral part of the third piece of the sacrum.

These ligaments, in conjunction with levator ani, act as supports to the uterine cervix and the vaginal vault. In uterine prolapse these ligaments are stretched.

Two other ligaments take attachment from the uterus:

1. The *broad ligament* is a fold of peritoneum on either side that connects the lateral margin of the body of the uterus to the side wall of the pelvis on either side (Figure 2.11). The uterus and its broad ligaments thus form a transverse partition across the pelvis, which defines an anterior compartment, the *uterovesical pouch*, containing the bladder, and a posterior compartment, the *recto-uterine pouch* or *pouch of Douglas*, which contains the rectum. The broad ligament contains or carries:

- the uterine tube in its free edge
- the ovary, attached by its mesovarium to its posterior aspect
- the round ligament on its anterior aspect
- the ovarian ligament crossing from the ovary to the cornu of the uterus
- uterine vessels, branches of the ovarian vessels, lymphatics, and autonomic nerves.

The ureter passes forwards to the bladder deep to the broad ligament and lateral to, and immediately above, the lateral fornix of the vagina (Figure 2.12).

2. The *round ligament*, which is a fibromuscular cord, passes from the lateral angle of the uterus in the anterior layer of the broad ligament to the internal inguinal ring. It then transverses the inguinal canal to the labium majus. Note that the round ligament, taken with the ovarian ligament, is the female equivalent of the male gubernaculum testis, along which the fetal testis descends to the scrotum.

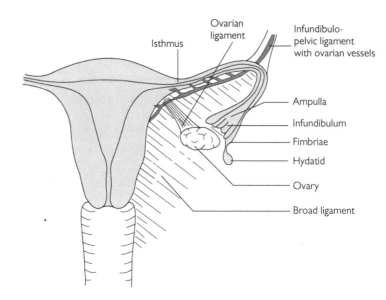

Figure 2.11 Uterus and adnexae.
Reproduced from Harold Ellis, *Clinical Anatomy: Applied Anatomy for Students and Junior Doctors*, figure 106, p. 152, Copyright Wiley, 2010, with permission.

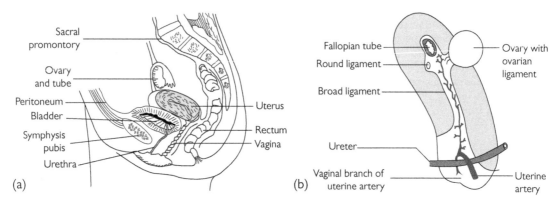

(a)

(b)

Figure 2.12 (a) Sagittal section of the uterus and its relations. (b) Lateral view of the uterus (schematic) to show composition of the broad ligament, the realtions of ureter and uterine artery, and the peritoneal covering of the uterus.
Reproduced from Harold Ellis, *Clinical Anatomy: Applied Anatomy for Students and Junior Doctors*, figure 101, p. 146, and figure 104, p. 150, Copyright Wiley, 2010, with permission.

The female genital tract

This comprises the vagina, uterus, and uterine (Fallopian) tubes, together with the associated ovaries.

The vagina

The vagina surrounds the uterine cervix, then passes downwards and forwards, traverses the pelvic floor, and opens into the vestibule. The cervix projects into the anterior part of the vault of the vagina, so that the continuous gutter that surrounds the cervix is shallow anteriorly, where the vaginal wall is some 7.5 cm in length, and deep posteriorly, where the wall is about 10 cm long. This continuous gutter is divided, for convenience of description, into the anterior, posterior, and lateral *fornices* (fornix = arch).

Relations

- The vagina is related anteriorly to the cervix above, then to the base of the bladder, and then to the urethra. The urethra is firmly embedded in the vaginal wall, opening in front of the vaginal orifice into the vestibule.
- The posterior fornix and the upper 2 cm of the posterior wall of the vagina is covered by the peritoneum of the recto-uterine pouch—the pouch of Douglas—and comes

into contact, usually, with loops of small intestine. It is here, of course, that collections of fluid such as blood or pus may be detected on bimanual vaginal examination. Below the pouch, the posterior vaginal wall lies against the anterior aspect of the rectum and then the anal canal, separated by the perineal body.

- Laterally—the levator ani, the pelvic fascia, and the ureter on each side, lying immediately above the lateral fornix—indeed, rarely an impacted ureteric calculus can be palpated at this side on vaginal examination!

The *arterial supply* of the vagina derives from the vaginal, uterine, internal pudendal, and middle rectal branches of the internal iliac artery, while a venous plexus drains via the vaginal vein into the internal iliac vein.

Lymphatic drainage (Figure 2.13) can be considered in thirds:

Upper third—to the external and internal iliac nodes

Middle third—to the internal iliac nodes

Lower third—to the inguinal nodes

The uterus

The uterus (Figure 2.14) is pear-shaped, about 7.5 cm in length, and comprises a fundus, body, and cervix.

- The uterine (Fallopian) tubes enter at each supero-lateral angle, termed the cornu, above which lies the fundus.
- The uterine body narrows to a waist, the isthmus, which continues as the cervix. This is clasped around its middle

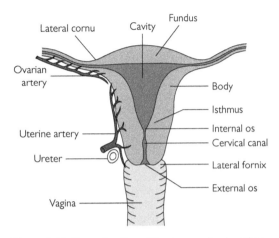

Figure 2.14 Coronal section of the uterus and vagina. Note the important relationships of ureter and uterine artery. Reproduced from Harold Ellis, *Clinical Anatomy: Applied Anatomy for Students and Junior Doctors*, figure 102, p. 148, Copyright Wiley, 2010, with permission.

by the vagina—this attachment defines the supravaginal and the infravaginal parts of the cervix.

- The isthmus is 1.5 cm in length. Its junction with the uterine body is marked by the internal os within the uterine cavity. It is the isthmus that becomes the lower segment of the uterus in pregnancy.
- The cavity of the body of the uterus is triangular in coronal section and slit-like in sagittal section. It opens into the cervical canal via the internal os and the cervical canal itself opens into the vaginal vault through the external os.
- In the nulliparous female the external os is circular, but it becomes a transverse slit, with an anterior and a posterior lip, after childbirth.
- The non-pregnant cervix is firm, with the consistency of the tip of the nose. In pregnancy it softens, and has the consistency of the lips.
- The fetal cervix is considerably larger than the body of the uterus. In the child the cervix is twice the size of the body (the infantile uterus). During puberty, the uterus enlarges, by relative overgrowth of its body, to reach adult size and proportions.
- In the adult, the uterus bends forward on itself at the level of the internal os—anteflexion of the uterus—while the cervix tips posteriorly with the axis of the vagina at roughly a right-angle—anteversion of the uterus. Thus, the uterus comes to lie in almost a horizontal plane (Figure 2.15).
- In *retroflexion of the uterus* the axis of the body passes upwards and backwards in relation to the axis of the cervix. In *retroversion of the uterus* the axis of the cervix passes upwards and backwards (Figure 2.15).
- In normal vaginal examination the anterior lip of the cervix is the lowermost part to be felt, while in retroversion

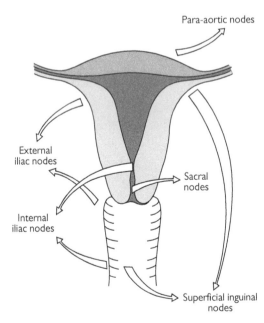

Figure 2.13 Lymphatic drainage of the pelvis. Reproduced from Harold Ellis, *Clinical Anatomy*, figure 105, p. 143, Copyright Wiley, 2002, with permission.

it is the posterior lip, or the os, which becomes the presenting part. These two conditions may often co-exist. They may be mobile and symptomless, as a result of a distended bladder or anomaly of development, and such mobile displacement may be found in up to 25% of women—it should be regarded as a normal anatomical variant. A fixed displacement of the uterus, in contrast, may result from a variety of pathologies, including endometriosis, pelvic inflammatory disease, adhesions, or a pelvic tumour.

Relations

- Anteriorly the uterine body relates to the uterovesical pouch of peritoneum and rests either on the superior aspect of the bladder or on loops of small intestine (Figure 2.12). The supravaginal cervix lies directly against the bladder, separated only by loose connective tissue. The infravaginal cervix lies immediately posterior to the anterior fornix of the vagina.
- Posteriorly lies the recto-uterine pouch (pouch of Douglas), which contains loops of intestine; the ovaries and adjacent tubes are often found to be prolapsed into the pouch.
- Laterally lies the broad ligament and its contents—the uterine tube, ovary, blood vessels, lymphatics, and autonomic nerves. The ureter passes below the broad ligament and uterine vessels and is situated 12 mm lateral to the supravaginal cervix, immediately above

the lateral vaginal fornix. It is here that the ureter may be accidentally damaged, divided, or tied when the uterine vessels are clamped during a hysterectomy, especially if the anatomy has been distorted by previous surgery, a mass of fibroids, pelvic inflammatory disease, or endometriosis.

Peritoneal relationships

The body of the uterus is covered with peritoneum of the pelvic floor except where it is reflected off at two sites—laterally at the broad ligament on either side and anteriorly onto the bladder at the level of the uterus isthmus. Anteriorly the peritoneum is only loosely adherent, to allow for bladder distension. Posteriorly the peritoneum continues inferiorly to cover the posterior wall of the upper quarter of the vagina, so that on vaginal examination, a finger in the posterior fornix of the vagina is only about 1 mm away from the peritoneum of the pelvic floor.

Blood supply

The principal arterial supply is from the uterine artery, a branch of the internal iliac artery (Figure 2.16). This runs in the base of the broad ligament and crosses immediately above and at right-angles to the ureter as it passes forward to the bladder. The artery reaches the uterus at the level of the uterine isthmus and the internal os. It is the only structure, apart from the broad ligament, to lie superficially to the ureter. The uterine artery then ascends in a tortuous

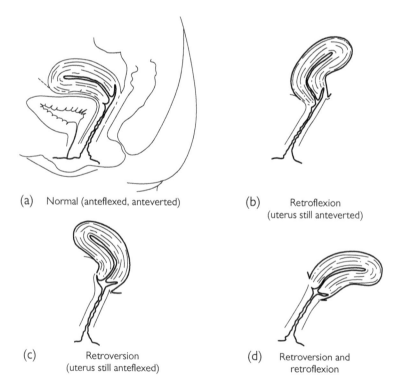

Figure 2.15 Positions of the uterus. Reproduced from Harold Ellis, *Clinical Anatomy*, figure 103, p. 141, Copyright Wiley, 2002, with permission.

(a) Normal (anteflexed, anteverted)

(b) Retroflexion (uterus still anteverted)

(c) Retroversion (uterus still anteflexed)

(d) Retroversion and retroflexion

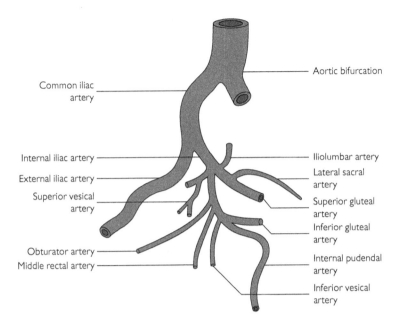

Common iliac artery

Aortic bifurcation

Internal iliac artery

External iliac artery

Superior vesical artery

Obturator artery

Middle rectal artery

Iliolumbar artery

Lateral sacral artery

Superior gluteal artery

Inferior gluteal artery

Internal pudendal artery

Inferior vesical artery

Figure 2.16 The aortic bifurcation and the right internal iliac artery. The internal iliac artery divides into anterior and posterior divisions. The latter gives rise to the superior gluteal artery, whereas the former gives off all the visceral branches. (Although the branches of the internal iliac artery are fairly constant, the arrangement of these branches is variable.) Reproduced from Harold Ellis, *Clinical Anatomy: Applied Anatomy for Students and Junior Doctors*, figure 111, p. 162, Copyright Wiley, 2010, with permission.

manner alongside the body of the uterus and anastomoses with terminal branches of the ovarian artery, which arises from the aorta below the level of the renal artery. The uterine artery also gives off a descending branch to the cervix and branches to the upper vagina, which anastomose with ascending twigs from the vaginal artery.

The uterine vein accompanies the artery and drains into the internal iliac vein. It also communicates with the ovarian vein and with veins of the vagina and bladder via the pelvic venous plexus.

Lymphatic drainage

There is a wide field of lymphatic drainage of the uterus (Figure 2.13).

- The fundus, together with the uterine tubes and the ovaries, drains along the ovarian vessels to the para-aortic lymph nodes.
- In addition, some lymphatic channels pass along the round ligament and then along the inguinal canal to reach the inguinal lymph nodes.
- The body of the uterus drains along the broad ligament to nodes lying along the external iliac blood vessels.
- The cervix drains in three directions: laterally, in the broad ligament, to the external iliac nodes; posterolaterally along the uterine vessels to the internal iliac nodes; and posteriorly along the recto-uterine fold to the sacral lymph nodes.

The uterine (Fallopian) tubes

The uterine tubes are about 10 cm in length. They lie in the free edge of the broad ligament on either side and open into the cornu of the uterus. Each is made up of four parts:

1. The *infundibulum* is the funnel-shaped lateral extremity, which extends distal to the broad ligament and opens into the peritoneal cavity by its ostium. The ostium is surrounded by a number of finger-like processes, the fimbriae, which usually flop over the ovary and obscure it from view at laparoscopy.
2. The *ampulla*, which is wide, tortuous, and comparatively thin-walled.
3. The *isthmus*, which is narrow, straight, and thick-walled.
4. The *interstitial part*, which pierces the uterine wall at the junction of the uterine fundus and body.

Apart from the interstitial part, the tube is covered with peritoneum. It is lined throughout by a ciliated columnar epithelium.

Blood supply: An arterial arcade lies in the broad ligament immediately below the tube, which is fed laterally by the ovarian artery and vein and medially by the uterine vessels.

Lymphatic drainage links with that of the ovary and passes to the para-aortic nodes. Some vessels from the medial part of the tube follow the uterine vein and pass to the internal iliac nodes, while others track along the round ligament to the superficial inguinal nodes.

The ovary

The ovary is an almond-shaped organ, on each side, roughly 4 cm in length. It is attached to the back of the broad ligament by a short peritoneal 'mesentery', termed the *mesovarium*. The ovary has two other attachments, the infundibulopelvic ligament (sometimes called the suspensory ligament of the ovary), in which pass the ovarian vessels, lymphatics, and autonomic nerves from the side wall of the pelvis, and the ovarian ligament, which passes to the cornu of the uterus.

The ovary is usually described as lying in the ovarian fossa, on the side wall of the pelvis. This is defined as the depression between the external iliac vessels anteriorly, and the internal iliac vessels together with the ureter posteriorly; it contains the obturator nerve. In fact, the ovary is very variable in its position and is frequently found to be lying in the pouch of Douglas.

Blood supply

The ovarian artery (Figure 2.14) arises from the aorta just below the level of the renal artery. The ovarian vein drains, on the right, into the inferior vena cava at the same level, while on the left it opens into the left renal vein. Lymphatics pass to the para-aorta nodes at the level of the renal vessels. This arrangement of blood vessels and lymphatics is explained by the development of the ovary (and, of course, the testis) from the genital ridge at the vertebral level of L1. The gonads then descend, dragging blood supply, lymphatic drainage, and autonomic nerve supply (T10) with them into the pelvis.

The external genitalia

The external genitalia in the female comprise the mons pubis, the labia majora and minora, the vestibule of the vagina, the clitoris, the bulb of the vestibule, and the greater vestibular (Bartholin) glands. The general term *vulva* (or pudendum) includes all these structures.

The mons pubis

This rounded eminence anterior to the pubic symphysis is formed by subcutaneous adipose tissue. At puberty it becomes covered with hair that has a horizontal upper limit, in contrast to the male, where the pubic hair extends upwards towards the umbilicus in and adjacent to the median line.

The labia majora and minora

The labia major are two folds of skin that meet anteriorly at the mons and posteriorly in the midline anterior to the anal orifice. They are more obvious anteriorly. The midline cleft between the labia majora is termed the *vulval cleft*. Within the cleft lie the thin, vascular folds of skin, the labia minora, which lack both hair and sebaceous glands. The space between these folds is termed *the vestibule*, into which opens the urethral orifice, 2.5 cm behind the clitoris, and behind the urethra lies the opening of the vagina.

The *bulbospongiosus muscle* runs on either side from its attachment to the perineal body in front of the anal canal beneath the skin of the vestibule to insert into the clitoris. Laterally, the *ischiocavernosus muscle* runs from the medial surface of the ramus of the ischium forward and medially to insert into the clitoris. The *superficial transverse perineal muscles* run laterally from the perineal body to the ischial ramus (Figure 2.9).

The clitoris

This is the female equivalent of the penis (Figure 2.9).

- It consists, like the penis, of three columns of erectile tissue but, unlike the penis, of course, it does not transmit the urethra, which opens behind it.
- The erectile tissue comprises the corpora cavernosa and the bulbs of the vestibule. The paired *corpora cavernosa*

lie deep to the ischiocavernosus muscle and arise from the ischiopubic ramus on each side. They meet in the body of the clitoris. The paired *bulbs of the vestibule* lie on each side deep to the bulbospongiosus muscle. Anteriorly each continues as a thin band of erectile tissue into the clitoris, uniting into a strand that expands into the *glans* at its tip.

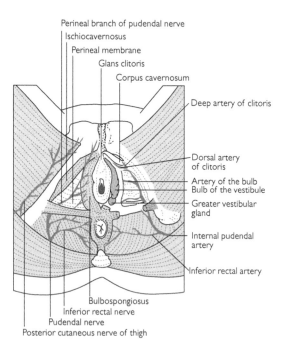

Perineal branch of pudendal nerve
Ischiocavernosus
Perineal membrane
Glans clitoris
Corpus cavernosum
Deep artery of clitoris
Dorsal artery of clitoris
Artery of the bulb
Bulb of the vestibule
Greater vestibular gland
Internal pudendal artery
Inferior rectal artery
Bulbospongiosus
Inferior rectal nerve
Pudendal nerve
Posterior cutaneous nerve of thigh

Figure 2.17 Dissection of the female perineum. Arteries are shown on the left, and nerves on the right. The superficial muscles have been removed on the left to show the bulb of the vestibule and the greater vestibular glands.
Reprinted from *Textbook of Anatomy*, A.W. Rogers, Figure 44.12, p. 668, Copyright Elsevier, 1992.

- The bulbs of the vestibule, together with the glans of the clitoris, are equivalent to the corpus spongiosum and glans of the male. The anterior ends of the labia minora split to surround the clitoris, providing it with a prepuce.

The greater vestibular glands of Bartholin

These comprise a pair of lobulated, pea-shaped, mucus-secreting glands that lie deep to the posterior parts of the labia majora. They are impalpable when healthy but become obvious when inflamed or distended. Each drains by a 2.5 cm-long duct, which opens into the groove between the vaginal orifice and the posterior part of the labium minus. Anteriorly each gland is overlapped superficially by the vestibular bulb.

Blood supply

The external genitalia have a rich blood supply (Figure 2.17) provided by branches of the *internal pudendal artery and vein*. These are derived from the internal iliac vessels and run forward on the lateral wall of the ischioanal fossa in Alcock's canal.

These vessels are:

- Posterior labial branches—which supply the labia and the superficial perineal muscles.
- The artery and vein of the bulb—supplying the bulb of the vestibule, the greater vestibular glands, and the clitoris, and contributing to the supply of the terminal part of the vagina.
- The deep vessels of the clitoris—supplying the corpus cavernosum.
- The dorsal vessels of the clitoris—supplying the clitoris and the glans.

These branches of the internal pudendal vessels anastomose with terminal branches of the superficial external pudendal vessels of the femoral artery and vein.

Nerve supply

The skin of the mons pubis and the adjacent anterolateral parts of the labia majora are supplied by spinal segment L1 through the *ilioinguinal* and *genitofemoral nerves*. The rest of the external genitalia are supplied by S3 via the *pudendal nerve* via its perineal branch (Figure 2.17).

Regional embryology

The genital tract

The *paramesonephric* duct develops, one on either side, on the posterior abdominal wall medial to the *mesonephric ducts*. All four tubes lie close together caudally and project into the anterior part of the cloaca (Figure 2.18).

- The paramesonephric ducts in the male and the mesonephric ducts in the female all but disappear, leaving behind congenital remnants that are of clinical interest.

- In the male the paramesonephric duct disappears, apart from the appendix testis (a tiny cystic structure perched on the upper pole of the testis, which may undergo torsion) and the prostatic utricle (a short sinus leading into the posterior aspect of the prostatic urethra).
- In the female the mesonephric duct system, which in the male develops into the epididymis and the vas deferens, persists only as small cystic remnants alongside the genital

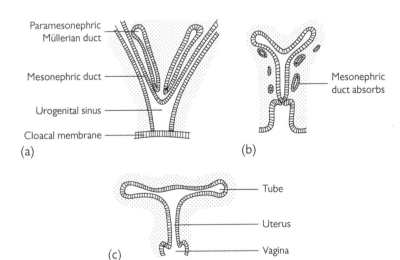

(a)

(b)

(c)

Paramesonephric Müllerian duct

Mesonephric duct

Urogenital sinus

Cloacal membrane

Mesonephric duct absorbs

Tube

Uterus

Vagina

Figure 2.18 The paramesonephric and the mesonephric duct systems lying side by side (a), resorption of the mesonephric duct (b), and the derivatives of the paramesonephric duct in the female species. Reproduced from Harold Ellis, *Clinical Anatomy*, figure 108, p. 149, Copyright Wiley, 2002, with permission.

tract termed the epoophoron, mesoophoron, and the ducts of Gartner.

- In the female the paramesonephric ducts cranially become the Fallopian tubes. More caudally, they sweep together and fuse in the midline to become the epithelium of the body of the uterus, the cervix, and the upper third of the vagina—at first a solid cord that then canalizes. The rest of the vaginal epithelium forms by canalization of the solid sinuvaginal node at the back of the urogenital sinus. (This accounts for the difference in the lymphatic drainage of the upper and lower vagina.)
- The musculature of the genital tract derives from the surrounding mesoderm, so that the cystic remnants of the mesonephric ducts in the female are found embedded in the myometrium, the cervix, and the wall of the vagina.
- As the paramesonephric ducts sweep together and fuse in their distal parts, they drag a peritoneal fold with them on either side—this becomes the broad ligament (Figure 2.19).
- Developmental anomalies of the genital tract can easily be deduced. All stages of the original double tube may occur, from a minor degree of bicornuate uterus to complete reduplication, with a double uterus and vagina. In contrast, there may be absence or poor development of the duct system on one or both sides.
- Failure of canalization of the solid caudal end of the developing duct system results, post-puberty, in accumulation of menstrual blood above the block. First the vagina, then the uterus, and finally the tubes may distend with blood (respectively haematocolpos, haematometra, and haematosalpinx).

The ovary

Both the ovary and the testis develop from a germinal ridge of mesoderm situated in the posterior wall of the abdominal cavity medial to the mesonephros at about the level of the first lumbar vertebra. This germinal ridge is attached to

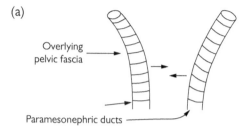

(a)

Overlying pelvic fascia

Paramesonephric ducts

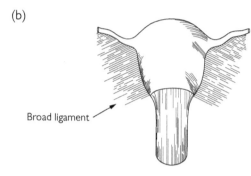

(b)

Broad ligament

Figure 2.19 Formation of the broad ligament in the female.

a strand of connective tissue termed the *gubernaculum*. It is along this strand that the testis in the male descends into the scrotum. The ovary too descends, dragging its blood supply, lymphatics, and nerve supply with it, but it impacts against the posterior aspect of the broad ligament. The gubernaculum persists as the *ovarian ligament*, which passes from the ovary across the posterior aspect of the broad ligament to the side of the uterus and, from there, as the *round ligament*, passing across the front of the broad ligament to the side wall of the pelvis to traverse the inguinal canal and end in the labium majus (Figure 2.12).

ADDITIONAL FACTS AND REVISION MATERIAL

Pelvic diaphragms

- The pelvic diaphragm (like other diaphragms in the body) consists of three layers: fascia on both sides of a middle layer of skeletal muscle. In the case of the pelvic diaphragm, the skeletal muscle is the levator ani.
- The anterior part of the pelvic diaphragm where the vagina and urethra pass through (the urogenital hiatus) lacks muscle support and is weak as a result. For this reason, the levator ani does not act on the urethra and does not contribute to its continence.
- The urogenital diaphragm is constructed on the anterior aspect and underside of the pelvic diaphragm to reinforce this deficient area (again, skeletal muscle

enclosed within two fascial membranes). It engulfs the urethra to form the sphincter urethrae muscle.

- The surface of the inferior fascia of the urogenital diaphragm (also known as the perineal membrane) provides attachment for the crura and bulb of the penis in the male. Whereas the crura have bony attachment, the bulb does not, being only attached to the perineal membrane. This lack of bony attachment leaves the bulb of the penis and the urethra travelling through it vulnerable to avulsion/detachment following severe pelvic trauma, leading to extravasation of urine into the scrotum and the anterior abdominal wall.

The erectile tissues and investing fascia

- The cavernous erectile tissues (the crura and the bulb), their surrounding skeletal muscles (ischiocavernosus and bulbospongiosus respectively), and the superficial transverse perineal muscles are all covered by Colles fascia, to create the superficial perineal pouch or space. Colles fascia is continuous with Dartos fascia of the scrotum and Scarpa's fascia of the anterior abdominal wall, but does not extend into the thigh, hence extravasated urine does not go into the thigh.

The breast

- This is a modified skin gland found entirely within the superficial fascia (i.e. between the skin and the deep fascia). Therefore, it can move relative to the body.
- The skin is connected to the deep fascia by suspensory ligaments of the breast (Cowper's ligament), which are responsible for skin 'puckering' in breast disease.
- The medial half of the breast drains its lymph to the parasternal chain of nodes, whilst the nipple, the areola, and the lateral half of the breast drains to the axillary lymph nodes. There is usually some cross drainage between breasts, a common route of metastatic disease.

CHAPTER 3

Physiology

The heart

General and electrical characteristics of the cardiac muscle cell

This section outlines the important aspects of cardiovascular physiology. The author presumes foundation knowledge level and recommends that the reader reviews the details of the physiology of the cardiac muscle cell and the differences between cardiac, skeletal, and smooth muscle cells. Within the heart differences also exist between the regular ventricular muscle cell and the specialized pacemaker tissues, and these should also be reviewed. In summary:

- Regular contracting ventricular fibres have a stable resting membrane potential (phase 4), unlike the specialized pacemaker and conducting fibres, which have unstable resting membrane potentials.
- Unlike the skeletal muscle, which has a short action potential, the action potential of the ventricular muscle cell is a long electrical event with a prolonged plateau phase, meaning there can only be one electrical event per mechanical event.
- The single electrical to mechanical event relationship ensures that, unlike the skeletal muscle, the cardiac muscle cell cannot be tetanized.
- Cardiac muscle cells have regions of low electrical resistance between fibres (junctional complexes between fibres including gap junctions) so that action potentials can move from cell to cell as a syncitium.

Membrane channels

The cardiac muscle cell membrane has channels for K^+, Na^+, and Ca^{2+} ions, which control the flow of ions in and out of the cell in response to the electrical events. The direction of flow of ions through these channels is governed by the large gradients in the concentrations of the ions and the status of the channels.

Un-gated K^+ channels

- These channels are always open and there is always an efflux of K^+ out of the cardiac muscle cell, as K^+ equilibrium potential is never reached.

Voltage-dependent (gated) K^+ channels

- These channels are open at rest.
- They are closed during the plateau phase of the action potential.
- They re-open with repolarization.

Voltage-dependent (gated) Na^+ channels

- These channels are closed at rest.
- They open quickly and close quickly.
- They are open during depolarization.

Voltage-dependent (gated) Ca^{2+} channels

- These channels are closed at rest.
- With depolarization they open and remain open during the plateau phase.

Cardiac muscle action potential

Phase 0 (depolarization)

- Fast Na^+ channels open.
- There is increased Na^+ conductance.
- The Na^+ influx into the cell causes the depolarization (Figure 3.1).

Phase 1 (slight repolarization)

- This is thought to be due to special K^+ rather than Cl^- channels.

Phase 2 (plateau)

- The slow voltage-dependent Ca^{2+} channels are open, resulting in Ca^{2+} influx into the cell.
- The Ca^{2+} influx participates in the contractile response and also triggers additional Ca^{2+} release from intracellular storage in the sarcoplasmic reticulum.
- Voltage-dependent K^+ channels are closed (only the un-gated channels are open, so K^+ conductance is low allowing just the usual efflux of K^+ but no more).

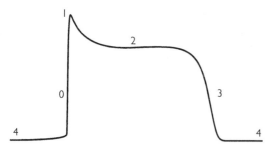

Figure 3.1 Phases of the cardiac muscle cell action potential.

- The Ca^{2+} influx balances the K^+ efflux, which produces the stable plateau phase and delays repolarization (Figure 3.1).
- The closure of the voltage-dependent K^+ channels ensures that there is no massive efflux of K^+, adding to the delay in repolarization (Figure 3.1).

Phase 3 (repolarization)

- The voltage-dependent Ca^{2+} channels close, thereby terminating the Ca^{2+} influx.
- Voltage-dependent K^+ channels re-open, thereby increasing K^+ efflux and causing repolarization (Figure 3.1).

Action potential characteristics of specialized cells (SA and AV nodes and Purkinje fibres)

- These cells have an unstable phase 4 (pacemaker potential or pre-potential) in that there is an intrinsic gradual depolarization towards threshold. This leads to the cell depolarizing automatically without the need for external stimuli (Figure 3.2).
- As there are not many fast channels, depolarization is not due to Na^+ influx through fast channels but probably to Ca^{2+} influx through slow channels.

- Repolarization is due to the efflux of K^+ like any other action potential.
- The SA nodal fibres are innervated by sympathetic and parasympathetic neurons.
- Sympathetic stimulation increases the slope of the pre-potential (phase 4) so that threshold is reached sooner, thus increasing the intrinsic firing rate.
- Parasympathetic stimulation decreases the pre-potential slope so that it takes longer to reach threshold, thus slowing down the intrinsic firing rate.
- SA nodal cells have the fastest intrinsic rate, with AV nodal cells being next fastest, and the Purkinje fibres have the slowest intrinsic rate.
- However, the Purkinje cells are the fastest conducting fibres, whilst the AV node cells are the slowest.

Cardiac muscle mechanics

- Preload is the stretch on the ventricular muscle at the end of diastole. Technically, it is equal to left ventricular end diastolic volume or pressure, but clinically it is more easily measured by the pulmonary capillary edge pressure.
- Left ventricular afterload is the force that the muscle must generate to eject the blood, measured by the mean aortic pressure. Afterload is increased in hypertension and decreased in hypotension.
- The overall force generated by the ventricular muscle during systole is the systolic performance and is determined by the number of actin–myosin cross-bridges that are cycling during contraction.
- The Frank–Starling relationship is simply the effect of preload on sarcomere length (Figure 3.3).
- Contractility measures a change in the force of contraction that is not explained by a change in preload (e.g. as occurs following the addition of adrenaline to contracting muscle in an organ bath).
- Acute changes in contractility are due to changes in Ca^{2+} ion dynamics; increased contractility implies more and quicker supply of Ca^{2+} to the contractile machinery.

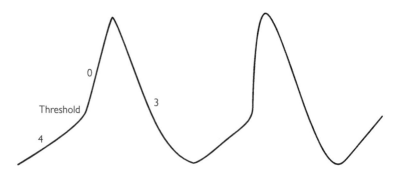

Figure 3.2 Action potential of specialized nodal cells and Purkinje fibres.

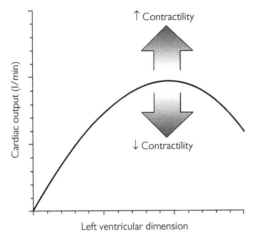

Figure 3.3 The Frank–Starling principle describes the relationship between stroke volume (cardiac output) and left ventricular end-diastolic volume or dimension (preload). Increased preload causes the stretch of cardiomyocytes, which results in increased force generation and, consequently, increased cardiac output. Thus, when the heart rate is constant, cardiac output is directly related to preload. However, at a certain point, cardiac output will not increase with any further increase in preload, but will decrease instead. An increase or decrease in cardiac contractility at a given end-diastolic volume shifts the curve up or down, respectively.

Reproduced from Srivastava and Yu, 'Stretching to meet needs: integrin-linked kinase and the cardiac pump', *Genes and Development*, **20**, pp. 2327–2331, Cold Spring Harbour Laboratory Press, with permission. Copyright 2006.

Control of heart rate

- The intrinsic heart rate is approximately 110 bpm without any sympathetic or parasympathetic input.
- Under resting conditions there is usually a parasympathetic tone to the SA and AV nodes through the right and left vagus nerves, which reduce the basal rate.
- Sympathetic stimulation leads to tachycardia and increased contractility.

Baroreceptor reflex and blood pressure regulation

- The carotid sinus stretch receptors are much more important than their aortic arch counterparts.
- The glossopharyngeal cranial nerve IX is under tonic activity and is continuously firing information on blood pressure into the CNS (Figure 3.4).
- If blood pressure (BP) increases (hypertension) or decreases (hypotension) then the afferent CNS input increases or decreases respectively and this is compared against a set point to determine the efferent output.
- The output targets the cardiac output and total peripheral resistance (TPR) via the autonomic nervous system.
- One arm of the output is the parasympathetic outflow, which runs only to the heart to alter the heart rate and thereby change the cardiac output (Figure 3.4).
- The sympathetic arm exerts a more complex series of effects on the:
  1. heart—increasing the cardiac output by raising the heart rate and contractility

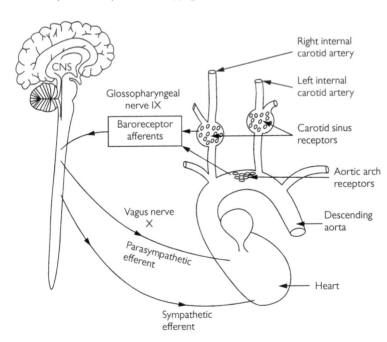

Figure 3.4 General characteristics of the baroreceptor reflex and control of blood pressure. Adapted from A.M. Davidson *et al.*, *Oxford Textbook of Clinical Nephrology* Third edition, 2005, chapter 15.1, pp. 2223–2224, Oxford University Press.

2. arterioles—increasing the TPR but only in non-essential tissues, e.g. skin, resting skeletal muscle, and kidneys (there is no effect on the brain or coronary circuits)
3. veins—venoconstriction and changing the amount of blood stored in the reservoir.

Peripheral circulation

The four main components of the circulation, namely the left side of the heart, the systemic circulation, the right side of the heart, and the pulmonary circulation, are all connected in series as a circuit. Thus, flow is the same at all points in the system. Therefore, if the cardiac output (CO) in the left ventricle is 5 l/min, the same is true of the right ventricle, and if the CO in the systemic circuit increases to 20 l/min, the same will apply to the pulmonary circuit. Although flow is the same, pressure, resistance, and capacitance differ significantly between the systemic and pulmonary circuits.

Although the systemic circulation is connected in series, the major organs in the systemic circuit (including the brain, heart, liver, kidneys, skin, and muscles) are connected in parallel, resulting in a low resistance system. In pregnancy, the placental circulation is also connected into the systemic circulation in parallel and further reduces systemic vascular resistance. This is reversed at delivery, resulting in an increase in resistance and thus blood pressure in the immediate postpartum period.

- One major advantage of the parallel connection of major organs to the systemic circulation is that flow can be independently controlled without changes in flow to other organs unless there are dramatic changes in the perfusing pressure.
- The perfusing pressure is the same for structures connected in parallel. Therefore, the structure with the greater flow (pulmonary circuit with 100% of the CO) must have the least resistance, and the structure with the least flow (coronary circuit with 5% of the CO) must have the highest resistance.

Other characteristics of the circulation include:

- The composition of the pulmonary venous capillary blood is the same as that of the systemic capillaries.
- Pulmonary arterial blood has the lowest pO_2 in the body, and is similar in composition to systemic venous blood.
- The major vessels are low-resistance pathways and so very little pressure is lost in pushing blood through them. Most pressure is lost pushing blood through the arterioles, which are high-resistance pathways.
- Blood pressure (BP) is the force or energy required to maintain flow to, and therefore perfuse, the tissues.
- The arterioles are used to control flow through the capillaries. Arteriolar dilatation results in increased flow in the capillaries downstream as well as an increase in pressure, since the arteriole now becomes a low-pressure system.
- With arteriolar constriction there is increased resistance and loss of pressure in the capillaries, but the flow downstream

is reduced. This is the situation in hypertensive individuals: the BP is high in the arteries upstream because of generalized vasoconstriction but the flow and pressure in the capillaries and organ beds are reduced.

- Vessel radius (r) is the chief determinant of vascular resistance. This is expressed in the Poiseuille's relationship: $Q = \dfrac{P_1 - P_2}{r^4}$ where Q = flow, and $P_1 - P_2$ = pressure gradient (i.e. flow is inversely related to the 4th power of the vessel radius). Thus, if the radius of an arteriole is halved, the resistance increases 16-fold, but reduces to a sixteenth of the original resistance if the radius is doubled. This relationship explains why arterioles are the main regulators of flow distribution and make up the greatest component of the systemic vascular resistance.
- Other determinants of vascular resistance include vessel length, blood viscosity, and turbulent flow.

Systolic, diastolic, and mean arterial pressure

The systolic blood pressure (SBP) is the peak pressure reached during systole, whilst the diastolic blood pressure (DBP) is the lowest pressure attained at the end of diastole. The mean arterial pressure (MAP) is the average pressure within the vessel. The MAP is closer to the diastolic than the systolic blood pressure, which is why DBP is a better index of MAP than SBP. MAP = DBP + ⅓(pulse pressure). Factors that increase SBP include increased stroke volume, reduced vascular compliance, and reduced heart rate. DBP is reduced by a reduction in any of SVR (more flow causes less pressure upstream), HR (more time available to empty the arteries), or SV (less blood pumped into the arteries), and increased by an increase in SVR, HR, or SV.

Application of the Poiseuille's equation to the systemic circulation

$$Flow(Q) = P_1 - P_2 / R$$

In the systemic circulation: flow (Q) = cardiac output; pressure gradient across the system ($P_1 - P_2$) = MAP (approximately); and R = resistance of all the vessels in the systemic circuit (SVR).

$$CO = MAP/SVR \text{ or}$$
$$MAP - CO \times SVR$$

In acute blood loss the CO falls as a result of volume loss, and the system compensates by vasoconstriction to raise SVR and maintain MAP. Otherwise, MAP would fall and compromise tissue perfusion. Thus, blood pressure measurement in this situation is not a good index of volume loss. During exercise there is arteriolar dilatation of the exercising muscles (i.e. a reduction in SVR), so the system compensates by increasing the CO to maintain MAP and avoid compromising tissue perfusion.

Regulation of organ blood flow

Generally, blood flow through the systemic circuit is regulated by constricting and dilating the smooth muscles of the arterioles. The factors that determine the degree of constriction of the smooth muscle surrounding the arterioles are divided into two categories, namely: intrinsic (or auto) regulation, in which the regulating mechanisms for arteriolar constriction are entirely within the organ itself; and extrinsic regulation, where the mechanisms of arteriolar smooth muscle regulation originate outside of the tissue. Autoregulated systems do not involve any nerves or circulating substances such as adrenaline.

Characteristics of autoregulating tissues

- In these tissues BP does not determine flow, and blood flow is independent of BP.
- Flow is maintained at a constant level across a wide range of BPs (Figure 3.5). If BP increases, the internal mechanisms constrict the arteriolar smooth muscles and reduce blood flow back to the constant level. If BP falls, the internal mechanisms relax the arterioles to increase the blood flow to the tissues back to the constant level. There are limits to the BP over which such regulation can maintain constant flow, as shown in Figure 3.5.
- Blood flow is independent of nervous reflexes such as the carotid sinus reflex.
- Completely autoregulating tissues include the cerebral circulation, coronary circulation, and exercising skeletal muscles (Table 3.1).

Characteristics of non-autoregulating (extrinsically regulated) tissues

- Extrinsically regulated tissues include the resting skeletal muscle and the cutaneous circulation.
- The main mechanism for the control of blood flow in all non-autoregulating tissues in the systemic circulation is the sympathetic nervous system, which releases noradrenaline onto the α-adrenoceptor under resting conditions.

- The β_2-receptor is not associated with nervous control but responds mainly to circulating adrenaline causing arteriolar dilatation and contributing to the regulation of blood flow in the resting skeletal muscle (Table 3.1).

Characteristics of the cerebral circulation

- The flow is directly proportional to arterial pCO_2, the vasodilatory metabolite.
- With hypoventilation, arterial pCO_2 rises and cerebral blood flow increases. During hyperventilation, arterial pCO_2 falls resulting in a fall in cerebral blood flow.
- Normal or high pO_2 do not affect cerebral blood flow, although a profound reduction in pO_2 will override this mechanism and increase cerebral blood flow regardless of the arterial pCO_2 level.
- Baroreceptor reflexes do not affect cerebral flow.

Table 3.1 Control of blood flow to resting *versus* exercising skeletal muscle

Resting skeletal muscle	Exercising skeletal muscle
blood flow is regulated mainly by sympathetic α-adrenergic activity through noradrenaline from nerve endings	switches to autoregulation and inactivates the α-receptors
β_2-receptors contribute to blood flow through circulating adrenaline	regulation of flow is mainly via vasodilatory metabolites
	β_2-receptors contribute to increased flow by vasodilatation
	significant contribution from the increase in cardiac output
	sympathetic nerves have no effect

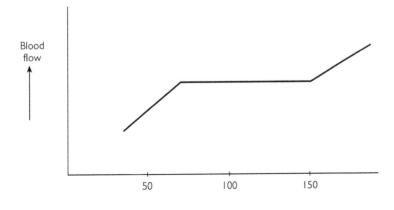

Blood flow

50   100   150

Figure 3.5 Autoregulation: Blood flow remains constant over a wide range of blood pressure values.

Characteristics of the coronary circulation

- There is severe mechanical compression of the left coronary vessels during systole so that there is little or no flow. Most of the blood flow to the left ventricle is during diastole. This makes severe tachycardia dangerous because of the shortened time interval available for coronary perfusion.
- The right coronary vessels are compressed only to a modest degree during systole so that some flow occurs. However, the greatest flow is during diastole.
- Oxygen extraction from this circuit is complete, a phenomenon that is not observed anywhere else in the body (the venous pO_2 is the lowest in the entire cardiovascular system).
- Flow matches metabolism.

Characteristics of the cutaneous circulation

- The cutaneous circulation is completely regulated extrinsically and almost entirely controlled by the sympathetic adrenergic nerves releasing noradrenaline, which acts on α- receptors. β_2-receptor effects do not have a physiological effect, although they can be demonstrated pharmacologically.
- There are large venous plexuses and arteriovenous shunts, which are heavily innervated by noradrenaline-releasing sympathetic nerve endings acting on α-receptors.
- Sympathetic stimulation of the skin produces a range of complex effects on the skin. These include: vasoconstriction of the skin arterioles, resulting in a reduction of blood flow to the skin; constriction of the venous plexuses, resulting in a reduction in the volume of blood within the skin and reduced heat exchange; and increased velocity of blood, resulting in reduced heat exchange.

Characteristics of the renal and splanchnic circulation

- Under normal conditions this is strongly autoregulated, but in emergency situations the generalized intense sympathetic vasoconstriction overrides the renal autoregulatory mechanism.
- With gentle falls in BP, the renal autoregulatory mechanism is maintained.
- The renal venous pO_2 is high because this tissue is normally over-perfused for its metabolic needs.

Characteristics of the pulmonary circulation

- This is a low resistance, low pressure (arterial 15 mmHg, venous 5 mmHg), and high flow circuit receiving the entire cardiac output.
- It is a passive circuit with very compliant arteries and veins. The total flow is unregulated as it is connected in series to the systemic circulation and there are no sympathetic nerves in the pulmonary vasculature.
- When there is low alveolar pO_2 a local vasoconstriction may follow, the so-called 'hypoxic vasoconstriction'. This facilitates the redistribution of flow to alveoli with better pO_2.
- Large changes in cardiac output produce very small changes in pressure within the pulmonary circuit because of its passive dilatation and profound low resistance.

Characteristics of systemic veins

- Compared to systemic arteries, the veins are 20 times more compliant.
- Small changes in pressure produce large changes in venous blood volume.
- Volume loss results in passive constriction and expansion of circulating volume.
- Increased sympathetic activity resulting from volume loss also causes an active venous constriction and contributes to maintaining the cardiac output.

Physiology of the capillary microcirculation

- Flow and pressure through the microcirculation are controlled by varying the resistance (radius) of the arterioles.
- Arteriolar dilatation causes an increase in flow and pressure in the capillaries downstream, whilst arteriolar constriction causes a reduction in flow and pressure.
- The microcirculation is permeable to all dissolved substances except plasma proteins.
- Proteins leak out slowly into the interstitium and are removed through the lymphatic channels.
- Individual substances such as glucose, K^+, Na^+, and O_2 exchange across the capillary membrane by simple diffusion, passing through the endothelial cells if lipid-soluble or between the endothelial cells if they are not lipid-soluble.
- Filtration is mainly due to the capillary hydrostatic pressure (P_c; 25 mmHg) that pushes fluid out into the interstitium, supported by a small interstitial osmotic pressure (π_{IF}; 1 mmHg) exerted by the small amount of filtered proteins (Figures 3.6 and 3.7).
- Reabsorption is mainly due to the capillary oncotic pressure (π_c; 20 mmHg) exerted by proteins that cannot penetrate the capillary membrane, supported by a small interstitial hydrostatic pressure (P_{IF}; 2 mmHg) (Figures 3.6 and 3.7).
- The net filtration force is therefore 4 mmHg (i.e. $(25 + 1) - (20 + 2)$).
- Capillary hydrostatic pressure (P_C), and therefore filtration, is increased by arteriolar dilatation (e.g. during exercise) and venous constriction (e.g. inferior vena cava compression in pregnancy). P_C is decreased by arteriolar constriction (e.g. essential hypertension and haemorrhage).
- Capillary oncotic pressure is increased by dehydration (sweating, diarrhoea, and raised plasma protein concentration) and reduced by liver disease (reduced protein

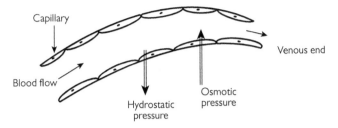

Figure 3.6 Capillary hydrostatic and oncotic pressures, and interstitial fluid.

synthesis), renal disease (increased protein loss), and saline infusion (dilution of blood and reduced protein concentration).

- Interstitial oncotic pressure is increased by chronic lymphatic blockade (e.g. lymphatic tumours, infestations) and factors that increase capillary permeability such as burns.

Pregnancy-specific changes in the cardiovascular system

- Plasma volume is increased by 45–50%
- Blood volume is increased by 40%
- Heart rate increases by 10–20 bpm (by 32 weeks)
- Cardiac output is increased by 30–50% (by 24 weeks)
- Systemic vascular resistance (SVR) is reduced by 20–30%
- Dilutional decrease in colloid oncotic pressure
- Central venous pressure is unchanged

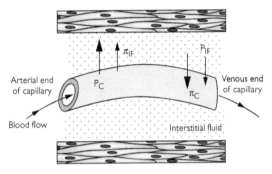

Figure 3.7 Filtration—hydrostatic pressure forces water and dissolved substances out of the capillaries into the intestial space. Reabsorption—mainly due to plasma oncotic pressure.

Respiratory physiology

Tables 3.2 and 3.3 and Figure 3.8 give an overview of the lung volumes and capacities involved in breathing.

Dead space and the respiratory zone

- 'Anatomical dead space' refers to the regions of the respiratory system that contain air but are not exchanging with blood. It includes the conducting airways and is approximately 150 ml in volume. The first 150 ml of the tidal volume (500 ml) fills the dead space and the rest (350 ml) is alveolar ventilation.
- The respiratory zone (theoretically in the alveoli) is approximately 2500 ml in volume and should be exchanging with blood. It is considered a constant environment.
- At the end of normal inspiration, the air within the dead space is the same as room air and is generally considered to lack CO_2.
- Following expiration, the air in the dead space has the same composition as that in the respiratory zone.

Mechanics of respiration

- When the main muscle of inspiration—the diaphragm—contracts, there is an increase in the negative pressure within the thoracic cavity from –5 mmHg to –8 mmHg, which is enough to overcome the forces of lung recoil.
- Lung recoil is the force that develops in the wall of the lung as it expands and always acts to collapse the lung. It increases with lung expansion and decreases as the lung gets smaller.
- As the lung expands, the recoil force increases progressively until it reaches +8 mmHg. At this point it equals the intrapleural pressure, therefore stopping further expansion of the lung.

Partial pressures and alveolar gas exchange

The main gases in the atmosphere, N_2, O_2, and CO_2, exert a combined atmospheric pressure of 760 mmHg. Oxygen makes up 21% of this mixture, or 160 mmHg of the total

Table 3.2 Average lung volumes in healthy adults and their measurements

Measurement	Definition	Approximate volume (ml) for an adult male	Approximate volume (ml) for an adult female
Tidal volume (TV)	Volume of air in and out of the lungs during a normal respiratory cycle	500	500
Inspiratory reserve volume (IRV)	Maximum volume of air that can be inspired beyond the normal tidal volume	3100	1900
Expiratory reserve volume (ERV)	Maximum volume of air that can be expired from the resting end-expiratory position	1200	800
Residual volume (RV)	Volume of air left in the respiratory system after a maximal expiration; this is the volume of air that you can never expire	1200	1100

Table 3.3 Average lung capacities in healthy adults and their measurements

Measurement	Definition	Approximate volume (ml) in an adult male	Approximate volume (ml) in an adult female
Total lung capacity (TLC)	Maximum amount of air contained in the lungs after a maximum inspiratory effort: TV + IRV + ERV + RV	6000	4200
Vital capacity (VC)	Maximum amount of air that can be expired after a maximum inspiratory effort: TV + IRV + ERV	4800	3100
Inspiratory capacity (IC)	Maximum amount of air that can be inspired after a normal expiration: TV + IRV	3600	2400
Functional residual capacity (FRC)	Volume of air remaining in the lungs after a normal tidal volume expiration: ERV + RV	2200	1800

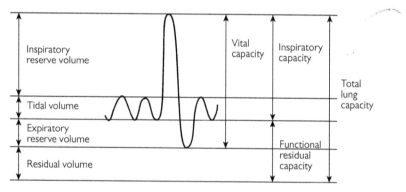

Figure 3.8 Lung volumes and capacities. Note that residual volume (RV) or any lung capacity containing RV (e.g. FRC or TLC) cannot be measured by simple spirometry. Reproduced from Jeremy Hull, Julian Forton, and Anne Thomson, *Oxford Specialist Handbook: Paediatric Respiratory Medicine*, 2008, Figure A4.1, page 821, with permission from Oxford University Press.

atmospheric pressure. However, when air is taken into the airway, water vapour is added and this reduces the partial pressure of oxygen from 160 mmHg to 100 mmHg (Figure 3.9).

Factors affecting alveolar pCO_2 and pO_2

A direct relationship exists between alveolar pCO_2 and the body's metabolic production of CO_2, whereas the relationship between alveolar pCO_2 and alveolar ventilation is indirect. If alveolar ventilation matches metabolism then pCO_2 remains constant. During exercise, if the body's metabolism trebles, then alveolar ventilation must treble, and if metabolic rate halves as a result of hypothermia, then alveolar ventilation must halve to match the body's metabolism.

- Under normal conditions the metabolic rate (MR) (metabolic production of CO_2) is constant, such that it is only alveolar ventilation that affects alveolar pCO_2. Alveolar pCO_2 decreases with hyperventilation and increases with hypoventilation.
- Three main factors affect alveolar pO_2:
  1. Atmospheric pressure (normally 760 mmHg at sea level but may be increased in hyperbaric chambers or decreased with increasing altitude)
  2. Fractional concentration of O_2 (21% in room and alveolar air, but increased by increasing the concentration of O_2 in the inspired air)
  3. Alveolar pressure of CO_2 (pCO_2) (normally 40 mmHg, but if pCO_2 is increased it decreases pO_2, whereas a change in pO_2 does not necessarily change pCO_2)
- The rate of gas transfer is directly proportional to the surface area, the solubility of the gas, and the concentration gradient across the membrane, which is the net force driving the diffusion of the gas (60 mmHg (i.e. 100 – 40) for O_2 and 7 mmHg (i.e. 47 – 40) for CO_2) (Figure 3.9).
- The rate of gas transfer is indirectly proportional to the thickness of the membrane across which transfer occurs.

Oxygen transport

Oxygen is carried in two forms in the bloodstream: (i) dissolved in plasma (up to 0.3 volume%); and (ii) carried by haemoglobin (19.4 volume%). 'Oxygen content' refers to the concentration of oxygen in the blood expressed in volume%; in the arterial blood the total oxygen content is 19.7 volume%. Although oxygen is very poorly soluble in plasma, it is the dissolved oxygen that creates pO_2. pO_2 is the force that keeps oxygen attached to the haemoglobin molecule because haemoglobin does not have sufficient affinity to bind oxygen in the absence of a pO_2.

Characteristics of binding sites for O_2 on the Hb molecule (oxyhaemoglobin)

Each haemoglobin molecule contains four iron (Fe^{2+}) ions, each providing an attachment site for an oxygen molecule. Therefore, each haemoglobin molecule can carry a maximum of four oxygen molecules. In the lungs haemoglobin combines with oxygen to form oxyhaemoglobin (HbO_2) with the saturation of the Hb molecule dependent on the amount of oxygen in the alveolar air. The four binding sites on the Hb molecule are specific and ranked from 1 to 4 depending on the strength of their affinity (the higher the affinity of the binding site, the smaller the PO_2 required for binding).

- Site 1—oxygen is usually attached to this site under physiological conditions.
- Site 2—minimum pO_2 for oxygen to bind to this site is 26 mmHg, which is also the P_{50} for oxygen binding to Hb (pO_2 required for 50% of the Hb to be saturated with oxygen).
- Site 3—minimum pO_2 for oxygen binding to this site is 40 mmHg, which is also the pO_2 of systemic venous blood. Venous blood is thus 75% saturated under resting conditions, meaning only one molecule of oxygen is extracted from the Hb molecule in the tissues.
- Site 4 has the least affinity for oxygen and therefore needs the greatest pO_2 to keep oxygen attached to the haemoglobin molecule. The pO_2 for binding to this site is 100 mmHg and thus Hb is 97% saturated when leaving the lungs.

Oxygen–haemoglobin dissociation curve

This is a graph that shows the percentage saturation of haemoglobin at various partial pressures of oxygen, or the equilibrium between oxyhaemoglobin and the non-bonded haemoglobin ($Hb + O_2 \Leftrightarrow HbO_2$) at various partial

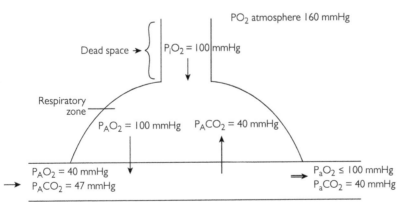

Figure 3.9 Pulmonary capillary blood flow and gas exchange.

pressures of oxygen (Figure 3.10). The sigmoid shape of the oxygen dissociation curve is a result of the cooperative binding of oxygen to the four binding sites of haemoglobin. Thus, haemoglobin is most attracted to oxygen when three of the four binding sites are bound to oxygen.

Factors affecting the oxygen–haemoglobin dissociation curve

Several physiologic or pathologic states may shift the oxygen–haemoglobin dissociation curve to the right or left (Figure 3.10). If the curve is shifted to the right, the P_{50} moves to the right, meaning that a higher pO_2 is required to keep oxygen attached to the haemoglobin molecule. In other words, there is a loss of affinity and systemic tissues will find it easier to get oxygen from the haemoglobin molecule. Factors that shift the curve to the right are mostly associated with tissue metabolism and include:

- *Temperature*—increasing the temperature denatures the bond between oxygen and haemoglobin.
- *Carbon dioxide and acidity (pH)*—CO_2 decreases the pH and this causes oxyhaemoglobin to dissociate and release O_2. A very small decrease in the pH results in a large decrease in the percentage saturation of the haemoglobin with O_2. The shift of the dissociation curve to the right when the pH is low even with a relatively high pO_2 is called the *Bohr effect*.
- *2,3-Diphosphoglycerate (DPG)*—the primary mammalian organic phosphate binds to haemoglobin and rearranges the haemoglobin molecule in a way that decreases its affinity for oxygen, and shifts the curve to the right.

If the curve is shifted to the left, there is a gain in haemoglobin affinity for oxygen. Therefore, it is easier to load haemoglobin with oxygen in the lungs but more difficult for the tissues to extract oxygen. Factors that shift the oxygen dissociation curve to the left include:

- Reduced temperature, reduced pCO_2, reduced 2,3-DPG, reduced H^+ (or raised pH), fetal haemoglobin, and myoglobin (Figure 3.10).
- Carbon monoxide—this shifts the curve to the left because it increases haemoglobin affinity for oxygen, but also shifts it downwards because it reduces saturation of the haemoglobin.

In simple anaemia, the oxygen saturation is normal but the overall oxygen content of the blood (oxygen-carrying capacity) is reduced because of the reduced Hb concentration. With polycythaemia there is more oxygen contained per unit volume. In both anaemia and polycythaemia, the curve does not shift.

Carbon dioxide transport

Carbon dioxide, unlike oxygen, is very soluble in plasma and is carried in three forms:

1. dissolved carbon dioxide
2. carbamino (protein) compounds ($HbCO_2$)
3. bicarbonate (HCO_3^-) (most CO_2 is carried as plasma HCO_3^-).
   - Within the capillaries of systemic tissues, the CO_2 produced is picked up by the RBC, where the reaction $CO_2 + H_2O \leftrightarrow H^+ + HCO_3^-$ takes place, catalysed by the enzyme carbonic anhydrase (Figure 3.11). The H^+ is buffered by the Hb molecule whilst the HCO_3^- is transported back out of the cell into the plasma, where it is transported. Chloride ions (Cl^-) move into the RBC to maintain electrical neutrality. Around 95% of the CO_2 generated in the tissues is carried as bicarbonate in this way (Figure 3.11).
   - When the RBCs reach the lungs these reactions are reversed, with HCO_3^- entering the RBC to combine with H^+ to form water and CO_2 (Figure 3.12). Chloride ions exit the RBC to maintain electrical neutrality

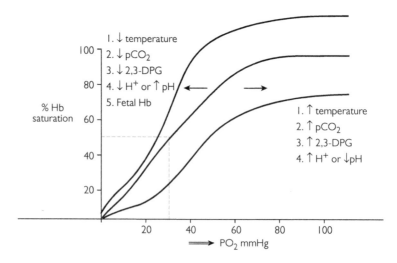

Figure 3.10 Oxyhaemoglobin dissociation curve.

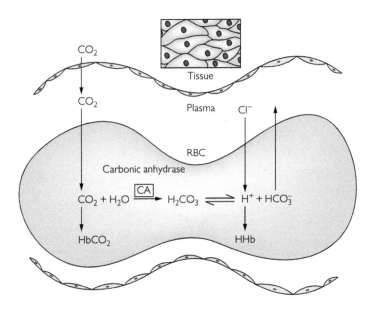

Figure 3.11 Carbon dioxide (CO_2) transport in systemic capillaries.

(chloride shift). The CO_2 is released to the air of the alveoli (Figure 3.12).

- Approximately 5% of the CO_2 generated in the tissues dissolves directly in the plasma (but if all the CO_2 generated were carried in the plasma, the pH of the blood would drop from 7.4 to a fatal 4.5).

Regulation of alveolar ventilation

Alveolar ventilation is affected mainly by pCO_2, pO_2, and H^+ concentration via the central or peripheral chemoreceptors. The blood–brain barrier (BBB) is very permeable to CO_2 and the receptors are very sensitive to increased systemic arterial (not venous) CO_2 tension. Increases in pCO_2 stimulate the central chemoreceptors and increase alveolar ventilation. A decrease in arterial pCO_2 causes a decrease in the stimulation of the chemoreceptor and therefore a decrease in the drive for alveolar ventilation. There are no oxygen receptors in the regulating centre and H^+ ions do not cross the BBB very easily, so CO_2 acting on the central chemoreceptor is the main drive for alveolar ventilation in a normal individual at sea level. H^+ in the CSF will also stimulate ventilation but arterial H^+ will not.

The peripheral chemoreceptors are located in the carotid and aortic bodies near to the carotid sinus and aortic arch respectively. They have H^+ and CO_2 receptors and directly monitor the chemical composition of the blood. However, they are less sensitive than the central chemoreceptors and therefore make a smaller contribution to the drive for alveolar ventilation. They monitor arterial pO_2 (dissolved

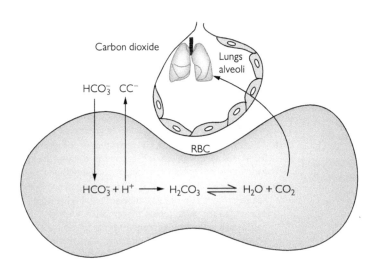

Figure 3.12 Carbon dioxide (CO_2) transport in the pulmonary capillaries.

oxygen) rather than the oxygen content of the blood and are very strongly stimulated by a dramatic drop in pO_2. Unlike the central chemoreceptors, which adapt to chronic hypercapnia, these receptors never adapt.

Pregnancy-specific changes in the respiratory system

- Oxygen demand is increased.
- Functional residual capacity (FRC) is reduced.

- Oxygen desaturation is more common.
- Minute ventilation is increased.
- Respiratory rate is increased.
- Mild respiratory alkalosis.

Renal physiology

Renal physiology in health and in pregnancy

The primary role of the kidney is to maintain a constant extracellular environment for effective cellular function. This involves the regulation of extracellular fluid volume and its composition, and removal of waste products of metabolism. The kidney regulates the excretion of water and solutes such as sodium, potassium, and hydrogen ions, and performs endocrine functions including the synthesis and secretion of renin, erythropoietin, and 1,25-dihydroxycholecalciferol (the active metabolite of vitamin D).

Normal pregnancy is associated with marked changes in renal physiology and anatomy characterized by alterations in renal handling of fluid and electrolytes.

Basic renal physiology

Nephron structure and function

The basic functional unit of the kidney is the nephron. Each kidney contains approximately 1 million nephrons. The nephron comprises a number of segments with specialized functions (Figure 3.13).

- The *glomerulus* is the tuft of specialized capillaries of the nephron, which sits over the Bowman's capsule. The primary function of the glomerulus is to produce a protein-free filtrate from blood via the uniquely specialized filtration barrier, formed by the capillary endothelium, basement membrane, and epithelial cells of the Bowman's capsule.
- The *proximal tubule* performs the bulk of solute reabsorption from the glomerular ultrafiltrate.
- The *loop of Henle* serves to generate the hyperosmolar interstitium that forms the basis of the nephron's concentrating capacity.
- Further solute reabsorption and secretion occurs in the *distal tubule*.
- The *collecting duct* allows the production of concentrated urine, under the influence of antidiuretic hormone (ADH; vasopressin).

Blood supply, haemodynamics, and glomerular filtration rate (GFR)

- The kidneys normally receive 20–25% of the total cardiac output.

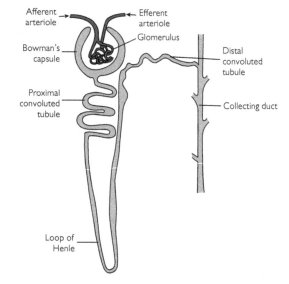

Figure 3.13 The nephron.

- The glomerular filtration rate (GFR) is the amount of filtrate produced from the blood per unit time. The GFR in non-pregnant individuals is 90–120 ml/min/1.73 m^2 of surface area and about 180 l of filtrate is produced each day.
- The filtration fraction is the proportion of renal plasma flow that gets filtered through the glomerulus, and in normal individuals it is approximately 20%.
- The glomerular filtrate normally contains no blood cells or platelets, and virtually no protein. The presence of significant protein or significant numbers of abnormal red blood cells in the urine is therefore suggestive of glomerular disease.
- As with any capillary bed, the formation of the glomerular filtrate in the Bowman's capsule is dictated by the hydrostatic and colloid osmotic (oncotic) pressures.
- *Autoregulation:* The cells of the distal nephron sense the solute composition of distal tubular fluid. Higher sodium delivery to the distal tubule triggers vasoconstrictor signals, which act on the afferent arteriole to reduce glomerular capillary hydrostatic pressure, thus reducing the GFR. This phenomenon, known as *tubuloglomerular feedback*, controls the GFR of each nephron.

- *The renin-angiotensin-aldosterone system:* Renin is released by cells of the juxtaglomerular apparatus (JGA) in response to reduced sodium delivery to this part of the nephron or a reduction in renal perfusion pressure (Figure 3.14). The effects of renin release are discussed in detail below.
- *Prostaglandins:* A decrease in the effective circulating blood volume triggers local prostaglandin synthesis within the kidney, and leads to arteriolar vasodilatation, thus increasing blood flow to the glomeruli.
- Other vasoactive peptides and substances such as atrial natriuretic peptide (ANP), dopamine, nitric oxide, kinins, and adenosine also help to regulate renal blood flow by exerting effects on renal blood flow and hence GFR.

Renal physiology in pregnancy

Anatomical changes

- The kidneys increase in size by up to 1.5 cm in bipolar diameter, due to increases both in vascular volume and interstitial space.
- The collecting system and ureters dilate, partly as a result of the high concentration of circulating progesterone, which reduces ureteral tone, peristalsis, and contraction pressure.
- Mechanical factors also contribute to the ureteral dilatation. Hydronephrosis is present in up to 90% of women by the third trimester and is typically more prominent on the right side because of the dextro-rotation of the uterus (which is believed to be at least in part due to the location of the sigmoid colon on the left side) and/or the kinking of the right ureter as it crosses vascular structures.
- Dilatation of the ureters may persist for several weeks postpartum.
- The dilated collecting system can hold 200 to 300 ml of urine, which can act as a reservoir for bacteria. There may be intermittent vesico-ureteral reflux during pregnancy. These factors lead to an increased risk of ascending infection.
- If untreated, 30% of pregnant women with asymptomatic bacteriuria will develop pyelonephritis with an increased risk of miscarriage or preterm delivery.

Changes in systemic haemodynamics

The altered renal haemodynamics in pregnancy is better understood in the context of the marked alterations in general cardiovascular physiology:

1. Increase in cardiac output

During normal pregnancy, the cardiac output (CO) rises by 30%–50% as a result of increases both in stroke volume (SV) and heart rate (HR). One half of this increase occurs by 8 weeks of gestation. Stroke volume increases early in pregnancy due to the combination of an increased preload (increased blood volume) and a reduction in afterload, which results from systemic vasodilatation. The baseline heart rate rises by 15 to 20 beats per minute and is the major

contributing factor to the increased cardiac output in late pregnancy.

2. Blood volume expansion

Salt and water retention leads to a 30%–50% expansion in plasma volume at term above non-pregnant levels. The high renin levels observed during pregnancy suggest that the increased plasma volume is a response to the relative under-filling that results from the profound systemic vasodilatation.

3. Reductions in blood pressure and systemic vascular resistance (SVR)

As cardiac output increases there is a marked decrease in systemic vascular resistance, resulting in a modest reduction in arterial blood pressure. The precise mechanism behind the vasodilatation is not fully understood. Contributing factors are likely to include a reduced responsiveness to the vasoconstrictive actions of angiotensin II, increased endothelial prostacyclin, and increased production of nitric oxide (see 'glomerular haemodynamics' below).

Changes in renal haemodynamics

Effective renal plasma flow (ERPF), as assessed by p-aminohippurate (PAH) clearance, increases by about 80% between conception and the second trimester, and then decreases to a level about 60% above the non-pregnant norm at term. In contrast, the blood flow to the brain and liver remains relatively constant.

Glomerular haemodynamics and glomerular filtration rate (GFR)

- GFR increases markedly during pregnancy, and peaks at about 50% above non-pregnant levels by 16 weeks gestation. A small decline may be observed during the third trimester.
- The increase in GFR is due to increases in single nephron GFR, as there is no change in the total number of nephrons.
- The rise in GFR is less than the rise in ERPF, implying a reduction in the 'filtration fraction' during pregnancy.
- Animal studies suggest that the increased GFR is due to increased glomerular plasma flow rate as a result of a balanced vasodilatation of both afferent and efferent glomerular arterioles, leading to increased flow. Furthermore, the ability of the kidney to maintain constant blood flow and GFR over a range of systemic blood pressure (renal autoregulation) remains intact during pregnancy, albeit with a higher 'set-point'.
- It is likely that the vasodilatation that underlies these increases in ERPF and GFR is a result of increased nitric oxide (NO) synthesis, since NO synthesis inhibitors reverse renal haemodynamic parameters in pregnant rats to non-pregnant levels.
- The stimulus for increased NO synthesis is unclear; a possible candidate is placental production of *relaxin* under the influence of human chorionic gonadotrophin.

- In pre-eclampsia the increases in ERPF and GFR associated with normal pregnancy are absent or markedly reduced. There is also a change in glomerular filtration characteristics leading to proteinuria.

- Other pathophysiological conditions where an increase in GFR (hyperfiltration) is caused by an increase in glomerular capillary pressure rather than increased glomerular plasma flow rate are associated with progressive glomerular damage. With no sustained glomerular capillary hypertension, normal pregnancy does not lead to kidney injury. However, where there is pre-existing kidney disease, hyperfiltration during pregnancy can accelerate renal damage.

Estimation of GFR during pregnancy

- In the steady state, creatinine (a product of muscle metabolism) is cleared by the kidneys when muscle metabolism is constant such that serum creatinine reflects renal clearance.

- Creatinine clearance (CrCl) is a measure of the volume of plasma cleared of creatinine per unit time and is an index of GFR in the non-pregnant state.

- Due to changes in ERPF and GFR, CrCl increases (i.e. serum creatinine concentration drops) by 25% in the first 4 weeks and by 40%–50% by the end of the first trimester of pregnancy. CrCl decreases by up to 20% in the third trimester and may increase slightly postpartum, returning to pre-pregnancy levels within 3 months of delivery. CrCl approximates renal function but is not an exact measure of GFR.

- These changes in GFR during pregnancy should alert clinicians that a serum creatinine in the normal range during pregnancy is likely to be abnormal and may indicate renal pathology.

Hormonal changes and alterations in electrolyte homeostasis

Salt and water balance in health

A schematic representation of the renin-angiotensin-aldosterone system (RAAS) in health is shown in Figure 3.14.

- Renin is a specific protease enzyme produced in and secreted by the granular cells of the juxtaglomerular apparatus (JGA) of the kidneys in response to reduced circulating volume (detected by the renal baroreceptors in the afferent arteriole), lowered sodium chloride in the ultrafiltrate (detected by the macula densa), and several neurohormonal factors (including sympathetic nervous system activity). The renal baroreceptors in the afferent arteriole are modified pressure-sensitive endothelial cells.

- Renin hydrolyses angiotensinogen, a circulating alpha-2 serum globulin produced by the liver, to the decapeptide angiotensin I. The function of angiotensin I is unclear and it appears to exist solely as a precursor for angiotensin II.

- Angiotensin-converting enzyme (ACE), a membrane-bound metalloproteinase located primarily on the endothelium of the pulmonary capillaries, catalyses the conversion of angiotensin I to angiotensin II. ACE can also be found in other parts of the body.

- Angiotensin II has a number of endocrine, autocrine/paracrine, and intracrine physiological functions:
  - Increased systemic vascular resistance (SVR) by:
    1. direct stimulation of arteriolar vasoconstriction
    2. indirect effect on the central nervous system to increase the sympathetic outflow by potentiating the release of noradrenaline from the postganglionic sympathetic fibres, and reduction of the response of the baroreceptor reflex.
  - Increased cardiac output (CO) by:
    1. increased sympathetic tone (increased HR)
    2. increased plasma volume through:
       i. Antidiuretic hormone (ADH) release from the posterior pituitary. ADH acts on the distal convoluted tubules and collecting duct epithelial cells to stimulate water reabsorption by the insertion of preformed water channels (aquaporins) into the apical membranes. It also has moderate direct vasoconstrictive effects.
       ii. Increasing aldosterone secretion from the adrenal cortex. Aldosterone acts on distal convoluted tubules and the cortical collecting ducts in the kidneys, enhancing sodium and water reabsorption in exchange for potassium.
       iii. Aldosterone and angiotensin II stimulate thirst (dipsogen) and salt craving centrally. Taken together, these effects increase BP.
- Angiotensin II also causes efferent renal arteriolar vasoconstriction to maintain glomerular filtration pressure (and GFR) during reduced renal perfusion.
- Once plasma volume and BP have been restored, increased perfusion of the JGA reduces renin secretion.
- Hypovolaemia leads to production of low volumes of urine that are highly concentrated (>350 mOsm/kg with specific gravity >1.020) but low in sodium (<10 mEq/l; fractional excretion of sodium, FeNa <1%). In contrast, if hypovolaemia continues and acute tubular injury supervenes, the effects of the RAAS are diminished and a salt-losing state with defective concentrating ability supervenes. Established acute tubular injury is, therefore, characterized by variable volumes of dilute urine (<350 mOsm/kg with specific gravity ≤1.010) that are high in sodium (>40 mEq/l; FeNa >2%).
- Excessive RAAS activity is a hallmark of long-term hypertension and is associated with pathological vascular changes. As a result, ACE inhibitors (ACEI) and angiotensin II receptor blockers (ARBs) have beneficial effects beyond mere reduction of BP.

Sodium and osmoregulation in pregnancy

- Renin activity and angiotensin II levels are increased in pregnancy but this is countered by reduced sensitivity to the vasoconstrictive effects of angiotensin II. The mechanism is

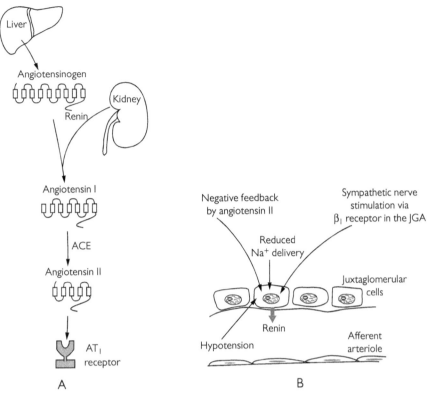

Figure 3.14 General organization of the renin-angiotensin-aldosterone system (RAAS) (A) and sensory inputs into the juxtaglomerular apparatus (JGA) for the regulation of renin (B).

unclear but increased local NO synthesis is likely to play a role.

- Aldosterone level reaches 4–6-fold non-pregnant levels in the third trimester. The effects of aldosterone (Na⁺ and H₂O retention, and increased K⁺ excretion) are believed to be antagonized by the high levels of circulating progesterone (see Table 3.4).

- Increases in renal plasma flow and GFR mean that the kidneys 'see' more solute and protein per unit time during pregnancy. Together with hormonal changes, these effects lead to considerable alterations in electrolyte physiology as follows:

1. Plasma osmolality drops by about 10 mOsm/kg during pregnancy. In a normal and healthy non-pregnant individual, this drop in osmolality should lead to inhibition of ADH and diuresis. However, the osmotic threshold for ADH release also drops during early pregnancy— the so-called 'downward' resetting of the osmostat. The drop in osmotic threshold correlates closely with levels of β-HCG, which is thought to act indirectly by inducing the release of the hormone relaxin.

2. The catabolism of ADH increases during pregnancy via placental degradation and the systemic effects of

the placenta-derived vasopressinase, which breaks down ADH even more. However, serum levels of ADH remain normal due to a fourfold increase in its production.

3. The increase in GFR and ERPF means that the daily filtered sodium load rises as the kidneys effectively 'see' more solute per unit time. Consequently, serum sodium drops by about 5 mEq/l during pregnancy. The hyponatraemia is not compensated for due to the 'downward' resetting of the osmostat and this resetting of the osmostat means that the lower serum sodium concentration will be maintained at this level despite marked daily variations in sodium or water intake.

4. Despite hyponatraemia, there is net sodium retention during pregnancy, distributed between fetal and maternal tissues, due to two or more mechanisms: an increase in sodium intake and reabsorption of filtered tubular sodium. The mechanism of increased sodium reabsorption is poorly understood.

5. The clinical sequelae of the changes in osmolality and serum sodium is that polyuria is uncommon, as most women can compensate for the higher catabolism of ADH by its increased production. However, polyuria

can occur in women with overt or subclinical central or nephrogenic diabetes insipidus in whom secretory reserve of ADH or renal responsiveness to ADH is impaired (exacerbated by the rise in GFR seen in pregnancy).

6. Generally, gestational hyponatraemia is usually mild and attempts to correct it are both unnecessary and ineffective.

Acid-base balance and potassium

- Dietary intake of proteins and homeostatic metabolism lead to generation of metabolic acids that are cleared by the kidneys under physiological conditions.
- The daily production of metabolic acids is increased in pregnancy due to an increase in basal metabolic rate, fetal metabolic load, and an increase in daily protein intake.
- Pregnancy is characterized by relative alkalaemia: a mean arterial pH of 7.44 (7.40 non-pregnant state) due to hyperventilation induced by progesterone on the respiratory centre and increased respiratory effort in response to the uterus splinting the diaphragm.
- There is an overall drop in arterial pCO_2 of about 10 mmHg (1.3 kPa) and a compensatory renal loss of

Table 3.4 Effects of physical and hormonal factors on sodium excretion in pregnancy

Factors	Effect on Na$^+$ excretion
Physical factors	
Increased intra-ureteral pressure results in effective arteriovenous shunting	↓
Decrease in mean arterial pressure leads to increased sodium reabsorption	↓
Supine and upright postures have exaggerated antinatriuretic effects in pregnancy	↓
Increased GFR causes increased sodium filtration at the glomerulus	↑
Decreased serum albumin reduces tubular reabsorption of sodium	↑
Hormonal factors	
Increased angiotensin II leads to increased sodium reabsorption	↓
Increased aldosterone has an antinatriuretic effect	↓
Increase in antinatriuretic hormones (e.g. oestrogen, cortisol, prolactin, placental lactogen, ACTH etc.	↓
Increased progesterone has a natriuretic effect	↑
Increased natriuretic hormones (e.g. atrial natriuretic peptide, ADH, oxytocin, neutrotrophins)	↑

bicarbonate, which partially compensates the pH but results in a lower serum bicarbonate of around 18–22 mmol/l during pregnancy. In acid-base terms, this could be described as a metabolic acidosis with respiratory alkalaemia.

- The renal handling of acid (excretion of H$^+$) and base (reabsorption of bicarbonate) are not altered during a normal pregnancy.
- The clinical consequence of the above changes in acid-base balance during pregnancy is that sudden metabolic acidosis is more dangerous because steady-state bicarbonate and pCO_2 are lower. Therefore, conditions such as acute kidney injury, lactic acidosis, and diabetic ketoacidosis should be treated with particular diligence.
- Potassium excretion is generally linked to acid-base balance. Acidosis is usually associated with hyperkalaemia and alkalosis with hypokalaemia. Acidosis is characterized by high concentrations of H$^+$ in the extracellular fluid compartment. Over time, H$^+$ flows into the intracellular compartment. To maintain electrical neutrality, K$^+$ ions are forced out of the intracellular compartment into the extracellular space, creating a state of hyperkalaemia. In alkalosis, the reduced H$^+$ concentration in the extracellular fluid compartment is compensated for by an efflux of intracellular H$^+$ into the extracellular space. K$^+$ flows into the cells to maintain electrical neutrality, creating a hypokalaemic state.
- Potassium excretion is reduced during pregnancy despite high aldosterone levels and relatively alkaline urine. The mechanism is not completely understood but it is likely to be related to the elevated levels of progesterone exerting anti-mineralocorticoid effects, probably through the inhibition of active potassium excretion in the distal tubule and collecting ducts. As a result there is net potassium retention, which, like sodium, is distributed throughout fetal and maternal tissues without causing hyperkalaemia.
- Clinically, changes in potassium homeostasis result in a relative resistance to kaliuretic drugs (e.g. mineralocorticoids) and protection against potassium-losing diseases in pregnancy (e.g. Conn's or Bartter's syndromes). Diseases that impair excretion of potassium, such as sickle cell disease, could become more dangerous in pregnancy.

Calcium

- Increased ERPF and GFR deliver an increased filtered load of calcium to the tubules, resulting in increased calcium excretion.
- Elevated levels of calcitriol (1,25-dihydroxy-vitamin D$_3$) suppress the counter-regulatory hormone, parathyroid hormone (PTH), but hypocalcaemia remains rare because calcitriol also stimulates calcium absorption from the gut.
- Renal stone formation is rare as urinary 'solubilizing agents', such as magnesium and citrate, are also high in pregnancy and maintain calcium in solution.

Tubular handling of other solutes and proteins

Glucose

- Under conditions of normal glucose load, the renal tubules reabsorb nearly all the filtered glucose and there is no detectable glucose in urine. During pregnancy, increased ERPF and GFR lead to the delivery of excessive amounts of glucose to the renal tubules. The tubular maximum (T_{max}) for reabsorption of glucose may therefore be exceeded, resulting in incomplete reabsorption of glucose and glycosuria.
- There are no abnormalities of carbohydrate metabolism in this setting and glycosuria resolves within a week of delivery.
- Glycosuria can be common in pregnancy and is not diagnostic of gestational diabetes. Clinically, there is a diurnal variation of glycosuria, being less in the morning and greater after meals.

Uric acid

- Reduced tubular reabsorption of uric acid (i.e. increased uric acid clearance) causes lowered serum levels of urate during early pregnancy. Often, serum uric acid levels are reduced by about 25%. As pregnancy progresses, uric acid levels rise again due to increased tubular reabsorption.
- Clinically, there is diurnal variation in serum urate levels and 'normal' values change as pregnancy progresses. Levels are higher with multi-fetal gestation, indicating that some maternal urate may be derived from by-products of fetal metabolism. There is sufficient variability in urate levels that some normal healthy women with uncomplicated pregnancies can have hyperuricaemia without clinical syndromes.

Proteins and amino acids

- Proteins are not normally filtered by the glomerulus because of their large size and charge. Increased GFR and glomerular permeability increase filtered levels of proteins during pregnancy. Consequently, both urinary total protein and albumin excretion increase. This is most apparent after about 20 weeks of gestation.
- In contrast, the excretion of many amino acids is increased during pregnancy (up to 2 g/day) but some return to lower levels of excretion as pregnancy progresses.
- Semi-quantitative proteinuria of 1+ is common on dipstick testing but not all of these patients have abnormal protein excretion. In general, serial measurements of urine for proteinuria are more useful than a single sample and quantification is important in cases where dipstick proteinuria is evident. Where proteinuria exceeds 300 mg per 24 hours it is considered to be abnormal.
- Although a timed sample of urine (usually over 24 hours) is the gold standard for urinary protein estimation, in practice the protein to creatinine ratio on a spot sample of urine is more convenient, saves time, and minimizes errors in sample collection. Accuracy with this method is high, especially if the sample has been collected after the first morning void and before bedtime.

Renal disease in pregnancy

Proteinuria

- Persistent proteinuria is often the first sign of renal disease and predates the development of overt renal impairment.
- Persistent proteinuria is a cardinal feature of pre-eclampsia or pre-existing renal disease, e.g. minimal change nephropathy, or secondary to systemic disorders such as diabetes or systemic lupus erythematosus (SLE). It can be difficult to distinguish between these conditions, as pre-existing renal disease is frequently associated with the occurrence of superimposed pre-eclampsia.
- The diagnosis of proteinuria can be made with a urine dipstick, but will also require a further method of quantification, such as the urine protein to creatinine ratio on a spot sample or a 24-hour collection.
- Proteinuria can be nephrotic (≥3 g per 24 h) or sub-nephrotic (<3 g per 24 h) in range. Quantification is essential as management of nephrotic-range proteinuria differs from that for sub-nephrotic proteinuria.

Nephrotic syndrome in pregnancy

- This is characterized by the triad of significant proteinuria, hypoalbuminaemia, and oedema. The proteinuria is often greater than 3 g per day and can be due to a primary glomerular disease (e.g. minimal change nephropathy), a systemic disease such as diabetes, or a manifestation of pre-eclampsia.
- There is loss of anticoagulant proteins in the urine and the risk of venous thromboembolic disease is high, especially if the albumin level falls below 20 mg/dl. Prophylactic anticoagulation should be considered.

Haematuria

- Macroscopic (visible) haematuria ensues with ≥5 ml of blood/l. Leakage of blood from glomeruli is often accompanied by leakage of protein (blood contains approximately 60 g/l of total protein, of which 40 g/l is albumin) so haematuria accompanied by significant proteinuria usually indicates a glomerular source for the haematuria. Lower quantities of haematuria are not usually visible to the naked eye (microscopic haematuria).
- Microscopic haematuria (non-visible) in pregnancy could be due to a urinary tract infection, glomerulonephritis, or pre-eclampsia. Macroscopic haematuria is more likely to be due to contamination from vaginal bleeding or a urinary tract infection, but can be seen in some glomerular diseases such as IgA nephropathy or Henoch-Schoenlein purpura (HSP).

Red blood cell physiology and haematology

Blood consists of 55% plasma and 45% cellular components (99% of which are red blood cells and 1% white blood cells and platelets).

Normal haematopoiesis

- Haematopoiesis is regulated by cytokines or haematopoietic growth factors.
- The site of haematopoiesis varies with age:
  - In the early embryo it is first seen in the yolk sac.
  - In infants it occurs in fetal liver and throughout the bone marrow (BM).
  - By adulthood it occurs in the BM of the central skeleton (vertebrae, ribs, sternum, skull, sacrum, pelvis) and in proximal ends of long bones (humerus and femur).
- The haematopoietic stem cell (HSC) is the earliest cell that can be identified in BM. It is pluripotent: capable of self-renewal and of differentiating into all cell lineages including red cells, white cells, and platelets.

Physiological changes in pregnancy

- Increased red cell mass by up to 30%.
- Increased plasma volume by up to 60%.
- Net increase in blood volume of up to 50%.
- Decreased haemoglobin concentration and haematocrit.
- Increased MCV.
- Decreased platelet count by up to 10%.
- Increased level of coagulation factors (see the section on 'Disorders of haemostasis associated with pregnancy').

Red blood cells (RBCs)

- They are large (about 6–8 μm) biconcave discs with no nucleus.
- There are about 4.5–5.8 million RBC/μl (with gender and racial variation).
- Their main role is to transport oxygen from the lungs to the body tissues, but they also transfer carbon dioxide from the tissues to be exhaled by the lungs.
- They do not contain DNA, RNA, or mitochondria and produce energy (ATP) from glycolysis through the reducing power of NADH and NADPH.
- The average life span of each RBC is 120 days.
- Production is regulated by the growth factor erythropoietin (EpO).

EpO

- EpO is produced in peritubular cells of the kidney.
- It is released at low O_2 tension (hypoxia, anaemia).
- It reacts with EpO receptors on RBC precursors to increase production ≥6-fold.
- Recombinant EpO is now available for the treatment of anaemia due to renal failure and for Jehovah's Witness patients who decline transfusion of allogenic blood components on religious grounds.

Haemoglobin

- This is a tetrameric molecule containing four haem groups and four globin chains. Haem is a ferrous iron molecule in a porphyrin ring structure and globin is a polypeptide chain containing two α chains and two non-α chains.
- Adult Hb (HbA) is made up of two α and two β globin chains.
- Fetal Hb (HbF) is made up of two α and two γ chains; the switch from HbF to HbA starts at birth and is complete by about 6 months.
- It is important for oxygen transport from the lungs, where there is a high partial pressure of oxygen (PO_2), to the tissues, with a low pO_2. On average, 1 g of Hb combines with 1.34 ml of O_2.

Haematinics: dietary substances essential for the production of RBCs and Hb

(a) Iron

- Plays a major role in several metabolic processes.
- Combines with protoporphyrin ring to form haem (there are four haem groups to each tetramer of Hb).
- Found in food as ferric hydroxide, ferric protein complexes, and haem protein complexes, with red meat being the best source available. Normal daily intake from a Western diet is 10–15 mg but only 1–2 mg (5–10%) is absorbed daily.
- Absorption occurs in the duodenum and jejunum, mainly in the ferric form, enhanced by acid and reducing agents, e.g. ascorbic acid.
- Transported in plasma combined with transferrin and stored as ferritin.
- Increased iron is required in pregnancy and lactation.

(b) Vitamin B_{12}

- Produced only by micro-organisms and found mainly in animal produce.
- Absorption occurs through the ileum in combination with intrinsic factor (IF), which is produced by gastric parietal cells.
- Minimum daily requirement of 1–2 μg; normal body stores of 2–3 mg last 2–4 years.

(c) Folic acid

- Natural folates in the polyglutamate form occur in most foods but especially liver, vegetables, and yeasts; however, they are easily destroyed by cooking.
- Absorption is through the duodenum and jejunum.
- Normal daily dietary intake of 600–1000 μg; daily requirement of 100–200 μg and body stores of 10–12 mg last for up to 4 months.

White blood cells (WBCs)

- These play an essential role in fighting infection by phago-cytosis, concentrating at the site of infection and ingesting bacteria, thereby preventing the spread of infection.
- Average life span of a few hours to a few days.
- WBCs include both granulocytes and agranular leukocytes.

Granulocytes (or polymorphs)

These have large, characteristic granules in their cytoplasm that can be seen under a light microscope. They are much smaller than the RBCs, averaging about 1/700 of a RBC. There are three types of granulocytes: neutrophils, eosinophils, and basophils.

(a) Neutrophils

- Average size is 10–12 μm in diameter.
- There is a dense nucleus made of two to five lobes connected by thin strands of chromatin, and the cytoplasm has very fine, pale lilac granules.
- Attracted to sites of infection/inflammation by chemotaxis, where they phagocytose and kill bacteria.
- Neutrophil leukocytosis or an increase in neutrophil numbers occurs mostly in infection but also in pregnancy, exercise, stress, steroid treatment, and myeloproliferative disorders.
- Neutropenia or a decrease in numbers occurs with bone marrow failure syndromes, drugs, viral infections, and autoimmune disorders. Severe neutropenia ($<1.0 \times 10^9$/l) can lead to life-threatening infections.

(b) Eosinophils

- Nuclei have up to three lobes and the cytoplasm contains coarser pink/red granules.
- Play an important role in specific defence against parasites and in response to allergic reactions.

(c) Basophils

- Have bi-lobed nuclei and contain large, dark-purple cytoplasmic granules.
- Involved in immediate hypersensitivity reactions (asthma, anaphylaxis) and in defence against allergens and parasites.

Agranulocytes

Agranulocytes do not contain visible granules. They include lymphocytes and monocytes:

- Lymphocytes produce antibodies including T cells, B cells, and NK cells.
- Monocytes are essential for active phagocytosis of bacteria.

Platelets

- Small (2–4 μm), non-nucleated cells with a complex infra-structure including numerous cytoplasmic granules.
- Production occurs in BM by fragmentation of the cytoplasm of their precursor, the megakaryocyte (very large, multi-nucleated cells found only in BM).

- Production is regulated by the growth factor thrombopoietin, which is produced mainly in the liver.
- Platelets play a vital role in the primary haemostatic process.
- Normal life span is 7–10 days.

Anaemia

Anaemia in pregnancy can be:

- dilutional anaemia (Hb rarely <10.0 g/dl)
- microcytic anaemia (low MCV) in iron deficiency anaemia, haemoglobinopathies
- macrocytic anaemia (high MCV) in folate deficiency (common), vitamin B_{12} deficiency (rare)
- anaemia due to other chronic underlying disorder.

Microcytic anaemia

(a) Iron deficiency anaemia

- Diagnosed on FBC by ↓ Hb, ↓ MCV, and ↓ MCH.
- Blood film shows microcytic, hypochromic red cells.
- Platelet count may be raised (secondary to bleeding).

Management

- Treat underlying cause.
- Replace with oral iron (ferrous sulphate; 67 mg elemental iron per 200 mg tablet) for up to 6 months to correct anaemia and replenish stores:
  - Expected Hb rise of about 2 g/dl every 3 weeks.
  - Side effects include diarrhoea or constipation.
  - Manage side effects by reducing dose or using preparation with a lower iron content, e.g. ferrous gluconate (37 mg iron/300 mg tablet).
  - Parenteral iron is available but may cause allergic reactions or anaphylaxis.
- Blood transfusion rarely indicated.

(b) Haemoglobinopathies

- Sickle cell disease: single amino acid substitution occurs on β chain (valine substituted for glutamic acid at position 6).
- Thalassaemias: mutations in one or more of the α or β globin genes cause a reduction in the amount of HbA produced (alpha thalassaemia is due to deletion or mutation in one or more of the four α globin gene copies and

Table 3.5 Iron deficiency anaemia

Iron studies	(Normal values)
Serum iron: ↓	(10–30 μmol/l)
Total iron binding capacity: ↑	(50–70 μmol/l)
Transferrin saturation: ↓	(>16%)
*Serum ferritin level: ↓	(12–150 μg/l)

(*best indicator of iron status; when <12 μg/l, indicates iron deficiency)

beta thalassaemia is due to mutations in one or both of the β globin genes).

Macrocytosis (raised MCV)

Macrocytosis can be caused by any of the following:

- reticulocytosis (acute bleeding)
- vitamin B_{12} or folate deficiency
- alcoholic liver disease
- hypothyroidism
- myelodysplasia.

Diagnostic tests

- Blood film
- Reticulocyte count
- Liver and thyroid function tests
- Serum B_{12} and folate assays
- Bone marrow aspirate: megaloblastic features occur in severe B_{12} or folate deficiency

Macrocytic anaemia

(a) Vitamin B_{12} deficiency

- May be caused by:
  - malabsorption
  - dietary lack (vegans)
  - pernicious anaemia: antibodies against intrinsic factor (IF)
  - blind-loop syndrome.
- Presents with macrocytic, megaloblastic anaemia but severe deficiency may cause neurological complications such as subacute combined degeneration of the cord.
- Pernicious anaemia (PA) is associated with other autoimmune disorders (e.g. myxoedema, Addison's disease) and an increased risk of gastric carcinoma.
- Investigations:
  - Radioactive vitamin B_{12} absorption +/− IF (Schilling test)
  - Serum gastric parietal and intrinsic factor antibodies
  - Endoscopy: gastric/duodenal biopsy
- Treat underlying cause; replace stores with parenteral B_{12} (hydroxycobalamin):
  - initial/loading dose of 1 mg every 3–4 days for up to 6 doses
  - maintenance dose of 1 mg every 3 months.

(b) Folic acid deficiency

- May be caused by:
  - inadequate dietary intake
  - malabsorption: coeliac disease, tropical sprue
  - increased requirements: pregnancy, haemolysis
  - drugs, e.g. anticonvulsants
  - excess alcohol intake.
- Investigations:
  - Serum folate levels (↓); serum B_{12} levels (N/↓)
  - Antigliadin and endomysial antibodies
  - Tests for malabsorption, e.g. duodenal biopsy

- Treat underlying cause and replace stores with oral folic acid (5 mg daily).
- Prior to replacement with folic acid, B_{12} deficiency must be excluded and treated to prevent development or exacerbation of neurological complications.
- Prophylaxis in pregnancy: deficiency in pregnancy is associated with neural tube defects in the fetus, although there is no clear correlation between maternal folate levels and the occurrence of defects. However, folic acid supplement in early pregnancy (400 µg daily from conception) reduces the incidence of spina bifida, anencephaly, and cleft lip and palate. The higher daily dose of 5 mg is recommended for women on antiepileptic drugs as these agents have antifolate properties.

Normal coagulation

(a) Primary haemostasis

- Coagulation is initiated almost instantaneously following vascular injury or endothelial damage, as this exposes collagen (normally underneath the endothelium).
- Circulating platelets bind to the collagen at the site of injury using the surface collagen-specific glycoprotein (Gp) Ia/IIa receptor to form a haemostatic plug.
- Platelet adhesion is strengthened further by the large multimeric circulating protein von Willebrand factor (vWF), which forms links between the platelet Gp Ib/IX/V and collagen fibrils.
- The platelets are then activated and release the contents of their granules into the bloodstream, attracting other platelets to aggregate at the injury site to form a haemostatic plug.
- The platelets undergo a change in their shape from discs to spheres and extrude long pseudopods, facilitating interaction between platelets. In addition, the shape change exposes a phospholipid surface for coagulation factors that require it. Fibrinogen links adjacent platelets by forming links via the glycoprotein IIb/IIIa. Furthermore, thrombin activates platelets.
- The platelet release reaction and aggregation are potentiated by the potent vasoconstrictor, thromboxane A_2.
- Platelet adhesion and aggregation are inhibited by prostacyclin (PGI_2), which is produced by vascular endothelial cells.
- Other substances increase platelet cyclic AMP levels, e.g. high levels of ADP.

(b) Secondary haemostasis

- Simultaneously, coagulation factors respond in a complex cascade to form fibrin strands, which strengthen the platelet plug.
- The coagulation cascade has two pathways that lead to fibrin formation:
  - the contact activation pathway (formerly known as the intrinsic pathway)
  - the tissue factor pathway (formerly known as the extrinsic pathway).

- It was previously thought that the coagulation cascade consisted of two pathways of equal importance joined to a common pathway. It is now known that the primary pathway for the initiation of blood coagulation is the *tissue factor* pathway.
- The pathways are a series of reactions, in which a zymogen (inactive enzyme precursor) of a serine protease and its glycoprotein co-factor are activated to become active components that then catalyse the next reaction in the cascade, ultimately resulting in cross-linked fibrin.

Disorders of haemostasis associated with pregnancy

(a) Disseminated intravascular coagulopathy (DIC)

- This is the result of intravascular deposition of fibrin and degradation of fibrin/fibrinogen leading to:
  - a coagulation defect due to consumption of coagulation factors and platelets and increased fibrinolytic activity
  - widespread bleeding, large and small vessel thrombosis, and haemorrhagic tissue necrosis.
- DIC can occur in a chronic compensated state or as life-threatening haemorrhage.
- In pregnancy it is associated with:
  - massive haemorrhage
  - septic miscarriage and intra-uterine infection
  - pre-eclampsia/eclampsia
  - abruptio placentae
  - retained dead fetus
  - amniotic fluid embolism
  - hydatidiform mole.
- Diagnosis is confirmed by haematological investigations:
  - ↓ platelet count
  - ↑ PT, APTT, TT
  - ↓ fibrinogen
  - ↑ fibrin(ogen) degradation products (FDPs)
  - ↑ cross-linked fibrin degradation products (D-dimers)

- Treatment includes the replacement of blood products (platelets, FFP, cryoprecipitate) (see Table 3.6) and urgent treatment of the underlying condition.

(b) HELLP Syndrome

- Microangiopathic haemolysis (H), elevated liver enzymes (EL), low platelets (LP).
- Occurs in severe pre-eclampsia.
- Laboratory findings as in DIC.
- Mainstay of treatment is delivery, although corticosteroids have been used.

(c) Thromboembolism

Pregnancy is a hypercoagulable state and pulmonary embolism (PE) remains a major cause of maternal death.
The following physiological changes in coagulation factors occur in pregnancy:

- ↑ levels of vitamin K-dependent factors (II, VII, IX, and X)
- ↑ factor VIII and von Willebrand factor levels
- ↑ fibrinogen levels
- ↑/N levels of coagulation inhibitors (protein C, antithrombin III).

Other risk factors for thromboembolism in pregnancy include:

- previous thrombotic history
- obesity
- caesarean section or other recent major surgery
- inherited pro-thrombotic states or familial thrombophilia due to deficiency of coagulation inhibitors (protein C, protein S, antithrombin III), factor V Leiden gene mutation, or activated protein C resistance and hyperhomocysteinaemia.

(d) Thrombocytopenia in pregnancy

- *Incidental* or *gestational* thrombocytopenia accounts for 75% of cases of mild to moderately low platelet counts ($70–150 \times 10^9/l$). Characteristically, there is no previous history and no clinical effect on the baby.

Table 3.6 Blood components available in the UK and their storage and clinical applications

	Storage	Shelf life	Dose	Outcome
Red cells	2–6°C	35 days	1 unit	Hb rise by 1 g/dl
Platelets	Keep on a special agitator rack at room temperature (22 ± 2°C)	5 days	1 adult dose or '1 pool' should contain $2.5–3 \times 10^{11}$ platelets	For a 70 kg adult, 1 pool typically gives a rise in platelet count of $20–40 \times 10^9$ ml
Fresh frozen plasma (FFP)	Frozen	12 months	12–15 ml/kg	Clinical assessment and by post-transfusion coagulation tests
Cryoprecipitate	Frozen	12 months	10 single donor units (containing 3–6 g fibrinogen in 200–500 ml)	Coagulation tests; expected rise in plasma fibrinogen level of about 1 g/l

- *Autoimmune thrombocytopenia* is caused by an antiplatelet autoantibody (IgG), which may cross the placenta and destroy fetal platelets.

Blood transfusion basics
Blood grouping
(a) ABO blood group
- This is the most important blood group system in human blood transfusion.
- Discovered in 1901 by Karl Landsteiner, an Austrian physiologist. He was awarded the Nobel Prize for Medicine for this in 1930.
- Each individual's ABO blood group is defined by the antigen on their red cells and corresponding natural antibodies present in their plasma (Table 3.7).

(b) Rhesus blood group
- Discovered by Karl Landsteiner and A.S. Wiener in 1941.
- The second most important blood group system in human blood transfusion.
- The most significant rhesus antigen is the RhD antigen because it is the most immunogenic of the five main rhesus antigens.
- RhD-negative individuals can produce IgG anti-RhD antibodies following a sensitizing event, possibly a fetomaternal transfusion of blood from a fetus in pregnancy or occasionally a blood transfusion with RhD-positive RBCs.

Transfusion transmissible infections
- Viruses: hepatitis A, B, and C; HIV-I and II; CMV
- Bacteria: *Treponema pallidum* (syphilis); Brucella; Salmonella
- Parasites: malaria; toxoplasma; microfilaria
- Prion protein: Creutzfeldt–Jakob disease (CJD) and new variant CJD (nvCJD)

Haemolytic disease of the newborn (HDN)
- This is transplacental passage of maternal red cell IgG antibodies resulting in haemolysis of fetal RBCs.
- The *most frequent* cause is ABO incompatibility, e.g. anti-A produced by a group O mother carrying a group A fetus. The disease is usually mild because ABO antibodies are IgM, which are large molecules and less likely to cross the placenta. Furthermore, maternal antibodies are partially neutralized by A and B antigens on other cells, plasma, and tissue fluids.
- The *most important* cause of HDN is anti-D, although other Rh antibodies (particularly anti-c and anti-Kell) are also implicated.
- Clinical features include anaemia, neonatal jaundice (resulting in kernicterus in severe cases), hydrops fetalis, and intra-uterine death (IUD).
- Treatment includes phototherapy in mild cases and red cell exchange transfusions for severe jaundice.
- Prophylactic anti-D IgG is given to Rh (D)-negative women within 72 hours of a potentially sensitizing event. The dose is adjusted according to the number of fetal cells detected in maternal circulation using the Kleihauer-Betke test.
- In the UK routine antenatal prophylaxis against rhesus disease is recommended. Intramuscular anti-D 1250 IU is routinely administered to all pregnant Rh D-negative women at 28 weeks and 34 weeks gestation.

Table 3.7 ABO blood group and corresponding plasma antibodies

Blood group	Antigen on red blood cells	Antibody in plasma
A	A	Anti-B
B	B	Anti-A
AB	A & B	No antibodies
O	No antigen	Anti-A & anti-B

General and reproductive immunology

The immune system

The role of the immune system is to eliminate pathogenic organisms and neutralize their toxins, and also to eliminate cells that have undergone or show the potential to undergo malignant transformation. Therefore, the immune system has to distinguish normal healthy cells ('self') from the 'non-self' (infected or malignant cells, and toxins), a major challenge given the infinite range of organisms, their toxins, and their capacity to adapt and mutate.

Components of the immune system

There are two functional units, namely the *innate* and the *adaptive* systems, which have extensive interactions and are required to mount an effective and efficient immune response.

Cells involved in immune reactions

- Lymphocytes and phagocytes, which originate from bone marrow stem cells, are the predominant cells of the immune system. They interact with each other and with other cells of the body to generate the immune response.
- Various leukocyte populations can be identified via their morphology and the molecules expressed on the cell surface (*markers*). A system of nomenclature (cluster of differentiation (CD)) has been devised for all the major molecules (Table 3.8).

Table 3.8 Key markers of lymphocyte populations

Marker function	Immunoglobulin antigen receptor	TcR/CD3 T-cell activator	CD4 MHC class II binding	CD8 MHC class II binding	CD8 MHC class I binding	CD5
B cells	+	–	–	–	–	+/–*
T_H cells†	–	+	+	+	–	+
T_C cells†	–	+	+	–	+	+

T_H : helper T cells; T_C : cytotoxic T cells; TcR: T-cell receptor; MHC: major histocompatibility complex.
*A minor subpopulation of B cells is CD+
† The great majority of helper T cells are CD4+ and the majority of suppressors and cytotoxics, CD8+; exceptions have been found.

- *B lymphocytes* are characterized by their expression of surface immunoglobulin (antibody), which acts as a receptor for antigen. These cells recognize native antigens in solution or on the surface of other cells. B cells, activated by contact with their specific antigen and triggered by cytokines released from T cells, divide and differentiate into antibody-secreting plasma cells. The secreted antibody is of identical antigen specificity to that on the surface of the original B cell, although it may become refined during the development of an immune response, resulting in an increasing affinity for the antigen.

- Antibodies are classified into different biochemical classes (see below). Virgin B cells initially express IgM with or without IgD on their surface. During B-cell differentiation, individual cells may switch to the production of IgG, IgA, or IgE, while retaining the antigen specificity.

- *T lymphocytes* mature in the thymus and three major events occur during thymic differentiation:

    1. The development of a repertoire of T-cell receptors (TcRs), and a preferential selection of cells carrying TcRs that may interact effectively with the individual's major histocompatibility complex (MHC) molecules during antigen presentation.

    2. The selective removal of cells that recognize the individual's own molecules (self antigens).

    3. The differentiation of different T-cell subpopulations.

T-cell precursors entering the thymus lack specific T-cell markers. They acquire CD2 at an early stage of development and this is retained in mature T cells. Immature thymocytes express both CD4 and CD8, but one of these markers is lost as the cells mature. Thus, T cells leaving the thymus express either CD4 or CD8. At least two major sets are described: helper T cells (T_H), predominantly CD4+; and cytotoxic T cells (T_C), mostly CD8+. T cells recognize antigens (as peptide fragments) on the surface of other cells, in association with molecules encoded by the MHC. The process by which cells express molecules recognizable by T cells is termed antigen presentation, and these cells are termed antigen-presenting cells (APCs). Many cell types are capable of presenting antigens in a recognizable form to both B and T lymphocytes, and are thus collectively described as APCs (Table 3.9). CD8+ T cells recognize antigen in association with MHC class I molecules and CD4+ T cells recognize antigen in association with MHC class II molecules. T-cell activation causes the cells to divide and secrete various cytokines that modulate immune responses. In addition, cytotoxic

Table 3.9 Characteristics of antigen-presenting cells

Cell type	Location	MHC Class II	Antigen presentation
Langerhans cell	Skin	+	Weak
Veiled cell	Afferent lymph	+	
Interdigitating dendritic cell	Lymph node, T-cell areas	+	Strong immunostimulation of resting T cells
Non-lymphoid cell	Connective tissues of most organs	+	? T cells
Follicular dendritic cell	Lymph node follicles	–	B cells
Mononuclear phagocytes and macrophages	Many tissues	0 → ++	B cells and primed T cells
Marginal zone macrophages	Marginal zone of spleen and lymph nodes	–/+	T-independent antigens to B cells
B cells	Lymphoid tissue	+ → ++	To primed T cells

T cells secrete molecules called perforins, which polymerize to form holes in the membranes of target cells.

- *Mononuclear phagocytes* are diverse and widely distributed throughout the body. They include blood monocytes, microglia of the brain, and the Kupffer cells of the liver. Blood monocytes can migrate into the tissues where they develop into macrophages. The latter express receptors for immunoglobulin and complement components, and may be activated by cytokines released from T cells. Their surface molecules facilitate binding to antigens and subsequent phagocytosis. Internalized material (e.g. viruses) is broken down within phagolysosomes (cytoplasmic vesicles) and converted into peptides, which can be recycled to the surface to be presented to T cells by MHC molecules. Macrophages are relatively long lived. Some return from the periphery to secondary lymphoid tissues, thereby transporting antigen from the periphery into the spleen and lymph nodes. An essential function of these cells is the internal destruction of pathogens and antigens.

Molecules involved in immune reactions

Three groups of molecules are involved in antigen-binding—antibodies, TcRs, and MHC molecules (Figure 3.15). Antibodies recognize antigen alone, while TcRs recognize antigen in association with MHC, and both are highly specific in their binding. MHC molecules bind peptides, which they present to T cells. Other molecules involved in immune responses include complement and cytokines.

Antibodies

- Antibodies (or immunoglobulins) have a basic structure consisting of four polypeptide chains—two identical heavy chains and two identical light chains—that are linked by disulphide bonds and non-covalent interactions

(Figure 3.16). Each of these chains is formed from a number of globular domains connected by less tightly folded regions of polypeptide chains.
- Light chains have two domains and heavy chains have four or five, depending on the class of antibody.
- Each four-polypeptide unit has two antigen-combining sites, formed by the N-terminal domains, which is very variable between antibodies, the greatest variability being clustered at the extreme ends of the domains where antigen binds. These domains are thus called variable or V domains, while the segments of polypeptide that show the greatest variability (three per V domain) are called hypervariable regions. These hypervariable regions are not contiguous in the polypeptide chain, but are brought into proximity at the antigen-binding site by the overall folding of the polypeptide chain within the domain. With six different hypervariable regions of different amino acid sequence at the paratope (antigen-binding site; three from the heavy chain, three from the light), the molecular surfaces of different antibodies are highly variable in shape, charge, and amino acid residues, thus giving them their antigen specificity.
- The remaining domains are less variable between antibodies and are called constant or C domains, but even here there is some variability.
- Light chains may be one of two different types, namely kappa (κ) or lambda (λ). These are generated from two different gene loci. The heavy chain gene locus of humans can generate nine different types of heavy chain that vary in their three domains (in addition to the huge amounts of variation seen in the V domains) and there is a gene for each of these chains. This allows for the formation of antibody isotypes, termed μ, $\gamma1$, $\gamma2$, $\gamma3$, $\gamma4$, $\alpha1$, and $\alpha2$, and the heavy chain isotype present in an antibody determines the class and subclass of that antibody. Any one of these isotypes can be produced in a membrane-bound

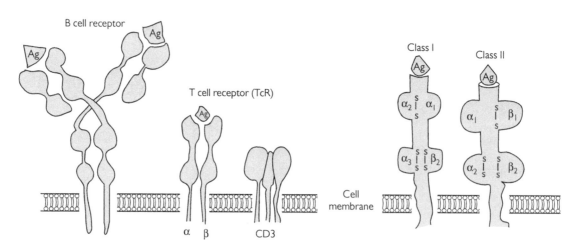

Figure 3.15 Molecules that bind antigens. Note the domain structure and the similarities among the molecules belonging to the immunoglobulin supergene family.

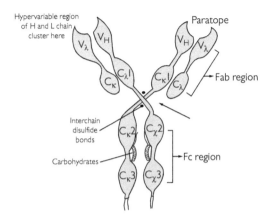

Figure 3.16 The structural details of an IgG molecule are illustrated with the names of the domains and different areas of the molecule noted. Interchain disulphide bands are marked in. In this example the light chains on λ.

form to act as a B-cell antigen receptor, or in a secreted form to become part of the effector arm of the immune response.

- Antibodies can be divided into five classes, or nine subclasses, corresponding to the nine isotypes (Table 3.10). The immunoglobulin G (IgG) class has four isotypes (IgG1, IgG2, IgG3, and IgG4) and the IgA class has two subclasses (IgA1 and IgA2). The IgD, IgM, and IgE classes are not usually subdivided.
- While all antibodies can bind antigen, each antibody class, and indeed subclass, has a different set of functions. These functions relate to the capacity of the constant regions of antibody to interact with different tissues expressing Fc receptors, or with C1q of the complement

system. Antibodies are therefore bifunctional molecules in which the V domains are responsible for antigen binding, while the C domains allow interaction with various effector systems.

The T-cell receptor

The TcR is an integral membrane protein consisting of a pair of polypeptide chains linked by a disulphide bond. Four genetic loci (α, β, γ, δ) encode these polypeptide chains, and a T cell may have either an αβ pair (TcR2) or a γδ pair (TcR1). Most mature peripheral T cells have TcR2, while TcR1 receptors are seen on a population of thymic T cells and on some T cells located in the peripheral lymphoid tissues such as those in the gut. The functional significance of there being two different types of TcRs is not known.

- The polypeptide chains each have two extracellular domains, of which the N-terminal domains are variable (V) and form the MHC-antigen recognition site.
- Each TcR is associated with a number of other polypeptide chains in the cell membrane. These associated polypeptides (denoted γ, δ, ε) appear to be involved in transducing the activation signal to the cell via calcium, and are referred to as the CD3 complex.
- The CD3 chains are monomorphic and distinct from the chains that form the TcR.

The major histocompatibility complex (MHC)

The MHC is the human leukocyte antigen (HLA) locus on chromosome 6, and its products are termed MHC antigens or molecules (synonymous with HLA). The MHC can be divided into three distinct regions encoding three classes of molecules (Figure 3.17). The A, B, and C loci (class I genes) encode class I molecules; the DP, DQ, and DR loci (class II genes) encode class II molecules; and the class III genes encode a variety of other molecules with diverse functions.

Table 3.10 Antibody characteristics and functions

Class	H_2L_2 subunits	H-chain domains	Isotypes	C1q binding	Placental transfer	Cellular binding	Serum concentration in adult (mg/ml)
IgE	1	4	IgG1	++	+	Neutrophils, MOs	9
			IgG2	+	(+)	Neutrophils, MOs weak	3
			IgG3	+++	+	Neutrophils, MOs	1
			IgG4	+	–	Neutrophils, MOs weak	0.5
IgA	1 or 2	4	IgA1	–	–	Neutrophils	3
						Neutrophils	0.5
IgM	5	5	IgM	+++	–		1.5
IgD	1	4	IgD	–	–		0.03
IgE	1	5	IgE	–	–	Mast cells, basophils, MOs weak	0.00005

MOs : mononuclear cells; H_2L_2 = heavy and light chains.

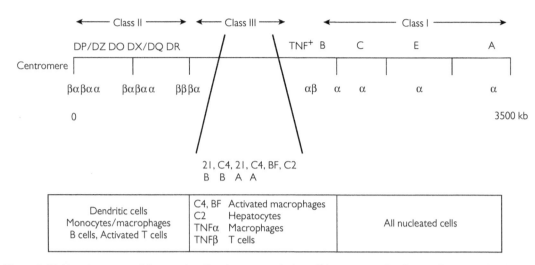

	C4, BF	Activated macrophages	
Dendritic cells	C2	Hepatocytes	
Monocytes/macrophages	TNFα	Macrophages	All nucleated cells
B cells, Activated T cells	TNFβ	T cells	

Figure 3.17 Major histocompatibility complex. Class I genes encode the α/β heterodimer. The β-chain (β$_2$-microglobulin) is on a different chromosome. The α- and β-chain genes for class II occur in pairs. Class III genes encode four components of the complement system but genes encoding 21-hydroxylase A and B are located in the same region. Tumour necrosis factor (TNF$^+$): α- and β-genes. BF: factor B. Issac T. Manyonda, *The Immunology of Human Reproduction*, Figure 5.3, Copyright © 2006 Informa Healthcare. Reproduced with permission from Informa Healthcare.

- The class I loci each encode the α-chain of a single class I molecule.
- Class II molecules have two polypeptide chains, and there are one or more genes for each pair of chains in each class II locus.

The MHC class I and II molecules share a common molecular ancestry with the domains of immunoglobulin and TcR, and are thus members of the immunoglobulin supergene family of molecules. They are cell surface glycoproteins, each of which has four external domains (Figure 3.18). Class I molecules have one polypeptide chain encoded within the MHC. Each chain folds into three extracellular domains, which are linked non-covalently to the molecule β$_2$-microglobulin, the latter making the fourth domain of the class I molecule. The two MHC class II polypeptides are non-covalently associated and both traverse the membrane. MHC molecules are highly polymorphic (i.e. there is a great deal of genetic variation between individuals).

MHC molecules are involved in presenting antigen to T cells. Different MHC molecules present different antigens more effectively than others. Consequently, it is advantageous to carry a wide range of MHC molecules that can present the numerous antigens that may be encountered. Analysis of the polypeptide structure of MHC molecules shows that the variability is concentrated in two particular regions: the α1 and α2 domains of class I molecules; and the N-terminal domains of the α and β chains of class II molecules. There is a considerable amount of structural similarity between the class I and II molecules, particularly with respect to the regions surrounding the binding site, and there is increasing evidence to suggest functional similarity between the two classes of molecule.

Complement

The complement system consists of more than 30 interacting proteins and their receptors, as summarized in Figure 3.19. There are two pathways by which complement can be activated. The classical pathway involves antibody–antigen complexes, and the alternative pathway involves the presence of activator surfaces.

- Activators in the alternative pathway include certain microbial cell walls, carbohydrates, and viruses. Activation can lead to the covalent attachment of a fragment of the

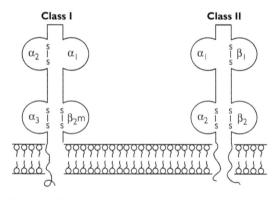

Figure 3.18 Schematic representation of class I and class II molecules of the MHC. Note the globular domain structure. Issac T. Manyonda, *The Immunology of Human Reproduction*, Figure 5.4, Copyright © 2006 Informa Healthcare. Reproduced with permission from Informa Healthcare.

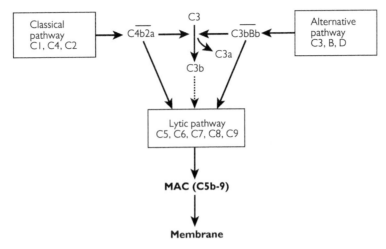

Figure 3.19 Complement pathways. Complement pathways may be activated by antigen-antibody complexes via the classic pathway or via the alternative pathway. Both routes generate a C3 convertase, which splits C3 into C3a and C3b. C3b deposited on an activator surface in association with a C3 convertase can initiate the lytic pathway to deposit membrane attack complexes (MAC) onto the target membrane. Issac T. Manyonda, *The Immunology of Human Reproduction*, Figure 5.5, Copyright © 2006 Informa Healthcare. Reproduced with permission from Informa Healthcare.

third component of the system (i.e. C3b) to the initiating agent. Mononuclear phagocytes and neutrophils express receptors (mainly CR1 and CR3) for this fragment; thus, complement deposition on particles or antigen–antibody complexes opsonizes them for phagocytosis. The binding of C3b to receptors on phagocytes increases their level of activation, thereby priming them to eliminate the material they have phagocytosed.

- The deposition of C3b on membranes can lead to the activation of the complement lytic pathway, which involves the assembly of a membrane attack complex (MAC) that contains components ranging from C5 to C9 and traverses the membranes of the target cell. If MACs become assembled on eukaryotic cells (e.g. on an erythrocyte), they cause osmotic damage and cell lysis.

- Other complement components are involved in the development of the inflammatory reaction, acting as anaphylatoxins, inducing smooth muscle contraction and mast cell degranulation, and being chemotactic for neutrophils and macrophages, thereby controlling their influx into sites of acute inflammation.

Cytokines

Cytokines are soluble proteins released by one cell that act on receptors on other cells to affect their functions. Many of the interactions between cells cooperating or participating in an immune response are controlled by cytokines. Cytokine actions are not confined to classical immune responses but are wide ranging, complex, and intertwined with other biological interactions. Several cytokines may have the same effect, or act synergistically, e.g. interferon-γ (IFN-γ) induces

MHC class II on many cells and this effect is enhanced by tumour necrosis factor-α (TNFα), while TNFα itself has no class II-inducing ability. Interleukin-1 (IL-1), released by macrophages and a number of other cells, enhances the level of IL-2 receptors on the T cell, while IL-2 maintains the T cells in cell cycle. Table 3.11 lists the known functions of the more important cytokines.

Effector functions in the immune response

The theory of clonal selection

The basis of an immune response is the stimulation and activation of clones of lymphocytes capable of recognizing the initiating antigen. Although there is only a modest number of genes for immunoglobulin and TcRs, a complex process of genetic recombination generates an enormous diversity of receptors. Since this occurs during lymphocyte ontogeny, antigen is not required to generate the repertoire of receptors.

- Each lymphocyte expresses only one specific receptor, and the entire repertoire is only present when one considers the total population of lymphocytes within the body. Therefore, the system generates receptors for a vast number of antigens, the great majority of which may never be encountered in a lifetime. One consequence of this diversity is that the proportion of lymphocytes expressing receptors for a particular antigen is relatively small. Thus, to mount an effective immune response, one of the first steps is the expansion of clones of antigen-reactive cells. In effect, antigen selects and activates those lymphocytes that recognize it. This is called the theory of clonal selection.

Table 3.11 Major cytokines and their functions

Cytokine	Sources	Targets	Principal effects
IL-1	Macrophages, LGLs, B cells	Lymphocytes	Activation and IL-2 receptor induction
		Macrophages	Activation
		Endothelium	Increased leucocyte adhesion
		Tissue cells	Numerous effects in inflammatory reactions
IL-2	T cells	T cells	T-cell division and differentiation; absolute requirement
		Active B cells	Promotes B-cell division
IL-4 and IL-5	T cells	B cells	Required for B-cell division and differentiation
IL-6	Lymphocytes	B-cells	B-cell differentiation
	Macrophages Fibroblasts	Hepatocytes	Acute phase protein synthesis
IFN-γ	T cells	Leucocytes	Macrophage activation
		Endothelium	Increased leucocyte adhesion
		Tissue cells	MHC induction
TNFα	Macrophages	Phagocytes	Activation
TNFβ	T cells	K and NK cells	Activation
		Endothelium	Promotes leucocyte adhesion
		Target cells	Increased susceptibility to cytotoxic cells
IL-3	T cells	Stem cells	Control stem cells division and differentiation pathways
M-CSF	Mononuclear cells	Stem cells	Control stem cells division and differentiation pathways
G-CSF	Endothelium		
GM-CSF	T cells	Stem cells	Control stem cells division and differentiation pathways
	Mononuclear cells		
	Endothelium		
	Fibroblasts		

IL: interleukin, LGLs: large granular lymphocytes; IFN: interferon; TNF: tumour necrosis factor; CSF: colony-stimulating factor; M: macrophage; G: granulocyte; GM: granulocyte-macrophage.

Cellular interactions in immune reactions

Figure 3.20 depicts an overview of events occurring during an immune response. The interactions of B cells and macrophages with T cells are particularly important in the development of the immune response. The critical events include:

- antigen uptake and processing by antigen-presenting cells
- antigen presentation to and recognition by antigen-specific B and/or T cells
- cooperation between T and B cells (Figure 3.21), with release of cytokines that subserve a variety of functions including induction of B-cell differentiation and macrophage activation
- the development of cytotoxic activity (Figure 3.22).

Antibodies produced by plasma cells may neutralize pathogens by direct binding (e.g. blocking viral receptors), but more often they link antigen to cells of the immune system, or activate the complement system. Many of the effects of antibodies occur via binding to Fc receptors, which bind to sites in the constant domains of the antibody.

Reproductive immunology

It is usually not possible to transplant grafts between genetically dissimilar individuals. Therefore, maternal tolerance of the genetically dissimilar fetus during pregnancy remains one of the main paradoxes of mammalian biology. In contrast to Medawar's original proposals, there is no anatomical separation of the fetus from the mother; fetal antigens can elicit an immune response even at an early stage, and the mother is not immunologically indolent. Other immunological paradoxes of pregnancy include:

1. Immunity to sperm and seminal fluid
2. How the pre-implantation embryo evades the maternal immune system

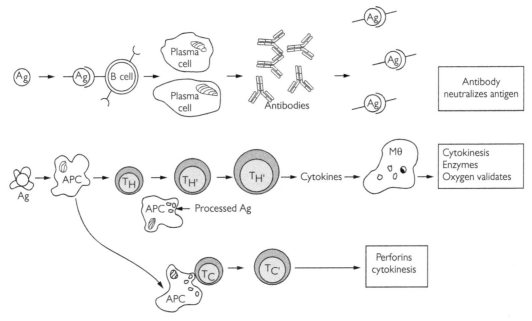

Figure 3.20 Overview of the immune response. Antigen (Ag) taken up by Ag presenting cells (APC) stimulates helper T cells (T$_H$) so that when they encounter the Ag again they proliferate and release cytokines. These are involved in the differentiation of B cells into antibody-producing plasma cells, the activation of macrophages (Mθ), and the proliferation and activation of cytotoxic T cells, which recognize Ag as APC and can kill them via perforins.

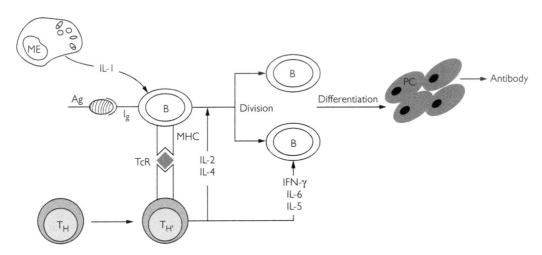

Figure 3.21 T cell–B cell cooperation. Activated T cells (T$_H$) can recognize processed antigen (Ag) and B cells (B) associated with MHC class II molecules. IL-2 released by macrophages (Mθ), in associated with IL-4 and IL-2 from T cells, promotes B cell division and additional cytokines then promote differentiation in plasma cells (PC) which release large amounts of antibody.

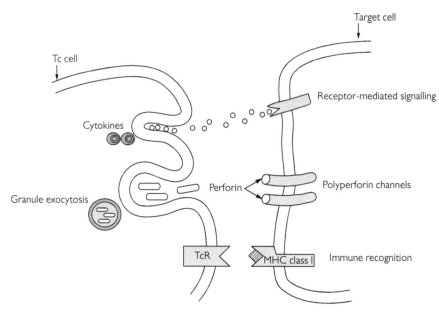

Figure 3.22 Actions of cytotoxic T cells (Tc). Tc recognize targets primarily by MHC-class I-mediated interactions. They can then damage the target cell by the release of perforins, which polymerize to form polyperforin channels, or via other molecules relased by the Tc, including some cytokines. TcR = T cell receptors.

3. Implantation and placentation: the nature of the maternofetal immunological interface
4. Maternal immunocompetence during pregnancy
5. Maternal immune responses to fetal antigens
6. Whether recurrent miscarriage represents failure of ill-defined immunoregulatory mechanisms that normally sustain successful pregnancy.

Sperm and seminal plasma

Antigenicity of spermatozoa

A multiplicity of antigens are localized to, and are specific for, particular areas of the spermatozoon. Some antigens may only be revealed after capacitation. Although some infertile men and women possess antibodies against all of these regions, antibodies against surface antigens of the acrosome and main tailpiece seem to be of the greatest pathological relevance because they cause immobilization and/or agglutination of sperm. Whether MHC antigens are or are not expressed on sperm is undetermined and the significance of sperm antigens in human reproduction is unclear.

Tolerance to self sperm antigens

Tolerance to self antigens occurs as a result of suppression and/or elimination of potentially self-reactive T cells in the thymus during fetal life. Since spermatogenesis does not commence until long after this self-recognition process is

over, spermatozoa should be particularly susceptible to the development of autoimmunity. This can arise and is a cause of male infertility, but among the mechanisms that prevent it from occurring more often are:

1. Physical contact between immunocompetent cells and developing spermatozoa is prevented by the tight junctions between Sertoli cells lining the seminiferous tubules.
2. These same tight junctions prevent the passage of circulating antibody into the tubules.
3. Autoreactivity against the highly immunogenic epididymal sperms may be prevented by suppressor T cells in the epididymal epithelium.
4. Once sperm leave the epididymis, they become coated with seminal plasma components including lactoferrin. This coating reduces their immunogenicity, probably relevant while the sperms are in the seminal vesicles and when they are deposited in the vagina.

Tolerance to sperm antigens in the female genital tract

Seminal plasma has a potent inhibitory effect on most cells of the immune system and impairs the activity of antibody and complement. The relevant studies are all *in vitro* and a biological significance cannot be assumed. The immunosuppressive components of seminal plasma include zinc-containing compounds, the polyamines spermine and spermidine, prostaglandins, transglutaminases, and a protein closely related to pregnancy-associated protein-A.

The pre-implantation embryo

As the zygote traverses the Fallopian tubes and enters the uterus, its protection depends on:

1. non-expression of paternal antigens at the two-cell stage, but expression from the six-to-eight-cell stage
2. a probable absence of MHC antigens at this stage of pregnancy, although the expression of these antigens increases with cellular division
3. hormone-dependent non-specific suppressor cells found in secretory-phase human endometrium.

Significant immunological problems are, therefore, not posed by the conceptus before implantation.

Immunology of implantation and placentation

To understand the intimate anatomical and immunological relationships between the mother and the fetus (Figure 3.23), several issues must be considered.

There is no vascular continuity between the fetal and maternal compartments. However, implantation and trophoblastic invasion result in an intimate interaction between trophoblast and decidua (Figure 3.24). The syncytiotrophoblast, the non-mitotic outer layer of the chorionic villi, is bathed in maternal blood, which also lines the intervillous spaces. Beneath the syncytiotrophoblast is the cytotrophoblast, whose cells are metabolically more active. Some cytotrophoblast cells push through the syncytiotrophoblast to make the cytotrophoblast columns, which help anchor the villi to the maternal tissue. Other cytotrophoblast cells break away to form the cytotrophoblast shell, with some of

these cells subsequently migrating into the myometrium where they are called the interstitial cytotrophoblast cells. Still other cytotrophoblast cells invade the spiral arterioles of the uterus and line the vessels as endovascular trophoblast. The cytotrophoblast and syncytiotrophoblast comprise the villous trophoblast. The non-villous trophoblast comprises the rest of the trophoblast tissue, from which the chorion laeve and chorionic plate, the marginal zone, and the basal plate of the placenta form. The trophoblast thus represents a continuous frontier over a considerable surface area, up to 15 m² at 20 weeks' gestation. It has therefore long been the prime candidate for the role of an immunologically protective or insulating barrier.

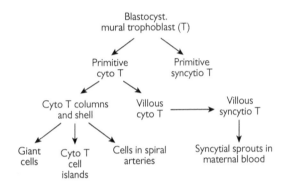

Figure 3.24 Possible interrelations between the various trophoblastic subpopulations. T = trophoblast.

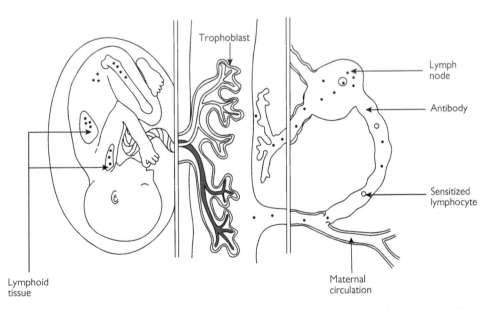

Figure 3.23 The immunological relation of mother and fetus. Issac T. Manyonda, *The Immunology of Human Reproduction*, Figure 5.10, Copyright © 2006 Informa Healthcare. Reproduced with permission from Informa Healthcare.

Antigen expression by the trophoblast

HLA-G: evolutionary vestige or shield against natural killer cells?

Most if not all of the HLA molecules expressed on the trophoblast are HLA-G, although the exact function of this molecule is unknown. Why, for instance, does it only occur predominantly on trophoblast, and why only in certain subsets of trophoblast? If it were simply redundant, it might be expressed on a wider range of tissues along with classical MHC antigens. It has been proposed that HLA-G may play a role in the resistance to lysis by natural killer (NK) cells. The hypothesis is that while lack of classical MHC antigens confers resistance to lysis by allospecific T cells, total lack of MHC antigens would render trophoblast susceptible to lysis by NK cells, which are thought to lyse cells on the basis of recognition of altered self antigens or absence of self. A monomorphic antigen, such as HLA-G, would be recognized as self.

The endometrium and decidua

Cell types in the decidua

Decidualization is the response of the uterine endometrium to the implanting embryo, but as yet the nature or precise source of the stimulus is unknown. The site of implantation where the placenta forms is called the decidua basalis, while the rest of the decidua is designated decidua parietalis. The decidua contains conventional immunological cell types (lymphocytes, macrophages) and non-conventional cell types, most notably the uterine large granular lymphocytes (U-LGLs). Clearly, immunological responses within the decidua are likely to be crucial, as this is the definitive maternofetal interface.

MHC class II+ and CD14+ macrophages, capable of a range of immunological functions including antigen presentation,

phagocytic activity, and secretion of prostaglandins, occur in abundance in the decidua. Conventional T cells are also found, although the proportions of CD4 to CD8 cells appear to be an inverse of the proportions seen in peripheral blood, in that there appear to be relatively more CD8 than CD4 cells. The significance of this is unknown. Conventional NK cells are also found in the decidua, but their activity is less than that in peripheral blood. It is known that in the peripheral blood they decrease in number and activity during pregnancy. Their function in the decidua is unknown.

Natural killer cells in pregnancy

Natural killer cells are capable of killing some tumour cells spontaneously without prior sensitization. They do not seem to have immunological memory and can lyse cells that are syngeneic, allogeneic, or xenogeneic to the NK cell donor. During human pregnancy, NK activity decreases from 16 weeks until term, returning to control levels after delivery. Studies have shown that in addition to a decrease in NK cell numbers during pregnancy, the cells that remain have less lytic activity.

Maternal immunocompetence in pregnancy

There is some diminution in the maternal immune response in pregnancy, mostly attributable to the hormones of pregnancy. However, women remain sufficiently immunocompetent during pregnancy, and the degree of immunodepression could not account for failure to eradicate as powerful a stimulus as an allograft. All the immune downregulatory phenomena observed in the mother, which by themselves could not explain the survival of the fetal semiallograft, could be viewed as acting synergistically with the central mechanism of an immunologically inert trophoblast to ensure the continuation of the species. In this way, the immune system allows the propagation of the species without leaving the body open to attack by exogenous pathogens.

The autonomic nervous system—general organization

General characteristics of the autonomic nervous system

The autonomic nervous system (ANS) is made up of two limbs, namely the sympathetic and the parasympathetic nervous systems (see Table 3.12). In organs innervated by both systems, they characteristically exert opposite effects. The end organs innervated by the motor fibres of autonomic nerves are smooth muscles, cardiac muscle, or glands. This is the key feature distinguishing autonomic nerves from the somatic nerves, whose motor fibres innervate

the skeletal muscle as the sole end organ. Furthermore, in the somatic nervous system the cell body of the neuron resides in the CNS and the axon travels great distances to reach the skeletal muscle end organ, in contrast to the ANS, which is generally a two-neuron pathway. This consists of a preganglionic neuron whose cell body is also in the CNS (brainstem or spinal cord), and a postganglionic neuron, with which it synapses in a peripheral ganglion (Figures 3.25 and 3.26). The only exception to this arrangement is in the adrenal medulla.

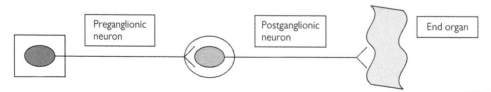

Figure 3.25 General organization and characteristics of the autonomic nervous system.

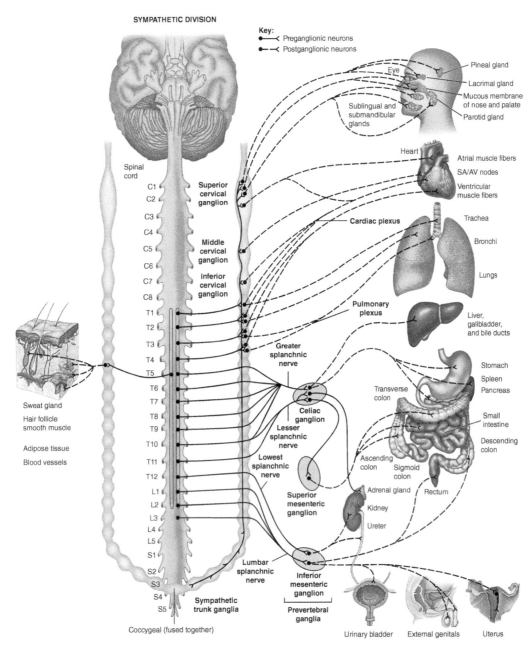

Figure 3.26 General organization and characteristics of the autonomic nervous system. Reproduced from G.W Jenkins, C.P. Kemnitz, G.J. Tortora, *Anatomy and physiology from science to life*, Wiley, figure 14.23, page 525, and figure 14.24, page 526. Copyright 2007 with permission.

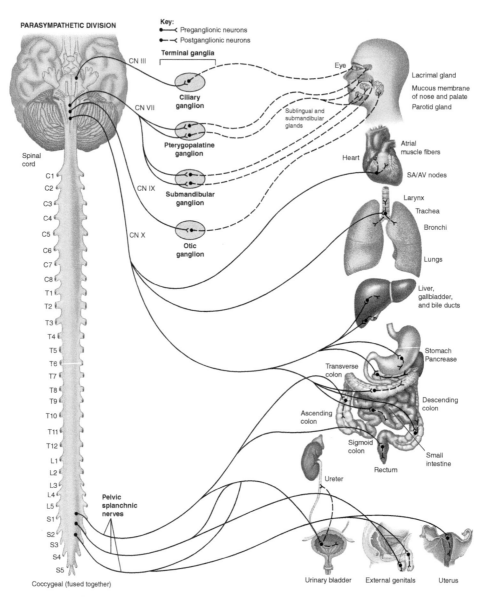

PARASYMPATHETIC DIVISION

Key:
- Preganglionic neurons
- Postganglionic neurons

Cell bodies of parasympathetic preganglionic neurons are located in brain stem nuclei and in the lateral horns of gray matter in the second through fourth sacral segments of the spinal cord.

Figure 3.26 (continued)

- The reader may recall that postganglionic neurons and the chromaffin cells of the adrenal medulla are both embryological derivatives of the neural crest cells. Therefore, in a developmental sense the chromaffin cells of the adrenal medulla are postganglionic cells in their own right, except that they did not continue their differentiation to become postganglionic neurons. However, they synthesize and release catecholamines (80% adrenaline and 20% noradrenaline (NA)) just like other sympathetic nerve terminals following stimulation.

- In the case of the adrenal medulla the catecholamines are released into the bloodstream and exert their effects through adrenergic receptors on the target tissues. Adrenergic neurons, on the other hand, synthesize catecholamines but release only noradrenaline as the neurotransmitter into the synaptic junction.

- During emergencies the sympathetic nervous system is stimulated, whilst the parasympathetic nervous system is activated during rest periods to restore energy, and during digestion of food.

Table 3.12 Comparison of the characteristics of the sympathetic and the parasympathetic nervous systems

	Sympathetic nervous system	Parasympathetic nervous system
Preganglionic neuron (cell bodies)	Resident in the spinal cord T_1–L_2	Resident in the brainstem and sacral segments $S_{2,3,4}$
Preganglionic neuron (axons)	Short	Very long
Postganglionic axons	Very long—nerve fibres have to reach above (T_1) and below (L_2) their origin	Very short—majority of them reside in terminal ganglia in or on the wall of the end organ
Distribution	Sympathetic nerves reach everywhere in the body! They are the sole innervation to the vascular smooth muscle, sweat glands, and erector pilae muscle in the skin.	Do not go everywhere in the body. Coverage is limited to the head, chest, abdomen, and pelvis. No innervation to body wall, sweat glands, or limbs
Routes of distribution	• The postganglionic fibres travel with the spinal nerves as they emerge from the spinal cord • The higher preganglionic fibres T_{1-3} ascend into the head and neck to reach and synapse in the cervical sympathetic ganglia before the postganglionic neurons travel in the spinal nerves • sympathetic innervation to the face (skin, sweat glands, smooth muscles etc.) is transmitted through the carotid vessel as there are no spinal nerves to the face and cranial nerves do not carry the sympathetics • compression or injury at the pericarotid plexus leads to Horner's syndrome—loss of sweating, pupillary constriction, and ptosis • Pre-aortic ganglia: a group of preganglionic fibres emerge from the spinal cord, bypass the sympathetic chain and continue on to the surface of the abdominal aorta where they synapse in the pre-aortic thoracic or lumbar ganglia. From here, they jump onto the blood vessels branching off from the abdominal aorta and are thus carried everywhere in the abdominal cavity	**Cranial nerve X (vagus)** • long preganglionic neuron • innervates the chest wall, airways, the heart, and most of the abdomen • does not innervate the head **Cranial nerves III, VII, & IX** • innervate the head • the preganglionic neurons synapse in parasympathetic ganglia (celiac, pterigoid, submandibular) in the head region instead of on the wall of the end organ • the postganglionic neurons leave these ganglia to supply the salivary and mucous glands $S_{2,3,4}$ **(pudendal nerve)** • the preganglionic fibres travel all the way to the pelvic organs and synapse with the postganglionic fibres on or in the wall of the end organ

Synthesis and release of noradrenaline (NA) at adrenergic nerve terminals

• The amino acid tyrosine is the precursor of all cate-cholamines including NA. Tyrosine is taken up into the nerve by an active transport system catalysed by nerve enzyme tyrosine hydroxylase. Tyrosine uptake is the rate-limiting step in the synthesis of NA. Tyrosine is converted to dihydroxyphenylalanine (L-DOPA), which is converted to dopamine by DOPA-decarboxylase (Figure 3.27).

• In some tissues (e.g. brain) dopamine is released as the neurotransmitter, but in almost all sympathetic nerve endings dopamine is just the precursor molecule for NA. Dopamine is converted to NA by dopamine β-hydroxylase. The accumulated NA is packaged in vesicles within the nerve terminal until their release in response to an excitatory event (Figure 3.27).

• Depolarization causes an influx of calcium into the nerve ending, resulting in the release of NA by fusion of the vesicles with the presynaptic membrane.

• The released NA acts on the effector cell where it exerts its biologic effects depending on the adrenergic receptor types.

• The action of NA on the effector cell is terminated by various mechanisms that regulate the removal of NA from the synaptic junction.

Mechanisms of termination of the action of NA on the neuroeffector cell

• The uptake-1 NA transporter system: This is the most important mechanism for the termination of NA action. The system removes NA from the synaptic junction, bringing it back into the presynaptic nerve ending.

- Metabolism by catecholamine-O-methyltransferase (COMT) enzyme within the surrounding tissues.
- Diffusion of NA away from the synaptic junction.
- Metabolism of NA to inactive forms by monoamine oxidase (MAO) in the presynaptic membrane: MAO metabolizes only the NA in the mobile pool of the presynaptic membrane and has no effect on the NA

packaged in vesicles. Dopamine is also a substrate for MAO.
- Alpha 2 (α_2)-adrenoceptor activation: α_2-receptors are present on the presynaptic membrane and are activated by NA to exert an autoregulatory and inhibitory effect on further synthesis (inhibits tyrosine hydroxylase) and release of NA from the granules (Figure 3.27).

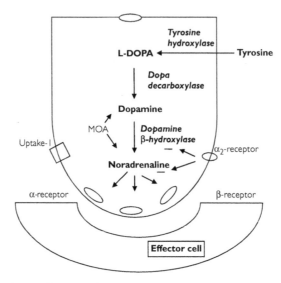

Figure 3.27 Synthesis and metabolism of noradrenaline at adrenergic nerve terminals.

ADDITIONAL FACTS AND REVISION MATERIAL

Blood pressure regulation

- The carotid and aortic baroreceptor systems control acute changes in blood pressure via neural (and therefore instant) reflexes modulated by the vasomotor centre in the brainstem.
- The renin-angiotensin system controls blood pressure in the long term. It is mediated via hormonal mechanisms and therefore takes time to exert its effect.
- ACTH may stimulate an early and transient release of aldosterone, but ACTH is not considered a significant regulator of aldosterone release.
- The juxtaglomerular apparatus is innervated by sympathetic neurons via β_2 receptors.
- Carotid sinus receptors monitor 'stretch' in the vessel and therefore BP. The carotid and aortic bodies are peripheral chemoreceptors and these monitor the chemical composition of the blood directly via their CO_2 and H^+ receptors.

Regulation of alveolar ventilation

- Alveolar ventilation is regulated mainly by the central chemoreceptors under normal conditions.

- Raised pCO_2 and H^+ increase stimulation to the chemoreceptors and alveolar ventilation. Reduced arterial pCO_2 also reduces the drive for alveolar ventilation.
- The blood-brain barrier is readily permeable to CO_2 but not so much to H^+. Central chemoreceptors are sensitive to arterial but not venous CO_2.

Glomerular filtration and renal function

- Substances that are filtered freely include:
  1. major monovalent electrolytes: Na^+, Cl^-, K^+, HCO_3^-
  2. metabolic waste products: urea and creatinine
  3. amino acids, glucose, ketone bodies, and other organic acids
  4. inulin, p-aminohyppuric acid
  5. low molecular weight proteins and peptides (e.g. insulin).
- Substances that are not filtered include:
  1. plasma proteins including albumin
  2. lipid-soluble substances bound to proteins (cortisol, thyroxine, oestrogen, testosterone, bilirubin).

CHAPTER 4

Molecular Biology

Fundamentals of molecular biology

Molecular biology deals with the detailed residue-by-residue transfer of sequential information during the processes of replication, transcription, and translation of genetic material. This information cannot be transferred back from protein to nucleic acid (Figure 4.1). Molecular biological techniques are increasingly used to insert, alter, or remove genes from cells to treat diseases, giving rise to the new and growing clinical specialty of gene therapy.

There are three main classes of biopolymers in living organisms:

- DNA
- RNA
- proteins.

The transfer of sequenced information between these biopolymers occurs via the processes of:

- DNA replication—duplication of DNA sequence
- transcription—formation of mRNA from DNA
- translation—formation of protein from RNA
- reverse transcription—transfer of information from RNA to DNA
- RNA replication
- direct translation from DNA to protein.

The first three of these, replication, transcription, and translation, together constitute the process of protein synthesis.

Biochemistry of genes and protein synthesis

The blueprint for each cellular protein is contained within a distinct region of DNA, the 'gene', which encodes the

sequence in which amino acids must be assembled to construct that particular protein. The nucleotides that constitute a gene can be subdivided into exons (conventionally considered as 'coding regions') and introns (or 'non-coding regions'). Converting the genetic code into a protein sequence is a two-step process whereby the DNA must first be transcribed into RNA, and then the RNA must be translated into a specific sequence of amino acids (Figure 4.2). Transcription initially requires the DNA duplex to separate and multiple proteins and enzymes must then bind to the exposed DNA template (around the sequence TATA or CAAT) to form the 'pre-initiation complex'. The subsequent polymerization of the RNA strand relies on complementary base pairing (Table 4.1) whereby the sequence of deoxyribonucleotide bases in the DNA template dictates the ribonucleotide base sequence in the growing RNA strand. This transcript elongates in the direction from the 5′ carbon to the 3′ carbon by the sequential addition of nucleotides to the free hydroxyl group on the 3′ carbon of the most recently added ribose sugar. These paired processes of transcription and translation give rise to a peptide, which is converted to a fully mature protein (with all of its structural and functional properties) through a series of post-translational modifications that might include:

- protein folding (into secondary and tertiary structures)
- cleavage (usually at the amino-/N-terminus, but sometimes in the middle of the protein)
- glycosylation (addition of carbohydrate groups)
- phosphorylation (addition of phosphate ions).

A common mistake is to assume that DNA only codes for mRNA. *All* RNA molecules (mRNA, rRNA, and tRNA) have to be transcribed from genes contained in the DNA.

- In the first instance, all of the nucleotides contained in the gene (including those in the introns) are transcribed into the RNA sequence (hence referring to introns as 'non-coding' can be misleading).
- Following transcription, the immature RNA strand is released from the DNA (which then anneals with the

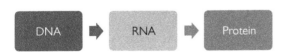

Figure 4.1 The transfer of sequenced information (DNA is transcribed to RNA; RNA is translated to protein).

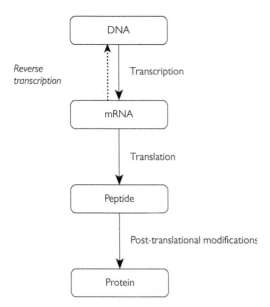

Figure 4.2 The 'central dogma' of molecular biology. Deoxyribonucleic acid (DNA) is transcribed into messenger ribonucleic acid (mRNA) transcripts, which are subsequently translated into a growing peptide chain.

contralateral strand to reform the DNA duplex) and the RNA undergoes post-transcriptional modifications. For mRNA, these include excision of the introns, addition of a reversed guanosine triphosphate (GTP) molecule as a 'cap' at the 5′ end of the mRNA transcript, and addition of a series of adenosine ribonucleotides (the 'poly-A+ tail') at the 3′ end of the strand.

- Having been processed, the mRNA transcript, which carries the same base sequence as the exons of the corresponding gene (with the exception that all thymines are substituted by uracils), is translated.
- The mRNA is bound by a ribosome (itself comprised of rRNA and accessory proteins), which interrogates the bases of the mRNA in triplet sequences, termed codons. The codon sequence AUG (corresponding to ATG in the genomic DNA sequence) serves as the start site for protein translation.
- Dependent on the sequence of bases in each codon, the appropriate tRNA molecule with the complementary anti-codon sequence binds into the ribosome, bringing with it one of 20 amino acids (Figure 4.3). (The composition of codons from three adjacent bases generates a total of 64 different codons, which are sufficient to code for the 20 different amino acids via corresponding anti-codons on the tRNA molecules.)
- The incoming amino acid is coupled (through a peptide bond) to the growing peptide chain, and the ribosome moves along the mRNA molecule (reading in the direction 5′ to 3′) to determine which aminoacyl-tRNA complex should be recruited to the next site. This continues, producing a peptide where the amino acids are threaded together like 'beads on a string' dependent upon the sequence of the mRNA codons (themselves dictated by the base sequence in the exons of the corresponding gene).
- When the ribosome reaches a 'stop' codon (typically with the base sequence UGA) the ribosome departs, leaving the peptide chain free to undergo post-translational modifications within the rough endoplasmic reticulum and/or Golgi apparatus.
- With the exception of cells that lack nuclei (e.g. erythrocytes), all cells carry the same DNA and hence the same genes. However, in different cells, different genes may be 'switched on' (expressed) and others will be 'switched off' (repressed). As different cells will have different genes expressed, they will produce different arrays of proteins, and it is this cell/tissue-specific pattern of gene expression that makes each tissue unique and specialized. The smooth muscle of the myometrium differs in several respects from the smooth muscle of the bladder, and the epithelium of the vagina is distinct from the epithelium lining the buccal cavity.

An important variation of this is observed in retroviruses such as HIV. Such viruses possess the enzyme 'reverse transcriptase', which confers on them the ability to literally reverse transcribe their viral RNA into DNA. This can then be incorporated (via their 'integrase' enzymes) into the patient's own genome. This makes it very difficult to eradicate

Table 4.1 Complementary nucleotide base pairing in nucleic acids

DNA Replication		Transcription		Translation	
Nucleotide base in:		Nucleotide base in:		Nucleotide base in:	
DNA template	Growing DNA strand	DNA template	Growing RNA strand	mRNA codon	tRNA anti-codon
Adenine (A)	Thymine (T)	Adenine (A)	Uracil (U)	Adenine (A)	Uracil (U)
Thymine (T)	Adenine (A)	Thymine (T)	Adenine (A)	Uracil (U)	Adenine (A)
Guanine (G)	Cytosine (C)	Guanine (G)	Cytosine (C)	Guanine (G)	Cytosine (C)
Cytosine (C)	Guanine (G)	Cytosine (C)	Guanine (G)	Cytosine (C)	Guanine (G)

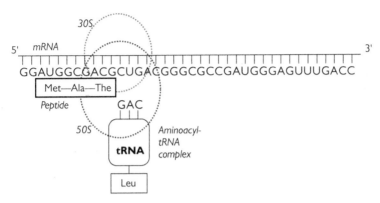

Figure 4.3 The mechanism of protein translation. The triplet codons of ribonucleotide bases in the messenger RNA (mRNA) transcript are translated by the 70S mammalian ribosome (of which the 30S and 50S subunits are depicted by the dotted, grey lines). The amino acid sequence of the growing peptide shown (represented by the sequence Met-Ala-The) is determined by the complementary nucleotide base pairing between the codons in the mRNA transcript and the anti-codons on the incoming transfer RNA (tRNA) molecules. Dependent upon the anti-codon sequence of the tRNA molecules, the aminoacyl-tRNA synthase enzymes ensure that the appropriate amino acid is coupled to the tRNA molecule, conferring fidelity on the process of protein translation.

a retroviral infection once the viral genome has been integrated into the host's own double-stranded DNA. These processes are described in detail in appropriate texts, and are only outlined here.

Molecular biology employs several techniques to identify the molecular component of cells including:

- expression cloning
- polymerase chain reaction (PCR)
- gel electrophoresis
- macromolecule blotting and probing
- arrays
- allele-specific oligonucleotide.

Polymerase chain reaction (PCR) is a technique for amplifying and copying DNA. PCR requires a set of basic reagents including:

- DNA template
- two primers
- DNA polymerase (commonly used is the Taq polymerase)
- deoxynucleoside triphosphate
- buffer solution
- divalent cations (Mg^{2+} is predominantly used)
- monovalent cations (K^+ is predominantly used).

The main principle of PCR is based on thermal cycling, the process by which repeated cycles of heating and cooling of the reaction results in DNA melting and enzymatic replication. There are six steps in the PCR procedure (Figure 4.4):

- Initialization: Consists of heating the reaction to a temperature of 98°C.
- Denaturation: Causes disruption of the hydrogen bonds between the complementary bases resulting in two

single-stranded DNA molecules. This process is also known as DNA melting.

- Annealing is the term used to describe the binding of a primer to a DNA strand. It occurs at temperatures of 50–65°C in the PCR. Annealing temperatures are usually 3–5°C below the melting temperature of the primer in the PCR.
- Elongation: DNA polymerase will polymerize a thousand bases per minute. The optimum temperature for this step is based on the DNA polymerase used (in the case of Taq polymerase it is 72°C). The quantity of target DNA is doubled by the end of this step.
- Final elongation: Occurs at 70–74°C for up to 15 minutes.
- Final hold: Occurs at a temperature of 4–15°C.

Macromolecule blotting techniques include:

- Southern blotting—used to detect DNA sequences
- Northern blotting—used to detect RNA sequences
- Eastern blotting—used to detect post-translation modification of proteins
- Western blotting—used to detect proteins in samples.

  - Southern blotting, named after its inventor Edwin Southern, is a method used to probe for DNA sequences within DNA. This method employs gel electrophoresis, membrane blotting, and exposure to a label DNA probe with a complementary base sequence to the target DNA. Southern blotting has widely been replaced by PCR today.

  - Western blotting allows detection and quantitative analysis of proteins. This method involves separation of proteins by size via gel electrophoresis followed by membrane blotting and antibody probing.

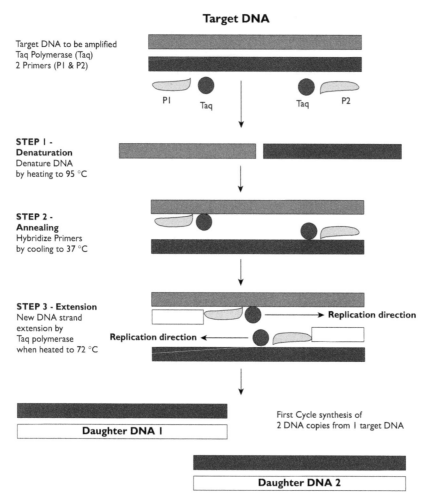

Target DNA

Target DNA to be amplified
Taq Polymerase (Taq)
2 Primers (P1 & P2)

P1   Taq   Taq   P2

**STEP 1 -
Denaturation**
Denature DNA
by heating to 95 °C

**STEP 2 -
Annealing**
Hybridize Primers
by cooling to 37 °C

STEP 3 - Extension
New DNA strand
extension by
Taq polymerase
when heated to 72 °C

Replication direction →

Replication direction ←

Daughter DNA 1

First Cycle synthesis of
2 DNA copies from 1 target DNA

Daughter DNA 2

Figure 4.4 Steps in the PCR reaction.
Reproduced with kind permission from Arisudhan Anantharachagan.

Cell

The cell (from *cellula*—Latin for a small room) is the basic functional unit of all living organisms, and the building block of all complex life. Two types of cell exist:

- prokaryotic
- eukaryotic.

Prokaryotic cells lack a nucleus and membrane-bound organelles. They include the archaea and bacteria domains of living organisms. Most prokaryotes contain a cell wall and are small in size (1–10 μm) compared to eukaryotes. Reproduction is by binary fission.

Eukaryotic cells contain a nucleus and membrane-bound organelles. They include protista, fungi, plants, and animals. The average size of a eukaryotic cell is 10–100 μm. Cellular division occurs by two processes that are distinct from those in prokaryotic cells:

- mitosis
- meiosis.

A eukaryotic cell is composed of the following components (Figure 4.5):

- A plasma membrane.
- The cytoplasm, which is bound by the cell's plasma membrane. It contains the cytosol, the organelles, and the cytoplasmic inclusions.
- The nucleus, which contains the cell's genetic material. It is enclosed by a nuclear envelope that has nuclear pores.
- The nucleolus, which is a non-membrane-bound structure within the nucleus. RNA is transcribed within the nucleolus.

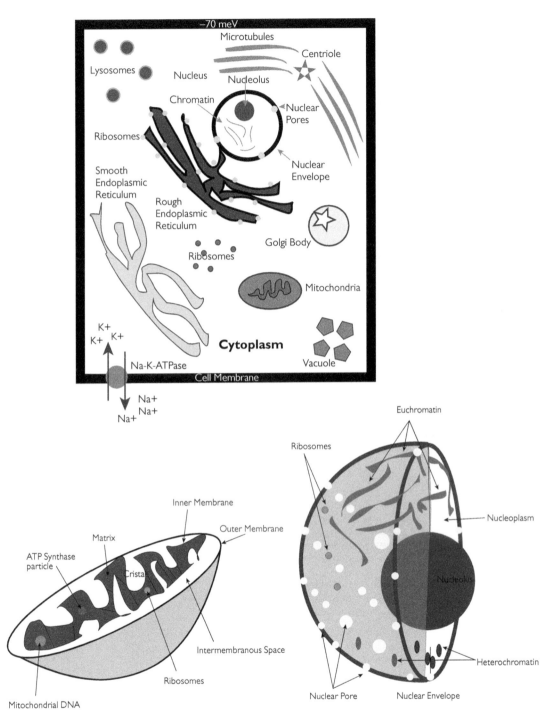

Figure 4.5 The human cell.
Reproduced with kind permission from Arisudhan Anantharachagan.

- The endoplasmic reticulum (ER), comprised of three kinds: rough, smooth, and sarcoplasmic. Rough ER is responsible for the synthesis of proteins. Smooth ER synthesizes lipids and steroids, and also regulates the intracellular calcium concentration. The sarcoplasmic reticulum's sole function is to regulate intracellular calcium levels.
- The ribosomes, which are the organelles responsible for assembling proteins from amino acids.
- The Golgi apparatus. This plays a crucial role in processing, modifying, and packaging proteins and lipids for cell secretion. It is composed of membrane-bound structures known as cisternae.
- Lysosomes and peroxisomes.
- Mitochondria, also known as the power house of the cell since they generate energy-rich ATP. The mitochondrial matrix contains specific mitochondrial genetic material in the form of DNA. This divides by binary fission and in humans is inherited through the maternal line.

Cell signalling

All living organisms communicate with each other and this is also true for cells. Cell signalling is important in governing basic cellular activities and maintaining normal tissue homeostasis.

There are four basic methods of cell signalling:

- juxtacrine
- paracrine
- endocrine
- autocrine.

Each of these methods requires a signalling molecule and a cell surface receptor.

Depending on the type and location of the signalling molecules (also known as ligands) they can be categorized as hormones, cytokines, chemokines, or neurotransmitters.

Cell surface receptors are specialized integral membrane proteins. There are three main classes of cell surface receptors:

- ion channel-linked receptors
- enzyme-linked receptors
- G protein-coupled receptors.

G protein-coupled receptors are also known as seven-transmembrane domain receptors. They are found on all eukaryotic cells and consist of three subunits: α, β, and γ. They include receptors for chemokines, bradykinin, opioids, leukotriene, relaxin, dopamine, histamine, glucagon, calcitonin, vasopressin, and glycoprotein hormones.

In most cases, ligand and cell surface receptor interaction is insufficient to elicit cellular response without an additional intracellular messenger. This intracellular messenger, known as a secondary messenger, is responsible for activating the intracellular receptors leading to gene transcription. The entire set of changes induced by the receptor activation is called signal transduction.

Receptors that are exclusively intracellular (necessitating the ligand to physically cross the cell membrane) include:

- steroid hormone receptors
- thyroid hormone receptors
- retinoic acid receptors
- vitamin D3 receptors.

Intracellular secondary messengers (where the ligand first interacts with a cell surface receptor) include:

- calcium
- nitric oxide
- diacylglycerol
- inositol triphosphate.

Nitric oxide is an intracellular messenger that causes smooth muscle relaxation. It is derived from L-arginine with a by-product of L-citrulline. Nitric oxide synthesis is catalysed by nitric oxide synthase (NOS). There are three types of NOS:

- Endothelial—This is calcium-calmodulin dependent. It is also expressed by the syncitiotrophoblast.
- Inflammatory—This is calmodulin independent. It is secreted by bacterial cell walls and neutrophils.
- Brain.

CHAPTER 5

Biochemistry

Biochemical and structural components of the cell

Four major classes of biochemical molecule (nucleic acids, proteins, lipids, and carbohydrates) form each cell in the body. Each type of molecule fulfils a different primary role (Table 5.1), but all contribute to cell/tissue structure and to key cellular functions.

Nucleotides consist of a pentose sugar (either ribose or deoxyribose) plus an organic, nitrogenous base (adenine, guanine, cytosine, thymine, or uracil) to form nucleosides (adenosine, guanosine, cytidine, thymidine, or uridine). These are converted to nucleotides by the addition of up to three phosphate groups to the 5′ carbon position on the pentose sugar (Figure 5.1A). While the polymerization of ribonucleotides forms ribonucleic acids (RNA), deoxyribonucleic acid (DNA) strands are formed by the polymerization of deoxyribonucleotides.

- Within nucleic acids, a purine base (adenine or guanine) always pairs with a pyrimidine (cytosine, thymine, or uracil) to maintain a uniform distance between the two nucleic acid strands. In DNA, adenine (A) pairs with thymine (T), whereas in RNA, adenine pairs with uracil (U). In both DNA and RNA, guanine (G) pairs with cytosine (C).
- Purine and pyrimidine nucleotides are all synthesized *de novo* in the body from amphibolic molecular intermediates.
- Purines are heterocyclic/double-ring structures (Figure 5.1B) constructed using the carbon skeleton of the amino acid glycine, combined with carbons derived from respiratory carbon dioxide (CO_2), N^{10}-formyl-tetrahydrofolate and N^5,N^{10}-methenyl-tetrahydrofolate, together with nitrogens contributed from aspartate and the amide groups of glutamine molecules.

Table 5.1 The major classes of biochemical molecules

Monomer	Polymer	Defining chemical groups	Major structural roles	Major functional roles
Nucleotide	Nucleic acid (DNA/RNA)	Nitrogenous base (G/A/C/T[a]/U[a]) + pentose sugars[b] with a phosphate backbone	DNA comprises chromatin in cell nucleus	Contain and relay the genetic blueprint for proteins in a cell-specific manner; ATP = cellular energy store
Amino acid	Peptide/protein	Amino (NH_2) groups and peptide bonds (-NH-CO-)	Cytoskeleton + majority of cellular enzymes and receptors	Catalyse reactions and mediate cellular signalling
Fatty acids	Phospholipids + triglycerides	Predominantly hydrophobic hydrocarbons + carboxylic acid groups (COOH)	Phospholipids for membrane bilayers around cells and organelles; triglycerides provide insulation and a long-term energy store	Restrict movements of hydrophilic ions to create specific micro-environments within cells and their organelles
Monosaccharide	Polysaccharide (glycogen[c])	Contain carbon, hydrogen, and oxygen in the same proportion as water: $C_nH_{2n}O_n$	Contribute to the structure of specific membrane lipids and of subcellular proteins	Provide both an immediate source and a short-term store of energy to power ATP synthesis

[a]Four bases in DNA are G, A, C, and T, but in RNA, U replaces T.
[b]In DNA, the pentose sugar is deoxyribose whereas in RNA, the pentose sugar is ribose.
[c]In plants, glycogen is replaced by cellulose, which has a different chemical bond structure that humans can only digest via bacterial enzymes in the gut.

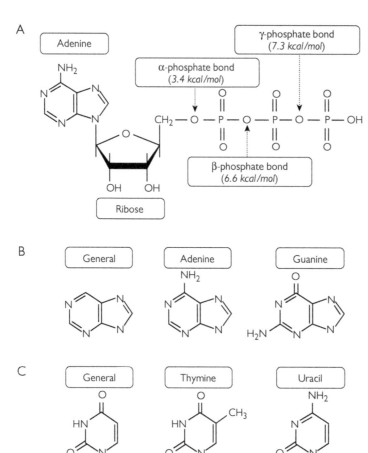

A

Adenine

B

General | Adenine | Guanine

C

General | Thymine | Uracil

Figure 5.1 Molecular structures of (A) adenosine triphosphate (ATP), (B) the purine bases, and (C) the pyrimidines. The cartoon structure of ATP as a typical nucleotide depicts the structural relationships between the nitrogenous base (adenine), the pentose sugar (ribose), and the three phosphate groups. Also shown in panel (A) are the energetic yields (in kilocalories) when a mole of ATP undergoes complete hydrolysis of the α, β, or γ phosphate bonds.

- A complex series of reactions, commencing with the synthesis of 5-phosphoribosyl-1-pyrophosphate (PRPP), produces inosine monophosphate (IMP), which can be converted to either adenosine monophosphate (AMP) or guanosine monophosphate (GMP). These monophosphates are metabolized to diphosphate and triphosphate derivatives (AMP→ADP→ATP; GMP→GDP→GTP) using phosphoryl transfer from adenosine triphosphate (ATP).

- In the liver, the synthesis of purine nucleotides is regulated by the availability of PRPP, which is suppressed (in a homeostatic negative feedback loop) by the accumulation of AMP/ADP and GMP/GDP.

- Pyrimidines are cyclic, six-membered rings (Figure 5.1C). Their synthesis starts with the combination of CO_2, glutamine, and a phosphate from ATP to form carbamoyl phosphate, catalysed by carbamoyl phosphate synthase (CPS)-II. This is then combined with the amino acid aspartate to form the cyclic ring structure of dihydroorotic acid (DHOA). Via a series of intermediates, DHOA is metabolized on to uridine diphosphate (UDP), which can either be reacted with ATP and glutamine to form cytidine triphosphate (CTP) or metabolized along an alternative pathway to generate deoxy-thymidine monophosphate (dTMP).

- The final reaction in the synthesis of dTMP requires a tetrahydrofolate derivative. Hence, synthesis of dTMP, vital for cell division, can be inhibited by agents such as methotrexate that inhibit dihydrofolate reductase.

- Pyrimidine nucleotide synthesis is stimulated (at the level of CPS-II) by the accumulation of PRPP but inhibited by purine nucleotides and by UTP.

- In the first instance, purines and pyrimidines are synthesized as ribonucleotides (ATP, GTP, CTP, and TTP), but each can be reduced to their 2′-deoxyribonucleotide counterparts (dATP, dGTP, dCTP, and dTTP) by the action of the ribonucleotide reductase complex (using thioredoxin as a donor of reducing equivalents).

The plasma membrane that surrounds each cell and the membranes that circumscribe each of the subcellular organelles (e.g. nucleus, mitochondria, endoplasmic reticulum, Golgi apparatus, and lysosomes) are comprised primarily of phospholipid bilayers (Figure 5.2). There are four major types of phospholipid (phosphatidyl-choline, -ethanolamine, -inositol, and -serine), each formed by esterification of two fatty acyl chains (typically one saturated and one polyunsaturated fatty acid) to a glycerol backbone with the polar/charged head group attached to the third carbon of that glycerol skeleton (Figure 5.3).

- Due to the hydrophobic nature of the fatty acyl tails, which form the core of the phospholipid bilayer, polar compounds (e.g. glucose) and charged ions (e.g. Na^+, K^+, Cl^-, and HCO_3^-) are unable to pass across the membrane bilayer without a protein-based transport mechanism. Hence, phospholipids effectively insulate cells (and their constituent organelles), allowing them to selectively take up or exclude specific hydrophilic molecules and ions, creating specific microenvironments within the cell. The typical cell membrane also contains two additional components: cholesterol and membrane proteins (Figure 5.2).

- Although it is a lipid, cholesterol increases membrane fluidity to the extent that the ultimate hydrophilic molecule, water, can pass through small spaces between neighbouring phospholipid molecules without destabilizing the membrane.

- By virtue of its molecular structure, at low to medium concentrations, cholesterol decreases the Van der Waal's forces and hydrogen bonding between adjacent lipid molecules, so increasing membrane fluidity (Figure 5.4). (At high concentrations cholesterol paradoxically decreases membrane fluidity, as the cholesterol molecules become organized into a stable, semi-crystalline structure).

Proteins either reside within the cell membrane ('integral' membrane proteins) or associate with the hydrophilic head groups of the phospholipid molecules ('peripheral' membrane proteins) (Figure 5.2). Membrane proteins typically serve as transport proteins, enzymes, or receptors. Cytoplasmic proteins that are not associated with the cell membrane

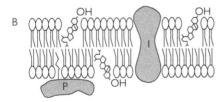

Figure 5.2 Cell membrane structure: panel (A) depicts the phospholipid bilayer on which all cell membranes are based, while panel (B) represents the fluid mosaic model of cell membrane structure, incorporating cholesterol molecules and membrane proteins. Peripheral membrane proteins (P) associate with the polar head groups of the phospholipids (by ionic interactions and hydrogen bonding), whereas integral membrane proteins (I) are embedded in the hydrophobic, fatty acyl core of the phospholipid bilayer.

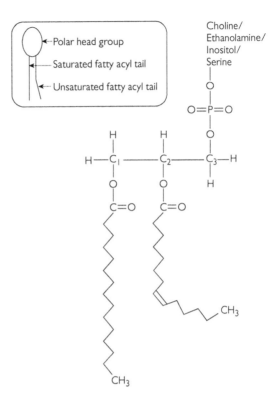

Figure 5.3 Molecular structure of a phospholipid (with the conventional schematic representation shown in the inset panel).

can make similar structural and functional contributions in the cytoplasm of the cell.

Carbohydrates are the preferred respiratory substrates from which cellular energy is derived and so make relatively limited contributions to cellular structure. In most tissues (except the liver), carbohydrates simply modify pre-existing sub-cellular structures by combining with lipids (to form glycolipids) or proteins (to form glycoproteins), altering the structure-function relationships of the modified lipid/protein molecules.

Functional components of the cell

Biochemistry is concerned with the reactions required to harness energy (ATP) from biological 'fuels' such as carbohydrates, lipids, and proteins, and the intracellular conversion of this energy orchestrated by nucleotides. There are, however, non-energetic functions of nucleic acids, lipids, proteins, and carbohydrates within cells.

- DNA and RNA carry the genetic blueprint of each cell. DNA (the foreman) instructs RNA molecules (the workers) to construct cellular proteins to the blueprint carried by the DNA via two distinct processes, whereby the DNA is first transcribed into RNA and the mRNA is then translated into proteins. This 'central dogma' of molecular

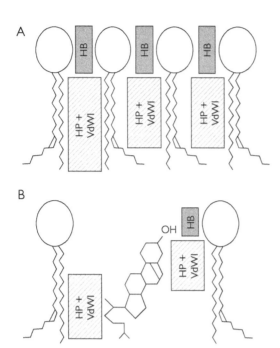

Figure 5.4 Effects of cholesterol on membrane fluidity. As depicted in panel (A), in the absence of cholesterol there are maximal opportunities for hydrogen bonding (HB) and ionic interactions between the polar phospholipid head groups, and for hydrophobic interaction (HP) and Van der Waal's interactions (VdWI) between the fatty acyl chains. However, with the intercession of cholesterol molecules (panel B), both sets of molecular interactions are decreased, which increases membrane fluidity.

biology is fundamental to creating specialization of cell structure and function.

- Lipid molecules form membranes that create the specialist cellular and sub-cellular microenvironments required for tissue- and cell-specific biochemistry (e.g. oligodendrocytes and Schwann cells serve to insulate the axonal membranes of neurons, accelerating the conduction of action potentials between the nodes of Ranvier). Lipid molecules also serve as signalling molecules (e.g. steroid hormones derived from cholesterol and inflammatory mediators, thromboxanes, prostaglandins, and leukotrienes, synthesized from the 20-carbon polyunsaturated fatty acid, arachidonate).

- Proteins serve three major functions within a typical cell: as components of the cytoskeleton, as enzymes, and as receptors. The arrangement of the actin, myosin, and tubulin proteins into the cytoskeleton confers a 3-dimensional shape on cells. The majority of intracellular enzymes are proteins with the exception of the ribozymes (RNA enzymes).

- Enzymes (E) are biochemical catalysts, which accelerate reactions by lowering the activation energy. The reaction

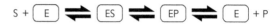

Figure 5.5 Biochemical equilibria for a single-step, enzyme-catalysed reaction. E = enzyme, EP = enzyme-product complex, ES = enzyme-substrate complex, P = product, and S = substrate.

centre of an enzyme (the 'active site'), is the region that binds the reaction substrate (S) and converts that substrate into the reaction product (P) (subsequently displaced from the active site by the binding of another substrate molecule) (Figure 5.5). Hence, any factor that changes the shape of an enzyme so as to alter the conformation of the active site will change the rate of reaction.

- The rate (or velocity) of an enzyme-catalysed reaction (V) can be accelerated by increasing the concentration of either the substrate (Figure 5.6) or enzyme. For a given amount of enzyme, when the maximal rate of reaction (V_{max}) is achieved, all of the available active sites are occupied by substrate and/or participating in the biochemical reaction such that the reaction velocity is unaffected by further increases in the substrate concentration. Assuming first order enzyme kinetics, the Michaelis-Menten constant (K_m) is the substrate concentration at which the reaction reaches a velocity equal to half of the maximal rate ($V_{max}/2$) (Figure 5.6).

- Since the molecular conformation of enzyme proteins is highly sensitive to both temperature and pH, the rate of reaction is affected by both of these variables. Hence, it is possible to define an optimum temperature (T_{opt}) and pH (pH_{opt}) at which a given enzyme operates (Figure 5.7). Most enzymes have evolved to function best at 37°C and any changes in body temperature (fever or localized inflammation) impair the biochemical reactions by denaturing the enzyme proteins. Likewise, except for specialist

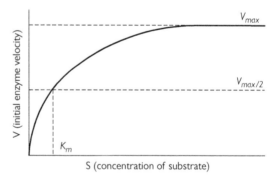

Figure 5.6 Michaelis-Menten kinetic plot showing the effect of substrate concentration (S) on the initial velocity (V) of an enzyme-catalysed reaction. V_{max} = the maximal velocity of the enzyme-catalysed reaction, $V_{max/2}$ = 50% of the maximal velocity, and K_m = the Michaelis-Menten constant (the concentration of substrate at which $V_{max/2}$ is achieved).

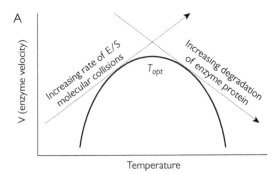

A

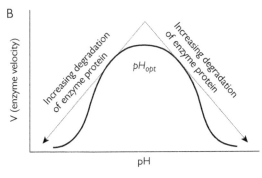

B

environments such as the stomach (normal pH <4.0) and vagina (normal pH range = 3.8–4.5), most enzymes operate optimally at pH 7.4. The efficiency of vaginal enzymes would decrease if the pH increased (e.g. in the presence of semen, due to decreased oestrogen action during menses, or in bacterial vaginosis).

- Proteins that are integral in the plasma membrane of the cell may function as 'receptors', binding extracellular signal molecules (e.g. gonadotrophins, prostaglandins, or growth factors) and initiating a signalling cascade that mediates the cellular response to the extracellular ligand (e.g. generation of a second messenger molecule and/ or activation of a protein kinase). Likewise, intracellular proteins, located in either the cytoplasm or nucleus, can serve as ligand-dependent transcription factors to regulate gene expression on binding a hydrophobic ligand (e.g. steroid or thyroid hormones).

Figure 5.7 The effects of temperature (panel A) and pH (panel B) on the initial velocity (V) of an enzyme-catalysed reaction. E/S = enzyme/substrate, pH_{opt} = pH optimum (the pH at which the maximal reaction velocity is achieved), and T_{opt} = temperature optimum (the temperature at which the maximal reaction velocity is achieved).

Fuel metabolism

The principles of processing respiratory substrates are the same irrespective of the class of biochemical fuel being metabolized. In each case:

- a respiratory substrate is oxidized
- a nucleotide co-factor is reduced
- the nucleotide co-factor is then reoxidized back to its oxidized state (via the mitochondrial oxidative phosphorylation pathway) leading to the generation of a high energy, γ-phosphate bond in ATP (Figure 5.1A).

While these principles are upheld for all fuels, the details of the metabolic pathways differ between carbohydrates, lipids, and proteins. In terms of the initial oxidative pathways, carbohydrates are metabolized by glycolysis, fatty acids by the β-oxidation cycle, and amino acids by transamination reactions. Under aerobic conditions, all respiratory substrates ultimately end up in the Krebs cycle (also known as the citric acid or tricarboxylic acid cycle), which yields far more reduced co-factor molecules (and hence more ATP) than the initial oxidative pathways (Table 5.2). Moreover, it is the Krebs cycle that unites the

metabolism of all biological fuels, and so facilitates the inter-conversion of different fuel types in the fed and fasting states (Figure 5.8).

Oxidative phosphorylation

The energy currency of the cell is the nucleotide triphosphate ATP, wherein the majority of latent biochemical energy is trapped in the terminal γ phosphate bond, with relatively low amounts of energy in the α and β phosphate bonds (Figure 5.1A). When respiratory substrates are oxidized, a relatively small proportion of their biochemical energy is harnessed directly as ATP in events referred to as 'substrate level phosphorylation' reactions. In most cases, the energy liberated from a single component reaction within a metabolic pathway or cycle is insufficient to power ATP synthesis directly, and instead results in the transfer of 'reducing equivalents' (hydrogen ions) to an enzyme co-factor such that:

- the oxidized form of NAD^+ is reduced to NADH
- the oxidized form of FAD is reduced to $FADH_2$.

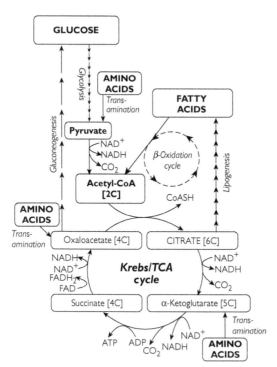

Figure 5.8 Overview of the biochemical pathways for the catabolism and oxidation of respiratory substrates, illustrating the central role for the Krebs/tricarboxylic acid (TCA) cycle. 4C/5C/6C = 4/5/6 carbon atoms; CoASH = coenzyme A; FAD/FADH$_2$ = flavin adenine dinucleotide (oxidized and reduced forms, respectively); and NAD$^+$/NADH = nicotinamide adenine dinucleotide (oxidized and reduced forms, respectively).

Oxidative phosphorylation is the biochemical process by which electrons pass (through a series of electron acceptors/donors) from the reduced nucleotide co-factors to oxygen, thereby recycling the oxidant co-factors and powering the synthesis of ATP within the mitochondria. The oxidative phosphorylation pathway comprises four sequential protein complexes, acting in concert with ATP synthase embedded in the inner mitochondrial membrane (Figure 5.9). As they oxidize the nucleotide co-factors, complexes I, III, and IV each export protons from the mitochondrial matrix into the aqueous space between the inner and the outer mitochondrial membranes in a process termed chemiosmosis. This establishes a concentration/pH gradient across the inner mitochondrial membrane and it is the flux of protons down this gradient back into the matrix via ATP synthase that drives the phosphorylation of ADP to ATP.

- Complex I (NADH dehydrogenase or NADH-coenzyme Q oxidoreductase), which has 46 distinct protein subunits, binds NADH and oxidizes this back to NAD$^+$ (and a proton). The abstracted pair of electrons passes via a flavin mononucleotide (FMN) prosthetic group to

iron-sulphur (Fe-S) centres in complex I and ultimately on to ubiquinone (coenzyme Q), which is reduced to ubiquinol. As the electrons pass through complex I, protons bind to the matrix face of the complex and are transferred across to be liberated into the intermembrane space.

- Complex II, which comprises four protein subunits and incorporates succinate dehydrogenase (succinate-coenzyme Q oxidoreductase), does not lie downstream of complex I, but instead represents an independent point of entry into the oxidative phosphorylation pathway (Figure 5.9). This complex contains FAD bound within the inner mitochondrial membrane, and as the dehydrogenase component oxidizes succinate to fumarate, the hydrogen ions pass to this nucleotide co-factor, reducing the FAD to FADH$_2$. Within complex II, the electrons again pass via Fe-S centres to coenzyme Q/ubiquinone, but because complex II does not span the inner mitochondrial membrane, any protons bound by this complex have to be returned to the mitochondrial matrix (rather than being exported into the aqueous intermembrane space).

- From complexes I and II, the electrons pass via ubiquinol to complex III (cytochrome c reductase): a dimeric assembly wherein each monomer contains 11 protein subunits associated with a single cytochrome c molecule and two b cytochromes (Figure 5.9). Each of the cytochromes contains at least one haem group in which the iron can either accept or donate electrons (transiting between the Fe^{2+} and Fe^{3+} states, respectively). As a consequence, complex III is able to receive electrons from complexes I and II (recycling the ubiquinol back to ubiquinone) and to pass those electrons on to cytochrome c. As the electrons pass through complex III, protons are bound on the matrix side of the complex and are exported into the intermembrane space (as for complex I).

- The final complex of the oxidative phosphorylation pathway, complex IV (cytochrome c oxidase), comprises 13 protein subunits, two haem groups, and ionic copper (Cu$^+$/Cu^{2+}), magnesium, and zinc. By virtue of its transition metal ions, complex IV can accept the electrons from the haem groups of cytochrome c (which then relax from their Fe^{2+} to the Fe^{3+} state). The electrons pass through complex IV to oxygen in the mitochondrial matrix, which splits into oxide ions and recombines with protons to form water molecules (Figure 5.9). As complex IV transports electrons and forms water, it also provides the third opportunity for protons to be exported from the mitochondrial matrix into the intermembrane space.

- Like complexes I, III, and IV (but not complex II), ATP synthase also spans the inner mitochondrial membrane. More specifically, the F$_0$ region of ATP synthase spans the membrane while the globular F$_1$ domain, which contains the synthase enzyme, protrudes into the mitochondrial matrix. As the protons exported into the intermembrane space of the mitochondrion by complexes I, III, and IV re-enter the matrix along the proton channel in the F$_0$ domain, they provide energy to the F$_1$ domain required

Table 5.2 ATP yields of oxidative biochemical pathways for different respiratory substrates

	Aerobic glycolysis	Anaerobic glycolysis	PDH[a]	β-oxidation cycle	Krebs cycle
Respiratory substrate	Glucose	Glucose	Pyruvate[b]	Fatty acyl-CoA (e.g. palmitoyl-CoA)	Acetyl-CoA (+ various amino acid C-skeletons)
ATP yield due to: Substrate-level phosphorylations	4×1	4×1	0×1	0×1	1×1
NAD^+/NADH	2×3	0×3[c]	1×3	8×3	3×3
FAD/$FADH_2$	0×2	0×2	0×2	8×2	1×2
ATP requirement	2×1	2×1	0	0	0
NET ATP yield (moles of ATP per moles of respiratory substrate)	8	2	3	40[d]	12[e]

[a]PDH = pyruvate dehydrogenase.
[b]Pyruvate is usually derived from glucose as the end product of glycolysis, but can also be derived from amino acids by transamination or deamination reactions.
[c]Under anaerobic conditions, glycolysis yields two molecules of NADH, but both of these are oxidized back to NAD^+ by lactate dehydrogenase without any attendant synthesis of ATP.
[d]The yield of ATP from the β-oxidation cycle depends on the nature of the fatty acyl-CoA substrate; the figure provided relates to palmitoyl-CoA, and following the lipolysis of a typical molecule of triglyceride, three molecules of palmitoyl-CoA would enter the β-oxidation cycle.
[e]The Krebs cycle turns twice (yielding 24 moles of ATP) during the complete oxidation of a molecule of glucose, and eight times (yielding 96 moles of ATP) during the complete oxidation of a molecule of palmitoyl-CoA.

to power the synthesis of the high-energy, terminal γ phosphate bond in ATP. Some antibiotics, such as oligomycin, inhibit the F_0 domain of ATP synthase, which contributes to the lethargic side effects of such drugs.

- Since NADH enters the oxidative phosphorylation pathway at complex I, there are three opportunities to export protons from the mitochondrial matrix (via complexes I, III, and IV) such that each molecule of NADH produced in the metabolism of a respiratory substrate generates up to three molecules of ATP. However, when succinate is oxidized by succinate dehydrogenase in complex II, protons can only be exported via complexes III and IV. Consequently, the oxidation of $FADH_2$ back to FAD can only power the synthesis of two molecules of ATP (Table 5.2).

Krebs/TCA cycle

The Krebs cycle (or tricarboxylic acid/TCA cycle) operates in the mitochondrial matrix only under aerobic conditions. The two-carbon (2C) molecule acetate is combined with the four-carbon (4C) molecule oxaloacetate to yield the ionized form of the symmetric six-carbon (6C) molecule citrate (Figure 5.10—reaction 1).

- In the initial rate-limiting formation of citrate, the 2C acetate molecule does not exist in free solution, but is attached to coenzyme A (CoA) via a sulphurous thioester linkage as acetyl-CoA (Figure 5.10). This is important since cleavage of the high-energy thioester bond in acetyl-CoA provides the energy for the formation of the new carbon-carbon bond when the acetate is combined with the oxaloacetate by the enzyme citrate synthase to form citrate.

- The fact that citrate is a symmetrical molecule is problematic, so in the next reaction of the cycle, aconitase converts citrate to isocitrate via the metabolic intermediate, aconitate (Figure 5.10—reaction 2). Once in an asymmetric form, this isocitrate can be oxidized by isocitrate dehydrogenase (ICDH) to form the five-carbon (5C) metabolite, α-ketoglutarate (α-KG) (Figure 5.10—reaction 3). Not only does this reaction liberate a molecule of CO_2, but it is the first reaction in which a nucleotide co-factor, specifically NAD^+, becomes reduced (to NADH), which will ultimately contribute to the ATP yield of this metabolic cycle (Table 5.2). Likewise, in the very next reaction, catalysed by α-ketoglutarate dehydrogenase (α-KGDH), a second carbon is lost as CO_2 and a second molecule of NAD^+ is reduced to NADH. The 4C product of this reaction is immediately esterified to CoA to form succinyl-CoA (Figure 5.10—reaction 4), which liberates energy when hydrolysed by succinyl-CoA synthase to yield free CoA and succinate (Figure 5.10—reaction 5). The large amount of energy derived from hydrolysis of the thioester bond in this step of the cycle is sufficient to power addition of phosphate onto guanosine diphosphate (GDP) generating guanosine triphosphate (GTP). As the GTP relaxes back to GDP, the energy from the third phosphate bond is transferred, by nucleotide diphosphokinase (NDPK), to adenosine diphosphate (ADP) generating a further molecule of ATP. This molecule of ATP is the only one to be generated in the Krebs cycle by substrate-level phosphorylation independently

A

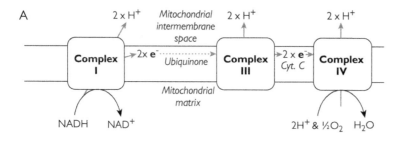

B

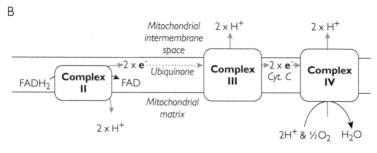

C

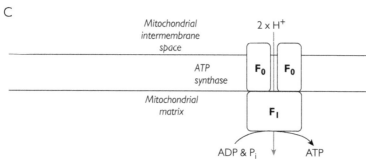

Figure 5.9 The oxidative phosphorylation pathway. Panel (A): The oxidation of NADH to NAD$^+$ by complex I, and the subsequent transfer of a pair of electrons (2 × e$^-$) to complex III (via ubiquinone) and complex IV (via cytochrome C/Cyt. C) powers the export of three pairs of protons via complexes I, III, and IV acting in sequence. Panel (B): The oxidation of FADH$_2$ to FAD by complex II, and the subsequent transfer of a pair of electrons to complexes III and IV (via cytochrome C/Cyt. C) powers the export of two pairs of protons via complexes III and IV only. Panel (C): The flux of each pair of protons from the aqueous intermembrane space back into the mitochondrial matrix via the F$_0$ and F$_I$ domains of ATP synthase drives the coupling of inorganic phosphate (P$_i$) to ADP to form a high-energy γ phosphate bond in ATP.

of the mitochondrial oxidative phosphorylation pathway (Table 5.2).

- Following the liberation of the succinate from succinyl-CoA, there follows a series of three reactions that see the 4C skeleton of succinate rearranged to form oxaloacetate with no further loss of CO$_2$ (Figure 5.10). Firstly, succinate is oxidized to fumarate by succinate dehydrogenase (SDH), reducing FAD to FADH$_2$ (Figure 5.10—reaction 6). While seven of the eight enzymes of the Krebs cycle exist within the matrix of the mitochondrion, SDH is unusual in being embedded in the inner mitochondrial membrane where it constitutes an integral part of complex II of the oxidative phosphorylation pathway. Fumarate is then hydrated by fumarase to form malate (Figure 5.10—reaction 7) and in the final reaction of the cycle, malate dehydrogenase (MDH) oxidizes the malate to oxaloacetate, reducing NAD$^+$ to NADH in the process (Figure 5.10—reaction 8).

In summary, each turn of the Krebs cycle can generate up to 12 molecules of ATP (Table 5.2). References to citric,

isocitric, α-ketoglutaric, succinic, fumaric, malic, and oxalo-acetic acid (rather than citrate, isocitrate, α-ketoglutarate, succinate, fumarate, malate, and oxaloacetate, respectively) often leads to confusion. These alternative names merely indicate whether the carboxylic acids are still capable of acting as proton donors or are in their ionized (basic) state. At the normal, physiological intracellular pH of 7.4, all seven acids are in their dissociated/ionized state, and so should properly be referred to as citrate, isocitrate, α-ketoglutarate, etc.

Glycolysis

Glycolysis relies on the cellular uptake of glucose from extracellular fluid/plasma. By virtue of its high proportion of polar hydroxyl groups, glucose is hydrophilic and so cannot diffuse freely across cell membranes. Instead, transport proteins are required to mediate monosaccharide flux into cells, and several different glucose transport (GLUT) proteins have already been identified. Following membrane

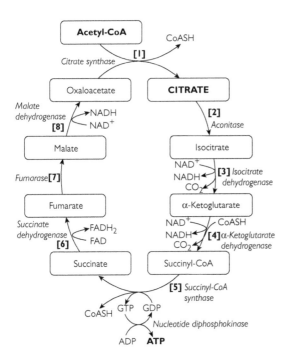

Figure 5.10 The Krebs (citrate/TCA) cycle.

uptake, glucose oxidation through the glycolytic pathway occurs in the cytosol.

- In fetal tissues, adult erythrocytes, and the brain, glucose uptake is mediated via the low affinity, high capacity GLUT1 protein.

- In skeletal muscle and adipose tissue, glucose uptake occurs via the insulin-sensitive GLUT4 transporter.

- Although glycolysis can occur in the absence of oxygen (i.e. under anaerobic conditions, and in cells that lack mitochondria such as red blood cells), this reaction series generates a relatively modest yield of reduced nucleotide co-factors, and hence of ATP. (Of the maximum net gain of 38 molecules of ATP generated through the aerobic oxidation of each molecule of glucose, only eight molecules are generated through glycolysis; this decreases to a net gain of only two molecules of ATP per molecule of glucose respired under anaerobic conditions.) (Table 5.2)

- Glycolysis is a nine-step pathway that commences with the hexose monosaccharide, glucose (Figure 5.11). The first reaction, catalysed in reproductive tissues by hexokinase (as opposed to the high K_m glucokinase enzyme expressed in the liver), is the ATP-dependent phosphorylation of glucose at carbon position C6 to yield glucose-6-phosphate (Figure 5.11—reaction 1). This has two effects: it decreases the effective intracellular glucose concentration, so maintaining a concentration gradient for further glucose uptake, and it traps glucose within the cell by the addition of a negative charged phosphate (PO_4^{2-}) ion. As a result, phosphate addition by the kinase

commits that glucose molecule to further metabolism by glycolysis, glycogen synthesis (in the liver or skeletal muscle), or the hexose monophosphate (HMP) shunt.

- In the second reaction, glucose-6-phosphate isomerase catalyses the rearrangement of the hexose skeleton, converting glucose-6-phosphate into fructose-6-phosphate (Figure 5.11—reaction 2). (Fructose, the sole monosaccharide in human semen, can also enter glycolysis directly at this point.) Subsequent ATP-dependent phosphorylation of the fructose-6-phosphate by 6-phosphofructokinase (PFK) generates fructose-1,6-bisphosphate (Figure 5.11—reaction 3), at which point the 6C molecule is cleaved by fructose bisphosphate aldolase into two 3C molecular fragments: dihydroxyacetone phosphate and glyceraldehyde-3-phosphate (Figure 5.11—reaction 4). There is isomerization between these two triose molecules, catalysed by triose phosphate isomerase, and the glyceraldehyde-3-phosphate (GAP) can be oxidized to 1,3-bisphosphoglycerate by glyceraldehyde-3-phosphate dehydrogenase (GAPDH), which reduces NAD^+ to NADH (Figure 5.11—reaction 5).

- Since each molecule of glucose (6C) gives rise to two molecules of GAP (2 × 3C), all downstream reactions occur twice for each molecule of glucose entering the glycolytic pathway. In this specific reaction, GAPDH will oxidize two molecules of GAP to two molecules of 1,3-bisphosphoglycerate, reducing two molecules of NAD^+ to two molecules of NADH in the process. Each molecule of 1,3-bisphosphoglycerate will then undergo reversible dephosphorylation to 3-phosphoglycerate by phosphoglycerate kinase with transfer of the liberated phosphate onto ADP to derive two molecules of ATP in a substrate-level phosphorylation reaction (Figure 5.11—reaction 6). Following a reversible molecular rearrangement of the 3-phosphoglycerate to 2-phosphoglycerate, catalysed by phosphoglycerate mutase (Figure 5.11—reaction 7), and oxidation of the 2-phosphoglycerate by enolase to yield phosphoenolpyruvate (PEP) (Figure 5.11—reaction 8), glycolysis ends with the dephosphorylation of PEP to pyruvate (Figure 5.11—reaction 9). This final reaction, catalysed by pyruvate kinase, again sees the liberated phosphate transferred onto ADP to generate ATP by substrate-level phosphorylation and occurs twice for each molecule of glucose entering the glycolytic pathway.

Alternative fates of pyruvate

After glycolysis, the fate of pyruvate (and hence the potential for further energy conversion into ATP) depends on the cellular provision of oxygen and the metabolic activity of the cell. Under normal aerobic conditions, pyruvate would enter the mitochondria and undergo further metabolism to enter the Krebs cycle. This allows each triose (3C) molecule to complete its respiration into three CO_2 molecules, ensuring the maximum conversion of biochemical energy from the respiratory substrate into ATP.

- The arithmetic of the Krebs cycle is very straightforward. The 4C molecule oxaloacetate combines with a 2C

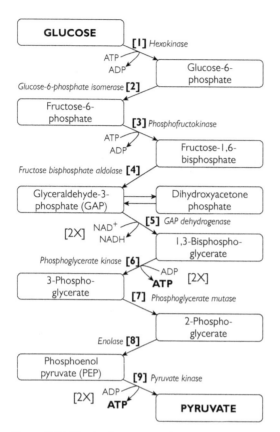

Figure 5.11 The glycolysis pathway. At reaction 4, the hexose (6C) monosaccharides are cleaved into interchangeable triose (3C) molecules (glyceraldehyde-3-phosphate and dihydroxyacetone phosphate), such that all downstream reactions (5 to 9 inclusive) occur twice for every hexose molecule entering the pathway.

- This series of reactions is often referred to as the 'link reaction' since the conversion of pyruvate to acetyl-CoA is not part of glycolysis (which ends at pyruvate), nor is it part of the Krebs cycle (which conventionally begins with the formation of citrate from oxaloacetate plus acetyl-CoA).

- In order for the Krebs cycle to run in balance, the amount of acetyl-CoA entering the cycle must match the amount of oxaloacetate available to combine with it and form citrate. If there is an excess of acetyl-CoA and/or a relative deficit in the availability of oxaloacetate, the PDH enzyme complex is inhibited (so preventing further conversion of pyruvate to acetyl-CoA) and pyruvate is instead metabolized by pyruvate carboxylase. As its name implies, this enzyme catalyses the addition of a CO_2 group onto the 3C pyruvate molecule to generate the 4C molecule oxaloacetate, which then combines with the excess acetyl-CoA, providing an alternative route of entry into the Krebs cycle.

- Under anaerobic conditions, the limited supply of oxygen to the mitochondria stops the oxidative phosphorylation pathway from regenerating the oxidant nucleotide cofactors NAD^+ and FAD. As the reduced forms of NADH and $FADH_2$ accumulate, the Krebs cycle is effectively rendered inoperative, and more importantly, the restricted provision of oxidized NAD^+ to the GAPDH enzyme would arrest the flux of carbon (and hence of energy) through the glycolytic pathway.

- In order for glucose to continue to be metabolized and yield at least some ATP under anaerobic conditions, in hypoxic/anaerobic tissues and cells that lack mitochondria, pyruvate has to be reduced to lactate by lactate dehydrogenase (LDH). This enzyme uses NADH as its reductant co-factor, and so regenerates NAD^+ in the cytoplasm independently of the mitochondria (Figure 5.12).

acetate molecule (derived from acetyl-CoA) to generate the 6C molecule citrate, and that 6C molecule then yields a total of 2 CO_2 molecules as it recycles back (via the 5C molecule α-KG and the 4C intermediates succinate, fumarate, and malate) to oxaloacetate. In the Krebs cycle there is no place for 3C triose molecules such as pyruvate, which must therefore be modified (either to a 4C or 2C metabolite) before it can enter the cycle. Provided there is sufficient oxaloacetate available in that cycle, the pyruvate will be oxidized to acetate (2C) and combined (through a high-energy thioester bond) with CoA to form acetyl-CoA (Figure 5.12). This requires a complicated sequence of biochemical reactions to be catalysed by the pyruvate dehydrogenase (PDH) enzyme complex, which has to remove the CO_2 (as the pyruvate becomes acetate), reduce NAD^+ to NADH (which can give rise to up to three additional ATP molecules via oxidative phosphorylation), and form the thioester bond between the acetate and the CoA acceptor molecule.

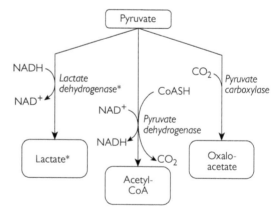

Figure 5.12 Alternative metabolic fates of pyruvate. Under anaerobic conditions (depicted by the asterisk) pyruvate is reduced to lactate, whereas under aerobic conditions pyruvate can either undergo oxidative decarboxylation to acetyl-CoA, or carboxylation to oxaloacetate.

β-oxidation cycle

The β-oxidation cycle, which occurs in the mitochondrial matrix, is the iterative cleavage of 2C fragments from a fatty acid chain to generate acetyl-CoA molecules that enter the Krebs cycle (Figure 5.13). In the case of fatty acids containing even numbers of carbon atoms, the β-oxidation cycle converts the fatty acid exclusively into 2C acetyl groups (seven, eight, or nine acetyl-CoA molecules per molecule of myristic, palmitic, or stearic acid, respectively). For odd-numbered fatty acids, 2C subunits are cleaved until the final 3C fragment remains as a propionyl-CoA molecule, i.e. the rare 17C fatty acid margaric acid would undergo the β-oxidation cycle to yield seven (rather than eight) acetyl-CoA molecules and a single propionyl-CoA molecule. The propionyl grouping has the same problem entering the Krebs cycle as pyruvate: the propionyl group has three carbons, and three is not a number favoured by the Krebs cycle. Therefore, any propionyl-CoA formed by β-oxidation of odd-chain fatty acids must be carboxylated to enter the Krebs cycle as the 4C component of succinyl-CoA (which decreases the ATP yield of propionyl-CoA to only six ATP

per turn of the Krebs cycle, as opposed to 12 ATP per turn for each acetyl-CoA molecule) (Figure 5.10).

- The β-oxidation cycle is preceded by esterification of a 'free' or non-esterified fatty acid (NEFA) chain onto the sulphydryl/thiol group of coenzyme A to form a fatty acyl-CoA molecule. (This is important since the thioester bond provides the energy to power this metabolic cycle.)

- There then follows a series of four reactions, and in each round the length of the fatty acyl-CoA molecule is decreased by two carbons.

- Two of these four sequential reactions are oxidation reactions, which reduce the oxidant nucleotide co-factors, FAD and NAD^+. This has two consequences. Firstly, it means that β-oxidation of fatty acids leads to the generation of ATP prior to the entry of the acetyl-CoA fragments into the Krebs cycle. Secondly, this requirement for FAD and NAD^+ to be recycled (via the oxidative phosphorylation pathway) explains why fat metabolism can only occur during aerobic conditions.

- The initial fatty acyl-CoA molecule for β-oxidation is formed from NEFA in the cytosol of the cell, whereas the β-oxidation cycle occurs within the mitochondrial matrix.

- In order to pass across the aqueous space between the mitochondrial membranes, cytosolic acyl-CoA molecules must combine with carnitine at the outer mitochondrial membrane, catalysed by the carnitine palmitoyl transferase (CPT) I enzyme, and then be released by the action of CPT II in the inner mitochondrial membrane (Figure 5.14).

- In the first step of the β-oxidation cycle, the fatty acyl-CoA is oxidized by acyl-CoA dehydrogenase to form trans-Δ^2-enoyl-CoA (with the attendant reduction of FAD to $FADH_2$). The trans-Δ^2-enoyl-CoA then undergoes hydration to form L-3-hydroxyacyl-CoA.

- Subsequent NAD^+-dependent oxidation, catalysed by hydroxyacyl-CoA dehydrogenase, forms the 3-ketoacyl-CoA molecule, and in the final reaction of the cyclic sequence, that 3-ketoacyl-CoA reacts with another molecule of mitochondrial CoA to liberate the acetyl-CoA and leave a shortened acyl-CoA, ready to commence the next round of β-oxidation (Figure 5.13).

- It is important to appreciate that through the β-oxidation cycle, the majority of carbon from a fatty acid molecule enters the Krebs cycle as acetyl-CoA. Since each fatty acid chain contributes carbon atoms to the Krebs cycle in pairs, and each turn of the Krebs cycle sees two carbon atoms oxidized to CO_2 (Figure 5.10), there is no net gain of carbon to the Krebs cycle via β-oxidation. It is as a consequence of this arithmetic that fatty acids cannot be converted into carbohydrates, whereas excess carbon (and calories) from carbohydrates can be converted into fatty acids and triglyerides. Therefore, questions suggesting the conversion of fatty acids to carbohydrates are trick questions and are false no matter what intermediate molecules are proposed to achieve this.

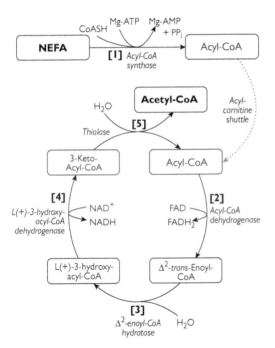

Figure 5.13 The β-oxidation cycle of fatty acids. In the first instance, a cytosolic non-esterified fatty acid (NEFA), liberated from triglyceride stores by lipolysis, is esterified to coenzyme A (CoASH) to form an acyl-CoA molecule that can be imported into the mitochondrial matrix via the acyl-carnitine shuttle. The initial formation of the acyl-CoA complex requires the hydrolysis of magnesium (Mg)-ATP to Mg-AMP and pyrophosphate (PP_i), where the spontaneous decay of the PP_i to two inorganic phosphate (P_i) molecules prevents the acyl-CoA synthase reaction from reaching equilibrium.

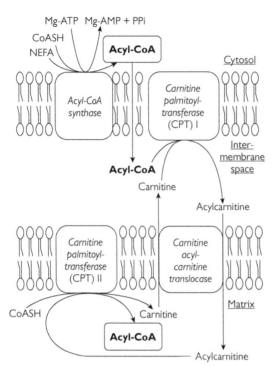

Figure 5.14 The acyl-carnitine shuttle. Acyl-CoA molecules, formed by the esterification of non-esterified fatty acids (NEFA) to coenzyme A (CoASH) molecules, are imported across the outer mitochondrial membrane. Within the aqueous intermembrane space, the fatty acyl chain is transferred onto carnitine by the action of carnitine palmitoyl-transferase (CPT) I. This acylcarnitine can then be imported across the inner mitochondrial membrane (by a translocase enzyme) before being cleaved back into carnitine and acyl-CoA (the substrate for the β-oxidation cycle) by the action of CPT II.

Unlike most tissues, the liver relies primarily for its acetyl-CoA (and thus its ATP) on the β-oxidation of NEFA. In specific metabolic conditions (e.g. starvation), hepatic β-oxidation generates more acetyl-CoA than can be incorporated into the Krebs cycle. Within the hepatic mitochondria, the excess acetyl-CoA molecules can be combined (by thiolase) to generate acetoacetyl-CoA molecules, which can be coupled with acetyl-CoA to synthesize 3-hydroxy-3-methylglutaryl-CoA (HMGCoA). Cleavage of this product by HMGCoA lyase liberates acetyl-CoA and free acetoacetate, where the latter can be reduced to 3-hydroxybutyrate by the reversible 3-hydroxybutyrate dehydrogenase enzyme. Acetoacetate and 3-hydroxybutyrate, collectively termed 'ketone bodies', are exported into the circulation and taken up by extra-hepatic tissues, most importantly the brain and skeletal muscle, where they serve as respiratory substrates. Hydroxybutyrate can be oxidized back to acetoacetate, which is converted to acetyl-CoA (via an acetoacetyl-CoA intermediate) to fuel the Krebs cycle.

Transamination and deamination of amino acids

There are 20 common amino acids, which are used to generate a wide repertoire of cellular proteins, but in starvation they can also sacrifice their amino (NH_3) groups in transamination and/or deamination reactions to generate α-ketoacid intermediates that enter the Krebs cycle as respiratory substrates.

- In the simplest reaction, the amino acid alanine is deaminated by alanine aminotransferase (also called alanine transaminase) transferring the NH_3 group from alanine onto either α-ketoglutarate or oxaloacetate. As a result, the α-ketoacids are converted into glutamate or aspartate, respectively, and the alanine is deaminated to form pyruvate, which enters the Krebs cycle as either acetyl-CoA or oxaloacetate (Figure 5.15A).

- The conversion of serine to pyruvate is slightly more complex: serine must first be metabolized to an aminoacrylate intermediate by serine dehydratase before the aminoacrylate is deaminated to yield pyruvate and a free ammonium ion (Figure 5.15B).

- In reactions that critically depend on the co-factor tetrahydrofolate (THF) to act as a donor/acceptor of single carbon methyl units, the amino acid threonine can also be metabolized (via glycine) to serine and thence on to pyruvate for entry into the Krebs cycle. The cleavage of threonine to glycine by threonine aldolase also liberates acetaldehyde, which can be oxidized (via acetate) to yield acetyl-CoA (Figure 5.15B).

- Glutamine, together with arginine, histidine, and proline, can be deaminated/transaminated to yield glutamate, which has two routes of conversion into the Krebs cycle 5C intermediate α-ketoglutarate. Glutamate can either be deaminated by glutamate dehydrogenase (liberating free ammonium that enters the urea cycle) (Figure 5.15C) or can be transaminated by an aminotransferase (transaminase) enzyme, which transfers the NH_3 group onto either pyruvate or oxaloacetate (generating alanine or aspartate respectively) (Figure 5.15D).

- The hydrophobic amino acids, isoleucine, valine, and methionine, can all be deaminated to form propionyl-CoA, which is subsequently carboxylated to enter the Krebs cycle as succinyl-CoA.

- In the presence of tetrahydrobiopterin, phenylalanine hydroxylase can oxidize phenylalanine to form the aromatic amino acid tyrosine. This can be catabolized to the 4C Krebs cycle intermediate, fumarate, accompanied by the formation of an acetoacetate ketone body (Figure 5.15E).

- The final pathway for amino acid entry into the Krebs cycle is via oxaloacetate. In addition to those four amino acids that can be converted to oxaloacetate via pyruvate (alanine, glycine, serine, and threonine), asparagine can be deaminated to form aspartate, and aspartate can be transaminated to remove its NH_3 group, so generating oxaloacetate (Figure 5.15D).

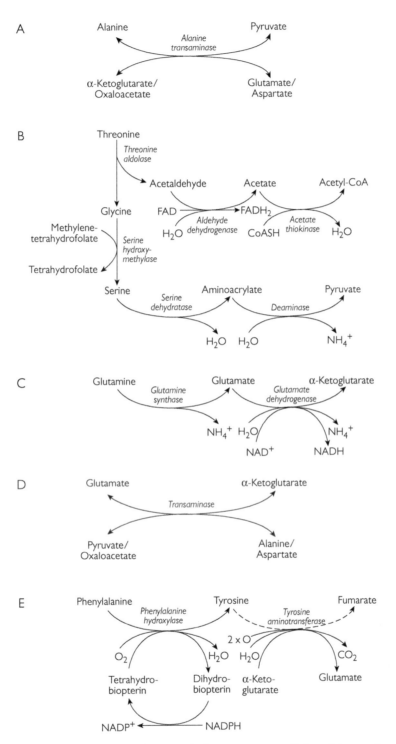

Figure 5.15 Transamination and/or deamination of amino acid substrates to generate Krebs cycle intermediates. Selected metabolic reactions for alanine/pyruvate (panel A), threonine/glycine/serine (panel B), glutamine/glutamate (panel C), glutamate/aspartate/alanine (panel D), and phenylalanine/tyrosine (panel E).

Transamination and deamination reactions liberate ammonium (NH_4^+) ions, which are potentially toxic and so must be converted into urea prior to their excretion in urine (or faeces). This is achieved in the liver by the urea cycle. Within hepatic mitochondria, CPS-I combines NH_4^+ ions with CO_2 and ATP-derived phosphate to form carbamoyl phosphate that combines with ornithine to form L-citrulline (Figure 5.16). Following export into the cytosol, and in the presence of aspartate plus ATP, the citrulline undergoes two sequential reactions to form the amino acid arginine (via arginosuccinate; Figure 5.16). In the final reaction of the urea cycle, the arginine is recycled back to ornithine by the arginase enzyme in a hydrolytic reaction that liberates urea. Deficiencies of urea cycle enzymes can result in hyperammonaemia and related conditions (i.e. citrullinaemia, arginosuccinicacidaemia, or hyperarginaemia).

Vitamins

Vitamins (or 'vital amines') are so named because they are vital for nutrition and cannot be synthesized within the body. Other essential nutrients that are not vitamins include the essential amino acids, essential fatty acids, and dietary minerals such as calcium, chloride, iron, potassium, phosphorous, and sodium.

- Vitamins are generally classified as either being 'fat-soluble' or 'water-soluble' (Table 5.3), where these have to be absorbed from the GI tract in the terminal ileum or colon, respectively.
- In the context of the oxidative metabolism of respiratory substrates, the most important vitamins are the B complex vitamins, which are precursors of several of the coenzymes (Table 5.3). Hence, deficiencies in any specific B vitamin can have potentially fatal consequences.
- In developed countries, vitamin deficiencies are rare due to adequate dietary intake and the fortification of common foods (e.g. bread) with additional vitamins. However, during pregnancy, women are often advised to take vitamin supplements (e.g. increasing their intake of

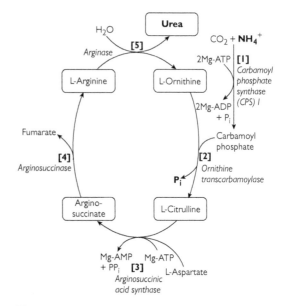

Figure 5.16 The urea cycle. Reactions [1] and [2], catalysed by carbamoyl phosphate synthase (CPS) I and ornithine transcarbamoylase, respectively, occur within the matrix of liver cell mitochondria, whereas reactions [3], [4], and [5] each occur in the liver cell cytosol.

vitamin B_9/folate) to ensure that the nutritional requirements of both the mother and the growing fetus can be met (folate deficiency can result in neural tube defects).
- While vitamins generally exert beneficial actions, overdose of any single vitamin can produce adverse side effects. Of these, the most relevant are the teratogenic actions of vitamin A (retinol) and its pharmaceutical derivatives (e.g. the acne treatment isotretinoin/13-cis-retinoic acid), which can induce serious birth defects if administered to pregnant women.

Table 5.3 The classification and roles of vitamins

(i) Fat-soluble vitamins

Vitamin	Chemical name	Biochemical roles	Deficiency diseases	Effects of overdose
A	Retinoids (retinoic acid, retinal, retinol, retinoids, and carotenoids)	Component of rhodopsin—required as the photoreceptor molecule in the eye	Night blindness	Hyper-vitaminosis A + teratogenesis
D	Calciferol (cholecalciferol and ergocalciferol)	Substrate for vitamin D_3—stimulates calcium absorption from the GI tract	Rickets (if pre-pubertal deficiency)/osteomalacia (if post-pubertal deficiency)	Hyper-vitaminosis D
E	Tocopherol (and tocotrienols)	Antioxidant	Mild haemolytic anaemia in newborns	None reported
K	Phylloquinone (and menaquinones)	Pro-coagulant (vital co-factor for the clotting cascade)	Bleeding diathesis/haemophilia	None reported

(ii) Water-soluble vitamins

Vitamin	Chemical name	Biochemical roles	Deficiency diseases	Effects of overdose
B_1	Thiamine	Component of pyruvate dehydrogenase (PDH) and α-ketoglutarate dehydrogenase (αKGDH) enzyme complexes	Beriberi	None reported
B_2	Riboflavin	Precursor of the co-factors FMN and FAD	Ariboflavinosis	None reported
B_3	Niacin (niacinamide)	Precursor of the co-factors NAD^+/NADH and $NADP^+$/NADPH	Pellagra	Liver damage
B_5	Pantothenic acid	Constituent of coenzyme A (CoA)	Paraesthesia	None reported
B_6	Pyridoxine (pyridoxamine and pyridoxal)	Production of erythrocytes and co-factor for the decarboxylation of aromatic amino acids (in synthesis of monoamine neurotransmitters)	Anaemia	Nerve damage and impaired neural function (specifically proprioception)
B_7	Biotin	Coenzyme R: co-factor for carboxylases (e.g. acetyl-CoA, propionyl-CoA, and pyruvate carboxylase enzymes)	Dermatitis and enteritis	None reported
B_9	Folate	Required for DNA replication and cell division, particularly in bone marrow and in the fetus	Megaloblastic anaemia; developmental neural tube defects	May mask or exacerbate deficiency of vitamin B_{12}
B_{12}	Cobalamins	Required for DNA replication and cell division, particularly in bone marrow and in the fetus; co-factor for methylmalonyl-CoA mutase	Megaloblastic anaemia; developmental neural tube defects	None reported
C	Ascorbate	Antioxidant	Scurvy	Diarrhoea; potential pro-oxidant and carcinogen

93

Fuel storage

The best way to understand the storage and balance of biological fuels in the fed and fasted states is by analogy to money. To avoid running out of funds, a person needs to earn new money, carry some ready cash in their purse or wallet, have easy access to cash stored temporarily in a current account, and have some funds in a savings account where the money performs better but is harder to access. In biochemistry:

- 'earning cash' is equivalent to taking in new calories (i.e. eating a meal)
- the 'ready cash' comes in the form of blood glucose—an abundant energy currency that can be converted into ATP by glycolysis in all cells, even those that are hypoxic or lack mitochondria
- the 'current account' is provided by glycogen—a labile polymer of glucose that is readily broken down to liberate more glucose into the plasma

- the 'savings account' takes the form of triglyceride stores in adipose tissue/fat—it is easy to deposit calories in this form but much harder to withdraw them at a later date.

As with money, calories are managed in a specific order: immediate needs are met first, then the glycogen stores ('current account') are topped up, and finally any remaining glucose is metabolized into fatty acids to be deposited into the adipose triglyceride stores. Before considering the management of glycogen and triglyceride stores in more detail, there are four important points to emphasize:

1. Some tissues, most notably the brain, rely on glucose (or, in starvation, on ketone bodies) as their energy source. This is why low plasma glucose concentrations (hypoglycaemia) result in coma.
2. Although it is possible to metabolize excess glucose into fatty acids (and hence to triglyceride), it is never possible

to reverse this reaction; fatty acids cannot be used to derive glucose.

3. Once glycogen stores have been depleted, the supply of plasma glucose for brain activity can be maintained by using the carbon skeletons of amino acids (never fatty acids).

4. The interconversion of excess glucose to fatty acids (lipogenesis) and of amino acids into glucose (gluconeogenesis) relies on intermediates in the Krebs cycle, underscoring the pivotal role for this cycle at the heart of metabolism.

Glycogen

Glycogen ('animal starch') is a polysaccharide formed by the sequential polymerization of glucose molecules primarily through α-1,4-glycosidic bonds. Approximately 8% of the glucose molecules are added via α-1,6-glycosidic bonds, which creates branch points in the glycogen molecule (Figure 5.17). The synthesis of glycogen is catalysed

by glycogen synthase, an anabolic enzyme that is stimulated after a meal by insulin (and inhibited in the fasting state by hormones such as glucagon and adrenaline).

● Glycogen is stored primarily in the liver (which receives the highest supply of glucose, via the portal vein) and skeletal muscle (where insulin stimulates glucose uptake via the GLUT4 glucose transporter). Significant levels of glycogen synthesis also occur in the vagina, uterus, and brain. The advantage of glycogen as a fuel store is that in the fasted state, glycogen can be rapidly mobilized to derive glucose for glycolysis. The disadvantages of glycogen are that:

1. it has a low calorific density (each glucose molecule can only generate a maximum net yield of 38 ATP molecules)

2. it has a high molecular mass, compounded by the fact that within tissues glycogen has to be complexed with a large volume of water

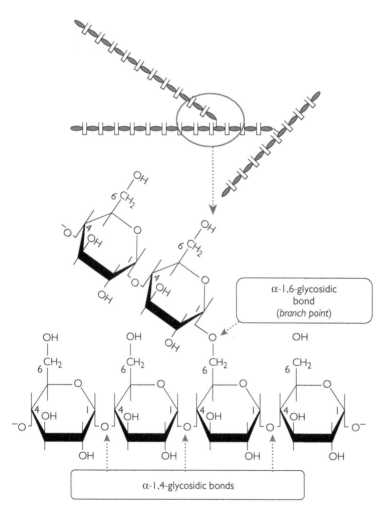

Figure 5.17 The molecular structure of glycogen. The upper part shows the macroscopic, branched, polysaccharide structure of glycogen while the lower part illustrates the role of α-1,4- and α-1,6-glycosidic bonds in the polymerization of the glucose subunits that comprise glycogen.

3. it is asymmetrically distributed around the body with the largest store confined to the liver.

- The catabolism of glycogen, termed glycogenolysis (not to be confused with 'glycolysis'), is catalysed by the enzyme glycogen phosphorylase, which acts sequentially to liberate glucose-1-phosphate molecules from the glycogen, shortening the glycogen polymer by 1 glucose subunit. The glucose-1-phosphate is then isomerized to glucose-6-phosphate by phosphoglucomutase.

- Since the charged glucose-6-phosphate molecule cannot pass across the plasma membrane of the cells, in most tissues (including the vagina, uterus, and skeletal muscle) glucose-6-phosphate generated by glycogenolysis has to be metabolized (by glycolysis) within the very same cell that held the glycogen store.

- Only hepatocytes express the glucose-6-phosphatase enzyme required to remove the phosphate ion, and so only the liver can export glucose into the bloodstream to support glycolysis (and the Krebs cycle) at distant sites.

Triglyceride

Triglycerides are stored predominantly within adipose tissue as the lipid droplets of mature adipocytes. Each triglyceride molecule is comprised of three fatty acyl chains esterified to the three carbons of a glycerol backbone (Figure 5.18) such that lipolysis (the breakdown of triglycerides) has to commence with the hydrolysis of the fatty acyl ester bonds.

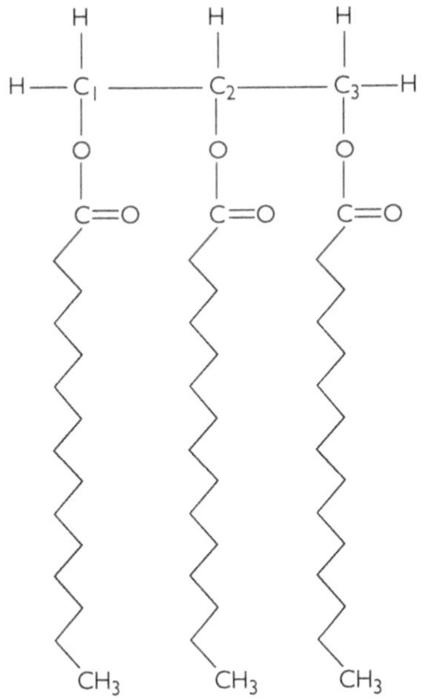

Figure 5.18 The molecular structure of a triglyceride. (Each triglyceride molecule can have any one of a number of fatty acyl chains esterified to the three carbons of the glycerol skeleton; in this example, palmitate is esterified at all three positions.)

This initial step is catalysed by hormone-sensitive lipase, which is stimulated by the hormones of starvation (glucagon, adrenaline, and cortisol) but inhibited by insulin.

- Once each fatty acyl chain has been liberated, the non-esterified fatty acids (NEFAs) can enter the β-oxidation cycle to contribute acetyl-CoA (and possibly propionyl-CoA) molecules to the Krebs cycle. Oxidation of the 16C molecule palmitate, a typical long-chain fatty acid, will contribute eight acetyl-CoA molecules to the Krebs cycle and, in so doing, generate a further eight molecules of NADH and eight molecules of $FADH_2$ as the fatty acid chain undergoes β-oxidation. As a result, palmitate could generate a maximum net yield of 136 ATP molecules (Table 5.2) such that a typical triglyceride molecule could yield up to 408 molecules of ATP (as opposed to only 38 ATP molecules per molecule of glucose respired under aerobic conditions).

- It is this high calorific density, combined with their relatively low weight per unit volume and a diffuse distribution around the body in subcutaneous depots, which makes triglycerides the preferred form for storage of excess calories.

Managing fuel reserves in the fed state

Following a meal, the elevated plasma glucose concentration (and to a lesser extent increased levels of amino acids and gastrointestinal tract hormones) suppresses the secretion of glucagon (from pancreatic α cells) while triggering the secretion of insulin (from pancreatic β cells). Insulin exerts several distinct cellular actions to maximize glucose uptake and metabolism, which restore the plasma glucose concentration to the normal range: between 4 and 8 mmol/l.

1. In skeletal muscle and adipose tissue, insulin stimulates the recruitment of GLUT4 glucose transporters to the plasma membrane of myocytes and adipocytes, so maximizing the number of transport sites available to mediate glucose uptake.

2. Within all metabolically active cells, insulin stimulates the activity of glycolytic enzymes (e.g. glucokinase/hexokinase, pyruvate kinase, and PDH), which decreases the intracellular concentration of free glucose, so maintaining the concentration gradient for further glucose import.

3. Finally, insulin stimulates the activity of glycogen synthase and simultaneously inhibits the activity of glycogen phosphorylase to ensure that excess glucose is directed primarily to replenish intracellular glycogen stores, particularly in liver and skeletal muscle.

As noted above, glycogen is an inefficient energy store due to its low calorific density and relatively high molecular mass. Therefore, there is a finite limit to the body's ability to convert excess carbon (and calories) from glucose into glycogen. Once the body's glycogen stores have been refilled, any remaining glucose is converted into fatty acids and triglyceride as follows.

- All excess glucose is respired (via glycolysis) to pyruvate, and those excess pyruvate molecules then enter the mitochondrial Krebs cycle as either oxaloacetate or (more likely) mitochondrial acetyl-CoA.

- When these molecules combine, the citrate that they form can either remain in the mitochondria to pass around the Krebs cycle or, in the fed state, can be exported out across the mitochondrial membranes. Once in the cytosol, the citrate is acted upon by ATP-citrate lyase releasing oxaloacetate and cytosolic acetyl-CoA (Figure 5.19).
- It is crucial to note that while mitochondrial acetyl-CoA (synthesized by pyruvate dehydrogenase and the β-oxidation cycle) is a substrate for the Krebs cycle, cytosolic acetyl-CoA is the substrate for lipogenesis. In the

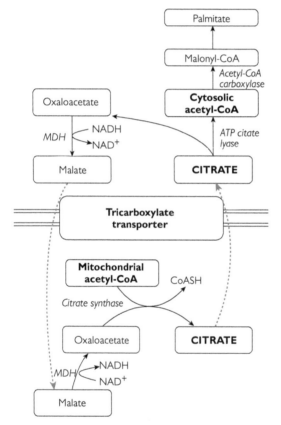

Figure 5.19 Mitochondrial exchange of malate and citrate as a precursor for lipogenesis. Excess citrate generated by the coupling of oxaloacetate and acetyl-CoA in the mitochondrial matrix is exported across the mitochondrial membranes by the action of the tricarboxylate transporter. Once in the cytosol, the citrate is split into cytosolic acetyl-CoA (the precursor for lipogenesis) and oxaloacetate. Since oxaloacetate cannot be imported back into the mitochondrion, it must be reduced to malate by the cytosolic malate dehydrogenase (MDH) enzyme. This malate can then be exchanged for citrate by the tricarboxylate transporter and the imported malate can be oxidized back to oxaloacetate in the Krebs cycle.

lipogenic pathway, the 2C acetate molecules from cytosolic acetyl-CoA are effectively polymerized (connected to an acyl carrier protein) to reconstitute a fatty acid that can be esterified to glycerol to form a triglyceride (completing the conversion of excess carbohydrate into 'fat').

- In the first reaction, a CO_2 group is added onto acetyl-CoA (by acetyl-CoA carboxylase) to form malonyl-CoA, which inhibits the mitochondrial CPT enzymes, so blocking mitochondrial uptake of acyl-carnitine and preventing futile cycling of carbon through the β-oxidation cycle.
- Elongation of the malonyl-CoA molecule occurs through a cyclic series of sequential reactions (effectively the reverse of the β-oxidation cycle), which ultimately generate a C16 fatty acid (palmitate) that can be cleaved from the acyl carrier protein by thioesterase and esterified onto glycerol to form a mono-/di-/triglyceride (Figure 5.20).

In the same way as insulin simultaneously inhibits glycogen phosphorylase while stimulating glycogen synthase, this anabolic hormone also acts in the fed state to inhibit hormone-sensitive lipase while simultaneously activating acetyl-CoA carboxylase to prevent futile cycling between lipogenesis and lipolysis.

Managing fuel reserves in the fasted state

In the moderately 'fasted' state (i.e. as the glucose concentration falls following a meal), the level of insulin falls accompanied by rises in glucagon and adrenaline, which act in concert to ensure that the plasma glucose concentration remains above 4 mmol/l (so avoiding a hypoglycaemic coma). Acute maintenance of plasma glucose is achieved by two mechanisms.

- Initially, acting through a common cell signalling pathway (the cyclic adenosine monophosphate-protein kinase A signalling system), glucagon and adrenaline activate glycogen phosphorylase while simultaneously inhibiting glycogen synthase, so inducing a net mobilization of glycogen to glucose. Because of the tissue-specific expression of glucose-6-phosphatase in the liver, only hepatic glycogen can be used to increase the plasma glucose concentration; in all other tissues, including the vagina and uterus, glycogen is hydrolysed to form glucose-6-phosphate molecules that must be used locally for glycolysis due to the absence of glucose-6-phosphatase.
- Once the major glycogen stores begin to run low (as would occur following an overnight fast), glucagon and adrenaline use the same second messenger system to activate hormone-sensitive lipase, so mobilizing fatty acids for β-oxidation.
- In tissues that can utilize fatty acids as respiratory substrates, this spares glucose metabolism, effectively increasing the amount of glucose available to cells and tissues that are glucose-dependent, such as the brain and erythrocytes.

On prolonged fasting and in other circumstances where calorific expenditure exceeds intake (e.g. in the later stages

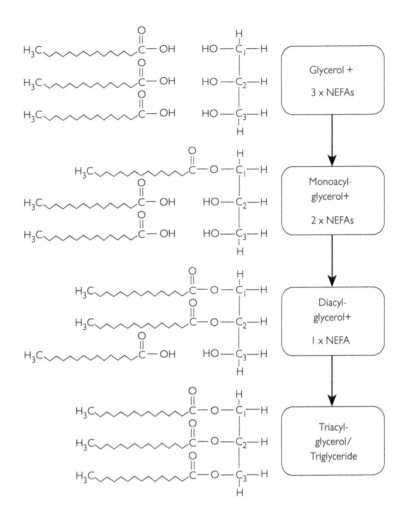

Figure 5.20 The synthesis of triglyceride (triacylglycerol) by the sequential esterification of three non-esterified fatty acids (NEFAs) to carbon positions 1, 2, and 3 in glycerol.

of pregnancy), the catabolic actions of glucagon and adrenaline are augmented by the chronic stress hormone, cortisol. This glucocorticoid steroid acts to change the expression of the genes encoding metabolic enzymes so as to maintain the plasma glucose concentration at a level required to support brain function. For example, cortisol up-regulates the expression of the lipolytic enzyme, hormone-sensitive lipase, required to mobilize triglyceride stores for β-oxidation in order to spare glucose metabolism by those tissues that can respire NEFAs. More importantly, with prolonged fasting, body glycogen stores will be depleted such that additional mechanisms are required to derive glucose. This takes the form of gluconeogenesis whereby the carbon skeletons of amino acids (derived by the breakdown of body protein) are converted into glucose in the liver.

- Gluconeogenesis starts with the 4C Krebs cycle intermediate, oxaloacetate, derived by the proteolytic breakdown of proteins to liberate free amino acids, which enter the cycle by multiple entry routes. The conversion of oxaloacetate into glucose occurs by 'reverse glycolysis' (Figure 5.21).
- This metabolic pathway is not as simple as the name implies, since three of the nine reactions in glycolysis (the steps catalysed by hexokinase/glucokinase, phosphofructokinase, and pyruvate kinase) are irreversible. Therefore, in the fasted state, cortisol must up-regulate the expression of three gluconeogenic enzymes:
  1. phosphoenolpyruvate carboxykinase (PEPCK)—required to metabolize oxaloacetate to phosphoenolpyruvate
  2. fructose-1,6-bisphosphatase—required to catalyse the dephosphorylation of fructose-1,6-bisphosphate to fructose-6-phosphate
  3. glucose-6-phosphatase—required to hydrolyse glucose-6-phosphate to free glucose (for export from the liver).
- In addition, cortisol increases the expression of pyruvate carboxylase (to increase the metabolism of pyruvate to

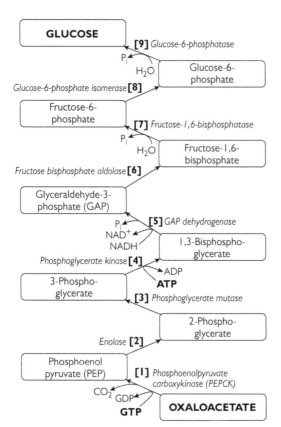

Figure 5.21 The gluconeogenic pathway of 'reverse glycolysis'. To facilitate comparison to the glycolysis of glucose to pyruvate, this pathway has been drawn running from oxaloacetate at the bottom of the figure to glucose at the top of the figure. Reactions 1 (catalysed by phosphoenolpyruvate carboxykinase/PEPCK), 7 (catalysed by fructose-1, 6-bisphosphatase), and 9 (glucose-6-phosphatase) represent those reactions that are irreversible in the glycolysis pathway (and so rely on enzymes that must be up-regulated for hepatic gluconeogenesis using oxaloacetate derived by protein catabolism and amino acid entry into the Krebs cycle).

oxaloacetate) and the enzymes of the urea cycle (required to process the ammonium liberated when amino acids are converted into α-keto acids for the Krebs cycle).

- Although fatty acids cannot be converted to glucose, in prolonged starvation the catabolism of triglyceride can liberate the 3C skeleton glycerol, which can be converted into dihydroxyacetone phosphate and glyceraldehyde-3-phosphate. These intermediates can give rise to glucose in the gluconeogenic pathway of reverse glycolysis.

- In starvation, the increased provision of NEFA to the liver for β-oxidation generates a surplus of acetyl-CoA molecules, which are converted into ketone bodies: acetoacetate and β-hydroxybutyrate. This is an important metabolic pathway since the brain can generate ATP by respiring ketone bodies in starvation when the mechanisms to maintain plasma glucose struggle to meet the brain's metabolic needs. However, prolonged ketosis, whereby the generation of ketone bodies exceeds the rate of their uptake and metabolism, can lower the plasma pH in the phenomenon of ketoacidosis, elaborated below.

Managing fuel reserves in the anaerobic state

In the anaerobic state, the Krebs cycle and β-oxidation cycle both slow dramatically due to their reliance on regeneration of oxidized NAD^+ and FAD by the oxidative phosphorylation pathway. Hence, under anaerobic conditions, the only effective metabolic pathway still to operate is the glycolytic pathway, and even then the net yield of ATP is dramatically decreased (as NADH has to be recycled to NAD^+ through the action of lactate dehydrogenase on pyruvate). To avoid a dangerous decrease in intracellular pH arising from excessive generation of lactate (lactic acidosis), this is exported into the bloodstream, transported back to the liver, and then oxidized back to pyruvate in the Cori cycle (Figure 5.22).

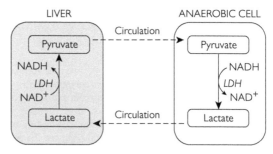

Figure 5.22 The Cori cycle; LDH = lactate dehydrogenase.

Acid-base balance

The respiration of biological fuels poses the threat of lowering plasma pH, either through the liberation of acidic biochemicals (ketone bodies and lactic acid) or by the generation of CO_2. Since significant changes in plasma pH affect the structure and functions of cellular proteins with potentially lethal consequences, multiple mechanisms exist to balance the plasma pH.

- The simplest buffering system is provided by the equilibrium between carbonic acid and bicarbonate ions in the blood (Figure 5.23). Excess CO_2 generated from the Krebs cycle combines with water in the plasma to form carbonic acid (H_2CO_3), which exists in equilibrium with dissociated bicarbonate ions (HCO_3^-) and free protons (H^+).

- Acidosis triggers an increase in the rate of breathing to exhale CO_2, displacing the carbonic acid-bicarbonate equilibrium such that HCO_3^- and H^+ combine to reform carbonic acid, so lowering the free proton concentration and increasing the plasma pH to the target pH of 7.4.
- The second major buffering system of the blood relies on the fact that the 20 different amino acids that comprise proteins each have different chemical side chains, and several of these side chains ionize at different pH values (Figure 5.24). When the plasma pH equals the pKa for a specific amino acid, the probability of that side chain being protonated will be the same as the probability of that side chain being ionized to liberate a proton. Hence, at the pKa, the ratio of protonated to ionized side chains for that specific amino acid will be 1:1 (Figure 5.24).
- If the plasma pH falls below the appropriate pKa (i.e. if there are excess protons in the plasma), the laws of chemical equilibrium will shift this balance to favour the protonated form of the amino acid side chain, whereas at plasma pH levels above the appropriate pKa, the amino acid side chain is more likely to exist in the ionized state, liberating additional protons and so lowering the plasma pH. Hence, each amino acid side chain can buffer small changes in plasma pH around the appropriate pKa value for the chemical group in its side chain.
- In blood, the major plasma protein, albumin, contains a mixture of all 20 amino acids such that it has effective buffering capacity across a wide range of plasma pH values, so maintaining the plasma pH around 7.4.
- In addition to binding protons, albumin can also bind calcium ions (Ca^{2+}). Consequently, as the pH of the plasma changes, and the demands on albumin to bind/release protons changes, so the free calcium concentration of the blood changes with physiological consequences.
- When the plasma pH is low, the excess of free protons effectively displaces Ca^{2+} ions from the albumin, increasing the free plasma calcium concentration (and so suppressing the parathyroid hormone and vitamin D_3/calcitriol endocrine systems). Conversely, with a sustained elevation in the plasma pH, albumin will ionize to liberate protons, increasing its capacity to bind Ca^{2+} ions, hence decreasing the free plasma calcium concentration and increasing the synthesis and secretion of parathyroid hormone and vitamin D_3/calcitriol.

$$H_2O + CO_2 \rightleftharpoons H_2CO_3 \rightleftharpoons H^+ + HCO_3^-$$

Figure 5.23 The carbonic acid-bicarbonate equilibrium. Carbon dioxide (CO_2) generated by the oxidation of respiratory substrates combines with water in extracellular fluid and plasma to form carbonic acid (H_2CO_3), which can then dissociate into bicarbonate ions (HCO_3^-) and free protons (H^+), so lowering the pH of the extracellular fluid or plasma.

Amino acid side chain	pH < pKa	pH > pKa
Sulphydryl (thiol) group (cysteine)	$\cdots CH_2—SH$	$\cdots CH_2—S^-$ & H^+
Hydroxyl (alcohol) group (serine, threonine & tyrosine)	$\cdots CH_2—OH$	$\cdots CH_2—O^-$ & H^+
Carboxylic acid group (aspartate & glutamate)	$\cdots C=O$ with OH	$C=O$ with O^- & H^+
Amino group (lysine, arginine & histidine)	$\cdots CH_2—NH_3^+$; $\cdots C=NH_2^+$ with NH_2 ; $\cdots CH_2$— (imidazole, N / NH)	$\cdots CH_2—NH_2$ & H^+ ; $\cdots C=NH$ & H^+ with NH_2 ; $\cdots CH_2$— (imidazole, N / N$^-$) & H^+

Figure 5.24 The buffering capacity of amino acid side chains. At plasma pH values below the pKa for the relevant side chain (i.e. when the concentration of free protons exceeds the pKa), the side chains will exist in the protonated state (as polar SH/OH/NH groups, or protonated amino groups), but when the plasma pH value exceeds the pKa for the relevant side chain (i.e. when the concentration of free protons falls below the pKa), the side chains will release their proton (and so will exist as deprotonated S^-/O^-/N^- groups, or as deprotonated NH_2/NH groups). When the plasma pH is exactly equal to the pKa value, the probability of any given side chain being in the protonated state will be exactly equal to the probability of that side chain being in the deprotonated state (i.e. half of those specific side chains will be protonated and half will be deprotonated).

ADDITIONAL FACTS AND REVISION MATERIAL

Glucose transporters

Glucose transporters (GLUT) are membrane protein molecules that facilitate the entrance of glucose into the cytoplasm of the cell from the extracellular fluid. There are four main types of GLUT:

- GLUT1 and GLUT3 have a high affinity for glucose and are present in most tissues. They bind glucose whenever it is available and are therefore responsible for basal tissue glucose uptake.

- GLUT2 are found only in the liver and the β-cells of the pancreas. They have a very low affinity for glucose, thus allowing absorbed glucose to pass through the portal system and the liver to the systemic circulation without most of it being metabolized by the liver.

- Since glucose is the stimulus for insulin release from the β-cells of the pancreas, the presence of the low-affinity GLUT2 transporters on these cells ensures that binding of glucose to trigger the release of insulin only occurs when there is abundant glucose. In between meals when the circulating glucose concentration is low, the low-affinity GLUT2 only bind/transport glucose into the β-cells at a low rate, thus ensuring that insulin release is not triggered in this state.

- GLUT4 are present on skeletal muscle cells and in adipose tissues. They are resident in the cytoplasm of the cell and only appear at the cell surface membrane following stimulation of transporter trafficking by insulin. GLUT4 are therefore highly regulated by insulin and are not expressed on the membranes of these tissues unless insulin is present (i.e. only in the fed state).

- Therefore, glucose uptake by skeletal muscle and by adipose tissue depends on insulin activation of GLUT4 transporters.

Glucose metabolism (glycolysis)

- Glucose enters the cell assisted by a tissue-dependent GLUT and it must be trapped within the cell by phosphorylation to glucose-6-phosphate by either of two enzymes—*hexokinase* or *glucokinase*.

- Hexokinase is constitutive, present in all tissues, and has a high affinity for glucose. Glucokinase is induced by insulin, present only in liver cells, has a low affinity for glucose, and is a major regulatory enzyme of glycolysis.

- The rate-limiting step of glycolysis is the ATP-dependent phosphorylation of fructose-6P to fructose-1, 6-bisphosphate, catalysed by *phosphofructokinase-1 (PFK1)*. PFK1 is induced by insulin and inhibited by glucagon.

- The conversion of 1,3-diphosphoglycerate (1,3-DPG) by *phosphoglycerate kinase* is an important reaction because it produces substrate-level ATP (i.e. in the cytoplasm). It is critical for cells that cannot operate the oxidative phosphorylation pathway due to lack of mitochondria or hypoxia.

- In cells without mitochondria (e.g. RBCs), NADH (produced in the first dehydrogenase reaction) is recycled back to NAD$^+$ by the action of *lactate dehydrogenase (LDH)*. Therefore, without LDH glycolysis will cease in cells that lack mitochondria or in hypoxic states.

- To enter the Krebs cycle, pyruvate must be converted into acetyl-CoA by *pyruvate dehydrogenase (PDH)*. Since PDH resides in the mitochondria, which are absent in the RBC, the RBC is totally reliant on a constant supply of glucose and glycolysis for ATP production at substrate level.

- In between meals, glucose supply to the brain and RBCs is maintained by glycogenolysis in the liver. In chronic starvation, the glucose supply is maintained by gluconeogenesis in the liver. This involves the conversion of lactate (from RBC metabolism), alanine (from protein degradation), and glycerol (from triglyceride breakdown) back to glucose.

Fatty acid synthesis, storage, and mobilization

- Accumulation of excess ATP inhibits the glycolytic enzymes and PDH, thereby slowing down ATP production from oxidative phosphorylation. Acetyl CoA accumulates and triggers fatty acid synthesis by the liver. Insulin induces *fatty acid synthetase*, the chief enzyme for fat synthesis.

- Insulin also activates *acetyl CoA carboxylase* by dephosphorylating it.

- Local regulation of fat synthesis is exerted by citrate: it signals liver synthesis of fat and inhibits PFK-1 leading to the accumulation of glucose-6-phosphate and its entry into the hexose-monophosphate pathway (HMP) to produce NADPH.

- Once synthesized, the fatty acid has to be transported away from the liver to adipose tissue to prevent its accumulation in the liver (which would lead to fatty liver, cirrhosis, and damage).

- Fatty acids are packaged in the liver as triglycerides (TG) (by the esterification of fatty acids onto a glycerol backbone), which can be transported in the bloodstream as very low density lipoprotein (VLDL).

- In peripheral tissues, the VLDLs are digested by the hormone-sensitive lipoprotein lipase enzyme, releasing glycerol. The glycerol is taken up and recycled by the liver (reaction catalysed by *glycerol kinase*) whilst the free fatty acids are deposited in the adipose tissue where they are reconstituted back into TG (catalysed by *phosphatidate phosphatase*, *monoacylglycerol*, and *diacylglycerol acyltransferases*).

- Glycerol kinase genes are only expressed in the liver and never in the adipose tissue. Hence, only liver cells can convert glycerol from fat breakdown into glucose.

Glycogen storage and metabolism

- Glycogen is the storage form of glucose retained mostly in the liver, cardiac and skeletal muscles, and the kidneys.
- Glycogen breakdown releases glucose-6-phosphate, which remains trapped within the cell unless it is released by glucose-6-phosphatase. Glucose-6-phosphatase is mainly expressed in the liver and ensures that glucose released from the breakdown of hepatic glycogen stores reaches the general circulation for use by the brain and RBCs.
- Unlike liver cells, muscle and renal cells lack glucose-6-phosphatase, so can only use the glucose from their glycogen stores locally and cannot export this glucose into the general circulation.
- In between meals the liver uses fatty acids rather than glucose for its own energy requirements, emphasizing the role of hepatic glycogen as a glucose store for the whole body.
- Deficiency of hepatic glucose-6-phosphatase leads to the accumulation of glucose-6-phosphate in the liver with severe hypoglycaemia, osmotic damage, hepatosplenomegaly, hyperlipidaemia, and hyperuricaemia (Type 1 glycogen storage disease (von Gierke's)).

Tissues in which glucose uptake is not affected by insulin

1. nervous tissue—brain, spinal cord, nerves
2. kidney—specifically the proximal convoluted tubule, secondary active transport of glucose linked to Na^+
3. intestinal mucosa
4. red blood cells
5. β-cells of the pancreas
6. insulin may accelerate but is not essential for glucose uptake in the liver.

CHAPTER 6

Endocrinology

Hormones

Hormones are chemical messengers that signal through their unique chemical structure, which is recognized by specific receptors on target cells.

Classification and general characteristics of hormones

There are three main chemical classes of hormones.

1. Protein and peptide hormones

- This is the most diverse and numerous group and includes hormones secreted by the hypothalamus, pituitary gland, pancreas, and parathyroid glands.
- Their half lives in the circulation are in the order of minutes and they generally circulate unbound and in free form *except for IGF-1*, which is strongly bound to the binding protein IGFBP-1 and so has a long half life.
- Protein and peptide hormones, catecholamines, and melatonin (biogenic amine hormones) are hydrophilic (water soluble) and do not cross the lipid bilayer of cell membranes.
- Their receptors are resident on the outer surface of the cell membrane and their intracellular actions are exerted by secondary messengers such as cAMP, which usually modify pre-existing proteins rather than generating new ones. For example, secondary messengers may phosphorylate or dephosphorylate protein enzymes to regulate their activity. Modification of already existing proteins allows water soluble hormones to act quickly, although they also have longer-term effects on gene transcription.
- They are stored within intracellular vesicles as prohormones.

2. Steroid hormones

- These are highly conserved and are derived from cholesterol.
- They are secreted from the adrenal cortex, ovaries, testes, and the kidneys (the active form of vitamin D).
- Their plasma transport involves binding to specific transport proteins and albumin, because unlike peptide

hormones they cannot dissolve in the aqueous medium of plasma. As a result their half lives are long and in the order of hours to days. The length of the half life is proportional to the affinity of the hormone for the binding protein. The very small unbound fraction is the biologically active form.

- Steroid and thyroid hormones are hydrophobic and readily cross the lipid bilayer of cell membranes.
- Their receptors are mainly intracellular and their biologic actions are exerted by generating brand new intracellular proteins, which in part explains why they take longer to act.
- Unlike protein and peptide hormones, steroid hormones are not stored in intracellular vesicles but are synthesized and released as required.

3. Hormones derived from an amino acid

- The catecholamines secreted by the adrenal medulla are tyrosine derivatives whilst melatonin secreted by the pineal is derived from tryptophan.
- Catecholamines circulate in free form and their half lives are in the order of seconds. Thyroid hormones are derived from two bound tyrosine molecules that are iodinated but like steroids they are mainly bound in the circulation and have long half lives.

Hormone receptors

- Most protein and peptide hormones act through G-protein coupled receptors (GPCRs), although a few, such as insulin, prolactin, growth hormone, growth factors, and cytokines, act through receptors with inherent tyrosine kinase or receptors associated with proteins that have tyrosine kinase activity.
- GPCRs are linked to enzymes that stimulate the production of second messengers such as cAMP or inositol triphosphate. These then activate intracellular kinases such as protein kinase A or C.
- Receptors with inherent tyrosine kinase activity or those linked with tyrosine kinases activate other cell-signalling pathways that are activated by tyrosine kinase or

TK-associated receptors. Such phosphorylated (activated) kinases can stimulate cytoplasmic processes (e.g. enzyme activation) or can activate transcription factors in the nucleus and thus induce gene transcription (Figure 6.1).

- Steroid and thyroid hormones interact with receptors that are either in the cytoplasm or in the nucleus. Cytoplasmic receptors are generally bound to heat shock proteins (hsps) in the cytoplasm. Upon hormone binding the hsps are released, the receptors dimerize, and then they translocate to the nucleus where they stimulate or inhibit gene transcription. Membrane or membrane-associated steroid and thyroid hormone receptors exist, which upon ligand binding can initiate rapid non-genomic actions within target cells (Figure 6.2).

The hypothalamic-pituitary axis—functional connections

The anterior pituitary gland is functionally connected to the hypothalamus by the hypophyseal portal capillaries.

Neurosecretory cells in the hypothalamus synthesize releasing and inhibiting hormones in their cell bodies and package them in vesicles, which are transported down their axons to the nerve terminals located on the hypophyseal portal capillaries. Hormones released into the portal system are transported to the anterior lobe of the pituitary gland. Here they stimulate or inhibit the release of hormone secretions of the anterior lobe (adenohypophysis) (Figure 6.3). Cells of the adenohypophysis are chromophils (acidophils and basophils, according to the histological dyes they take up) and chromophobes, which are generally considered to be non-secretory.

The posterior lobe of the pituitary gland originates from neural tissue and consists of the nerve terminals of neurosecretory cells whose cell bodies lie in the supraoptic and paraventricular nuclei of the hypothalamus. Here they synthesize and package oxytocin and vasopressin (VP), otherwise known as antidiuretic hormone (ADH). The secretory vesicles containing the hormones are transported down the axons that pass through the neural stalk, and are stored in the nerve terminals in the posterior pituitary gland.

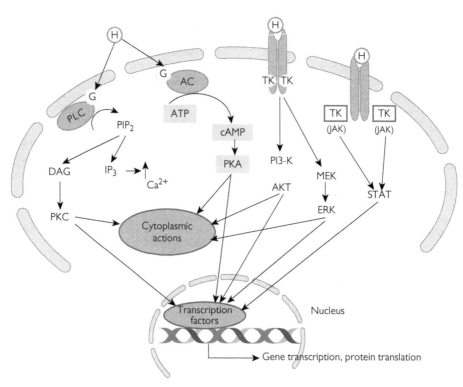

Figure 6.1 Major signalling pathways for protein and peptide hormones. (i) G-protein coupled receptors activate adenyl cyclase (AC) or phospholipase C (PLC). AC increases cAMP production and activates protein kinase A. PLC increases production of diacyl glycerol (DAG) and inositol triphosphate, which increase protein kinase C and a rise in intracellular calcium respectively. (ii) Receptors with inherent tyrosine kinase activity, such as the insulin receptor, activate (phosphorylate) downstream kinases. (iii) Receptors linked to proteins with tyrosine kinase activity, such as janus kinase (JAK), phosphorylate downstream kinases such as STAT. Growth hormone, prolactin, and cytokines use this signalling pathway. There is considerable cross talk between different signalling pathways.

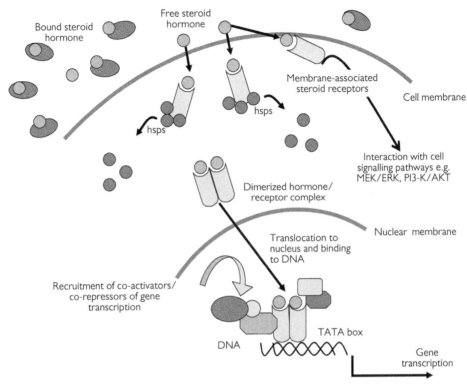

Figure 6.2 Signalling pathways for steroid hormones. For details see text.

The major secretions of the anterior pituitary gland, the cells from which they are secreted, and the proportion of these secretory cells in the adenohypophysis are:

- growth hormone (GH) from somatotrophs (acidophils)—50%
- prolactin (PRL) from lactotrophs (acidophils)—10–15% (increasing in pregnancy)
- thyroid-stimulating hormone (TSH) from thyrotrophs (basophils)—3–5%
- adenocorticotrophic hormone (ACTH) from corticotrophs (basophils—15–20%)
- gonadotrophins, luteinizing hormone (LH), and follicle-stimulating hormone (FSH) from gonadotrophs (basophils)—10%.

Growth hormone

This is a large protein hormone (192 amino acids) that is structurally similar to prolactin. Its synthesis and secretion are stimulated by growth hormone-releasing hormone (GHRH) and inhibited by somatostatin, both of which are released by neurosecretory cells in the hypothalamus. Their integrated actions result in the secretion of discrete pulses of GH throughout the day (approximately six pulses) with an increased pulse amplitude related to the onset of sleep.

GH pulse frequency and secretion is high during puberty and declines in senescence.

Control of GH secretion

- Stimulation – GHRH, hypoglycaemia, decreased free fatty acids, starvation, sleep exercise, stress, puberty oestrogens and androgens, α-adrenergic agonists, and dopamine agonists.
- Inhibition – somatostatin, hyperglycaemia, increased free fatty acids, insulin-like growth factors (IGFs), growth hormone (short loop feedback), progesterone, glucocorticoids, β-adrenergic agonists, and dopamine (DA) antagonists (see Figures 6.4 and 6.5).

Actions of GH

- GH has short-term (acute stress response) actions, which are direct, and long-term indirect (anabolic) actions.
- GH raises plasma glucose by directly stimulating gluconeogenesis in the liver and reducing the uptake of glucose in peripheral tissues. It mobilizes fat and increases circulating free fatty acids by stimulating the action of *hormone sensitive lipase*, a major mobilizer of fat from adipose tissues.
- Long-term anabolic GH actions are mediated through the stimulation of the synthesis and secretion of IGFs and

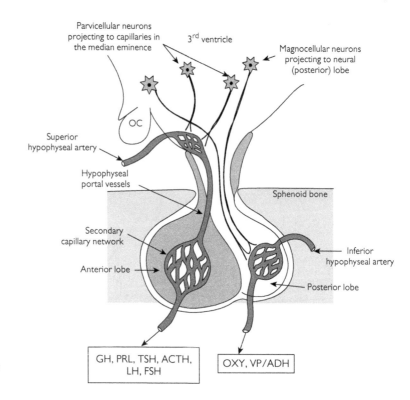

Figure 6.3 Hypothalamo-pituitary connections.

IGF-binding proteins (IGFBPs) from the liver. GH stimulates the uptake of amino acids for protein synthesis and increases lean body mass. IGFs stimulate somatic cell growth with an increase in the size and function of organs and tissues. IGFs have a (long-loop) negative feedback effect on GH secretion.

- IGF-1 is a relatively good index of plasma GH 24-hour secretion because GH itself is released in a pulsatile fashion and IGF-1 has a long half life.

Prolactin

- Unlike all other anterior pituitary hormones, the predominant hypothalamic control of prolactin secretion is inhibitory through dopamine (DA) secreted by neurosecretory cells (Figure 6.4).
- Secretion is stimulated by TRH, although other hypothalamic stimulatory factors have been proposed. Pregnancy, lactation (suckling), oestrogens, opioids, stress, and dopamine antagonists are also stimulatory (Figure 6.5).

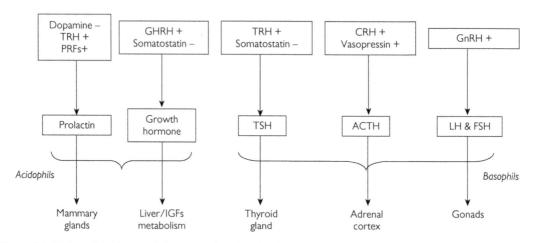

Figure 6.4 The hypothalamic control of secretions from the adenohypophysis.

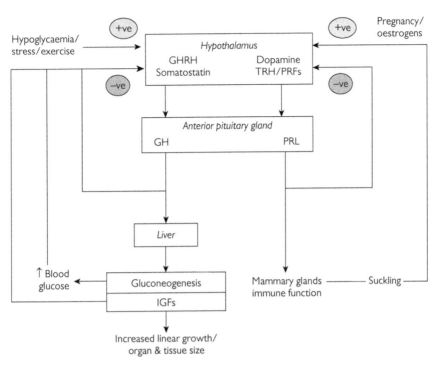

Figure 6.5 Actions of growth hormone (GH) and prolactin (PRL) and the feedback signals regulating their secretion.

- Prolactin is secreted in a pulsatile fashion and the amplitude of pulses increases with the onset of sleep.
- The major function of prolactin is the stimulation of breast development and milk production in females, although males have the same circulating concentrations of prolactin.
- Numerous other functions have been attributed to this hormone including salt and water balance, growth and development, metabolic actions, immunoregulation, and reproductive functions. Excess prolactin may cause infertility due to the inhibitory actions of prolactin on GnRH secretion.

Physiology of lactation

- The growth and development of mammary tissue (alveolar lobules) occurs throughout pregnancy and is stimulated by oestrogen and progesterone. Prolactin, GH, and cortisol must be present in the system for maximal growth.
- During pregnancy, the high concentrations of circulating oestrogens increase prolactin secretion, but along with progesterone block the synthesis of milk. After delivery oestrogen levels fall, withdrawing the blockade on milk synthesis. The numbers of prolactin receptors in mammary tissues increase and milk synthesis begins.
- Suckling is required to maintain milk synthesis and the high prolactin levels. If there is no suckling, prolactin levels fall.

Effects of suckling

Suckling stimulates the nerve endings (neural receptors) in the nipple, which are wired up to the CNS to set up three separate efferent effects:

1. The release of oxytocin from the posterior pituitary, which is delivered to the breast where it causes the contraction of the myoepithelial cell leading to milk ejection.
2. Reduction of the secretion of dopamine from the hypothalamus so that the output of prolactin from the pituitary is maintained and milk synthesis is increased.
3. Reduction of GnRH release leading to reduced output of FSH and LH and suspension of ovarian activity for approximately three months, although this is not universally observed in all women.

Thyroid hormones

Synthesis and secretion

The synthesis and secretion of thyroid hormones is stimulated by the anterior pituitary hormone TSH, and requires two substrates – I$^-$ and thyroglobulin (see Figure 6.6).

- Circulating iodide (I$^-$) is actively taken up by follicular cells through a Na$^+$/I$^-$ symporter. The gland takes up about 125 μg/day against an electrical and concentration gradient and can concentrate I$^-$ up to 30 to 50 times the concentration of the general circulation.

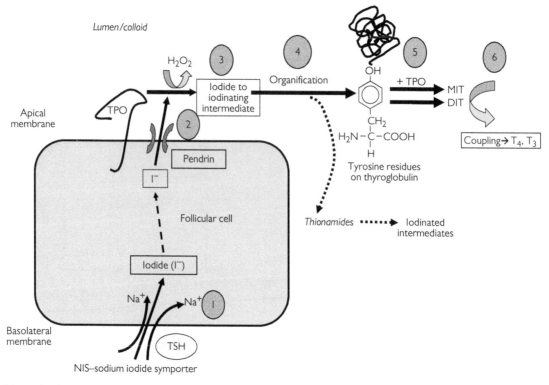

Lumen/colloid

Figure 6.6 Synthesis of thyroid hormones. For details see text. Thioinamides, important anti-thyroid drugs, inhibit organification of tyrosine residues.

- At the follicular colloid interface I^- is oxidized to iodine by H_2O_2, a reaction catalysed by thyroid peroxidise (TPO). The iodine is then incorporated into the tyrosine residues of the large thyroglobulin protein. A tyrosine residue can take up a maximum of two iodine molecules to form di-iodotyrosine (DIT), which is the most common form produced when iodine is readily available, in contrast to mono-iodotyrosine (MIT), which is produced in greater quantities in iodine deficiency states.

- Coupling of two DIT molecules forms thyroxine (T_4), and coupling of one DIT and one MIT forms tri-iodothyronine (T_3). The thyroglobulin with coupled iodinated tyrosine residues is stored in the lumen of the follicle.

- Secretion of thyroid hormones involves pinocytosis of thyroglobulin droplets at the apical surface, release of T_4 and T_3 by lysosomal enzymes, and secretion into the circulation and the basal surface of the follicle cell.

- The thyroid gland secretes approximately 20 T_4 molecules for every T_3 molecule released. However, there is 50 times more T_4 than T_3 in the general circulation because T_4 has a higher affinity for binding proteins, hangs around for much longer, and has a longer half life of six days (compared to only one day for T_3).

- On average approximately 100 µg of T_4 and 10 µg of T_3 are secreted daily. T_4 has little biological activity and about 80% is converted to T_3 in the liver and kidneys, the rest being converted to T_3 in target tissues, e.g. the pituitary gland. Small amounts of T_4 are converted to reverse T_3, which is inactive. Thyroid hormones exist in the circulation mainly bound to thyroid-binding globulin (TBG) with only a small fraction existing in free form and able to enter cells.

Control of secretion

The synthesis and secretion of T_3 and T_4 are controlled by TSH, which is released in response to TRH and inhibited by somatostatin secreted by hypothalamic neurosecretory cells (Figure 6.7). TSH rapidly increases all the steps in the synthesis and degradation of thyroid hormones, and in excess causes hypertrophy of the thyroid cells leading to increased size of the thyroid gland or goitre. Goitre is simply an enlarged thyroid gland and does not correlate with functional status. Although there are 50 T_4 for every T_3 molecule in the circulation, T_3 and T_4 exert equipotent negative feedback effects on the hypothalamic pituitary axis, because when T_4 is taken up by nerve cells or thyrotrophins, it is immediately converted to T_3, the biologically active form of the hormone.

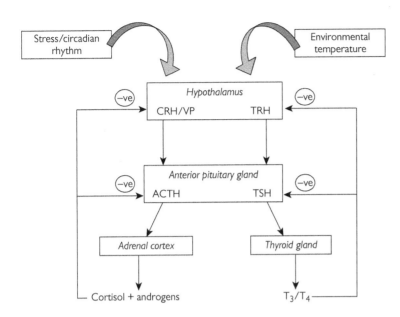

Figure 6.7 Control of the synthesis and secretion of cortisol and thyroid hormones.

Physiologic actions of thyroid hormones

Thyroid hormones act on virtually every cell in the body through nuclear receptors. Their main effects include:

- Stimulation of the basal metabolic rate (BMR) in most tissues (except the brain, spleen, and testis) by increasing the number of mitochondria and stimulating the respiratory chain by increasing membrane Na^+-K^+ ATPase.
- Chronotropic and inotropic effects on the heart, some of which may be mediated by non-genomic events and may involve changes in the number and affinity of β adrenergic receptors.
- Thyroid hormones are absolutely necessary for normal brain development and maturation. Deficiency of thyroid hormones in fetal, neonatal, and early childhood stages of development can result in impaired neuropsychological function and impaired growth. The most severe effects are caused by *in utero* deficiency, which leads to cretinism.
- Fetal growth rate may be normal in the absence of thyroid hormones; however, at birth thyroid hormone replacement must be initiated within 2 weeks to avoid irreversible nervous tissue damage.
- Thyroid hormone is considered a major anabolic hormone and is required for the synthesis and secretion of GH such that if a pre-pubertal individual is hypothyroid, growth, including bone ossification, is retarded.

- Clinical features of hyperthyroidism include heat intolerance, tachycardia, tremor, anxiety, and a warm, moist skin. Features of hypothyroidism include cold intolerance, fatigue, dry, scaly skin, and bradycardia.

Maternal and fetal thyroid function

During pregnancy there is an increased size and vascularity of the thyroid gland. Under the influence of increasing oestrogen during pregnancy, TBG levels increase during the first trimester and remain high until term. Thus, total T_4 and T_3 are increased and there may be a small increase in free T_4 and T_3. The increased glomerular filtration rate in pregnancy results in an increased loss of iodine but there is no reduction in serum iodide unless a woman is iodide deficient.

Fetal thyroid function begins at 10 weeks and this is important since very little maternal thyroid hormone crosses the placenta, although iodine is actively transferred. The secretion of fetal thyroid hormones and TSH reaches a peak at 20–30 weeks' gestation; thereafter TSH secretion declines whilst thyroid hormones continue to rise, although levels are always less than maternal levels. TSH secretion rises within minutes after birth and thyroid hormones consequently rise over the next 24 hours. Hormone levels return to normal adult levels after about 3 days. Neonatal thyroid function, along with phenylketonuria, is screened for in the Guthrie test. TSH concentration in capillary blood depends on the time after birth when the sample was obtained and other factors such as prematurity and illness.

The adrenal gland (steroids and catecholamines)

Embryology and functional anatomy

The fetal adrenal cortex develops from the coelomic meso-derm whilst the adrenal medulla is formed from an adja-cent sympathetic ganglion that is derived from neural crest cells. The fetal cortex engulfs the sympathetic ganglion and the cells differentiate into the secretory cells of the adrenal medulla. More mesodermal cells surround the fetal cortex and these will eventually form the permanent adult adrenal cortex. At birth there is still extensive fetal adrenal cortex but the glomerulosa and fasciculata layers are differentiated. After 1 year the fetal cortex has all but disappeared but the zona reticularis does not differentiate until the end of the third year after birth. The adrenal gland sits on the top of the kidney (ad-renal) and about 80–90% of the adrenal gland mass is comprised of the cortex, with about 10–20% adrenal medulla.

The adrenal cortex produces three major classes of steroids, each secreted from different layers of the cortex (Figure 6.8):

- aldosterone (a mineralocorticoid) from the zona glom-erulosa
- cortisol (a glucocorticoid) from the zona fasciculata
- androgens, mainly dehydroepiandrosterone (DHEA) and its sulphated form (DHEAS) and to a lesser extent androstenedione, from the zona reticularis.

This functional zonation of steroid secretions is, in part, related to steroidogenic enzymes expressed in different lay-ers and blood flow in the gland (from the outer cortex drain-ing inwardly to venules of medulla). The zona fasciculata and reticularis constitute a functional unit controlled by ACTH.

Therefore, ACTH can increase adrenal androgen output but cannot do so in the gonads, which are controlled by LH.

The adrenal medulla secretes adrenaline (80%) and nora-drenaline (20%) from the chromaffin cells.

Synthesis of adrenal steroids and their control

All steroids are derived from cholesterol (Figure 6.9).

- The synthesis and secretion of aldosterone is controlled by angiotensin II and independently by K^+. The sensory inputs and regulation of the renin-angiotensin-aldoster-one system (RAAS) functional unit is discussed in detail in the renal section. Although ACTH causes a transient in-crease in aldosterone secretion this is not an important or significant regulator of aldosterone secretion.

- The synthesis and secretion of cortisol is controlled by ACTH, stimulated by corticotrophin-releasing hormone (CRH) from the hypothalamus. In addition, vasopressin neurosecretory cells that terminate on the hypophyseal portal capillaries can potentiate the action of CRH on the corticotrophs of the anterior pituitary gland.

- ACTH secretion from the corticotrophs is controlled by negative feedback effects of circulating cortisol both at the level of the hypothalamus (CRH and VP) and pitu-itary gland (ACTH). This feedback loop, however, can be overridden by both internal and external factors such as stress (emotional or trauma), which increases ACTH/ cortisol secretion, and the internal 'biological clock', which produces a circadian rhythm of cortisol secretion with peak levels secreted in the early morning, declining to a nadir in the evening (Figure 6.7).

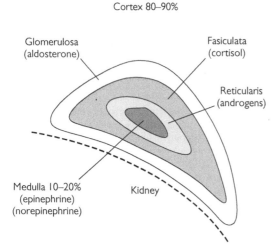

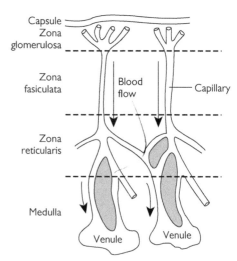

Figure 6.8 Gross anatomy of the adrenal cortex and functional zonation of the gland in relation to the blood supply draining from the capsule of the gland to the adrenal medulla. Reproduced from SS Nussey & SA Whitehead, *Endocrinology, an integrated approach*, Taylor and Francis, with permission. Copyright 2001.

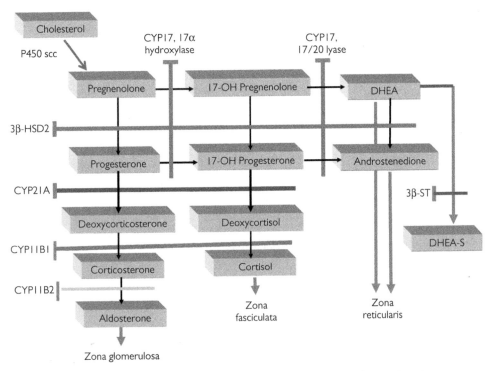

Figure 6.9 Steroid synthesis in the adrenal cortex. CYP, the family of genes coding for specific steroidogenic enzymes; HSD, hydroxysteroid dehydrogenase; ST, steroid sulphatase.

- Once released, cortisol is bound to cortisol-binding globulin (CBG) with a small fraction (<5%) being free to enter target cells and initiate glucocorticoid effects.

The secretion of adrenal androgens is also controlled by ACTH, although these control and feedback effects are less well defined compared with the control of cortisol. However, excess ACTH secretion resulting from a pituitary adenoma (2° Cushing's disease) is associated with excess androgen secretions.

Physiological actions of glucocorticoids (cortisol)

Glucocorticoid receptors are widely distributed in the body. Once activated by steroid binding they initiate transcriptional activity, although there is evidence that glucocorticoids can also initiate non-genomic events (Figure 6.2). The actions of glucocorticoids are diverse and these are summarized in Table 6.1.

- Cortisol is generally a stress hormone like adrenaline, GH, and glucagon. Its overall effect on metabolism is essentially anabolic in the liver and catabolic in muscle and adipose tissue, breaking down stored glycogen and triglycerides to raise circulating levels of blood glucose and fatty acids.
- Cortisol has important permissive actions on glucagon and catecholamines. Glucagon requires cortisol to promote

glycogenolysis in the liver. Without cortisol, fasting hypoglycaemia develops rapidly. Catecholamines promote glycogenolysis, lipolysis, bronchodilatation, and vasoconstriction. Without cortisol blood pressure falls.
- Glucocorticoids also have effects on the brain, bone, cardiovascular system, kidneys, skin, connective issue, and the fetus.
- Excess cortisol secretion (Cushing's syndrome/disease) caused by an endogenous source (e.g. ACTH-secreting pituitary adenoma or adrenal tumour) or by exogenous steroidal anti-inflammatory drugs results in proximal myopathy, bruising, scarring, and purple striae round the abdomen, loss of bone mass, hypertension, and depression.
- Primary adrenocortical deficiency—Addison's disease—causes low systolic blood pressure, weight loss due to reduced appetite, and skin pigmentation due to excess ACTH (reduction of negative feedback), which interacts with melanocortin receptors in the skin.

Maternal adrenocortical function

Total cortisol and its binding globulin increase during pregnancy, as well as an increase in the free fraction of cortisol. ACTH levels also rise during pregnancy and probably cause the pigmentary changes that occur.

Table 6.1 Major biological actions of cortisol

System	Specific target	Physiological function
Metabolism	Liver	Increased glycogen synthesis and gluconeogenesis
	Skeletal muscle	Increased proteolysis, decreased protein synthesis, increased glycogenolysis, decreased GLUT-4 mediated glucose uptake
	Adipose tissue	Increased lipolysis, decreased lipogenesis
Plasma glucose		Fasting state cortisol contributes to maintenance of plasma glucose. In stress, cortisol increases blood glucose at expense of muscle protein. Permissive effect on lipolytic actions of adrenaline and GH in adipose tissue
Cardiovascular system	Heart	Increased contractility
	Blood vessels	Maintenance of vascular tone. Increased vascular reactivity to catecholamines
Kidney		Increases GFR, decreases calcium reabsorption. In excess has mineralocorticoid action (Na^+ retention)
Skin/connective tissue	Fibroblasts	Inhibits proliferation
	Collagen	Inhibits formation
Bone, cartilage		Increases bone resorption, inhibits bone-forming activity of osteoblasts
Immune system	Inflammatory response	Inhibits phospholipase A_2, a key enzyme in prostaglandin, leukotriene, and thromboxane synthesis. Stabilizes lysosomes
	Immune response	Inhibits monocyte proliferation, decreases circulating T lymphocytes
Central nervous system	Psychiatric parameters	Maintains emotional balance, decreases REM sleep, induces hippocampal atrophy
Fetus	Development	Normal development of CNS, retina, skin, GI tract, and lungs
	Lung	Stimulates production of surfactant

Adrenal androgens and congenital adrenal hyperplasia (CAH)

- The effects of adrenal androgens are minimal except in post-menopausal women, where they provide a substrate for peripheral conversion to oestrogens.
- Fetal exposure to excess androgens can cause virilization of females and this occurs in CAH, an autosomal recessive syndrome resulting from defects in enzymes responsible for steroidogenesis in the fetal adrenal gland. The most common form is a defect in 21 hydroxylase (CYP21A2), although defects in 11β-hydroxylase (CYP11B1), 17α-hydroxylase (CYP17), and 3β-hydroxysteroid dehydrogenase (HSD) also occur very rarely. All enzyme deficiencies lead to a deficiency in cortisol and because cortisol is the main feedback signal to ACTH secretion, ACTH increases leading to adrenal hyperplasia and increased adrenal androgen production.
- Deficiency of CYP21A2 inhibits the synthesis of cortisol and aldosterone so that the pregnenolone and progesterone are shunted into the synthesis of androgens (Figure 6.9). Lack of cortisol feedback effects increases fetal ACTH secretion and this further stimulates androgen secretions.
- 11β-Hydroxylase deficiency affects only the adrenal cortical tissues of zona glomerulosa, and fasciculatareticularis. There is reduced aldosterone but the excess amounts of weak mineralocorticoids including deoxycortisone may lead to increased Na^+ and water reabsorption, expanded extracellular fluid compartment, and high blood pressure.
- 17α-Hydroxylase is absent in the zona glomerulosa tissue so its deficiency affects only the zona fasciculatareticularis of the adrenal, the Leydig cells of the testes, and the ovaries, resulting in reduced cortisol, adrenal and testicular androgens, and oestrogens from the ovaries, respectively.

Adrenal medulla—noradrenaline and adrenaline

- Noradrenaline (NA) is synthesized from tyrosine via dihydroxyphenylalanine (DOPA) and dihydroxyphenylethylamine (dopamine).
- NA is widely distributed in tissues associated with sympathetic innervation but the conversion of NA to adrenaline (A) occurs almost exclusively in the adrenal medulla.
- The secretion of NA and A from the adrenal medulla is stimulated by preganglionic sympathetic neurons, which release acetylcholine in response to a variety of stressful stimuli.
- Developmentally, the neural crest cells of the adrenal medulla are the postganglionic neurons that didn't quite differentiate completely into neurons but retained catecholamine secreting capability.
- There are two major classes of adrenoreceptors, α and β, which are further subdivided into $\alpha_{1A, 1B, 2A, and 2B}$ and $\beta_{1, 2, and 3}$.

- The physiological effects of catecholamines on their receptors have been characterized as preparing us for 'fight or flight' and overall they increase heart rate and stroke volume, increase blood pressure, mobilize glucose, and stimulate lipolysis through β adrenoceptors. Blood flow to the splanchnic bed is reduced by vasoconstriction mediated by α adrenoceptors. These same receptors can also cause vasodilatation in muscle.

Hormonal control of calcium and phosphate (parathyroid hormone and vitamin D)

These two hormones are important in maintaining circulating levels of calcium required for bone formation, secretory processes, muscle contraction, enzymic processes, stabilization of membrane potentials, and blood coagulation. Both hormones raise blood calcium levels (Figure 6.10). Calcium is very precisely regulated almost exclusively by PTH, whilst phosphate is primarily auto-regulated by the kidney, although its excretion can be increased by PTH.

- PTH is secreted from the parathyroid glands (four small glands sitting on each pole of the two lobes of the thyroid gland) in response to low levels of free unbound calcium. The only important physiological stimulus regulating the release of PTH is reduced free calcium.
- PTH rapidly stimulates the reabsorption of Ca^{2+} from the distal convoluted tubule (DCT) of the kidney, inhibits phosphate reabsorption from the proximal convoluted tubule (PCT), and increases the exchange of calcium from the interstitial fluid pool surrounding bone, which is saturated with calcium and phosphate.
- In the longer term PTH slowly increases the formation and activity of osteoclasts, the cells that reabsorb bone. This releases calcium and phosphate into the circulation. PTH also increases the formation of $1,25-(OH)_2-D_3$ (the active form of vitamin D) in the PCT.
- Excess PTH (e.g. primary hyperparathyroidism due to a tumour) causes bone resorption, hypercalcaemia, and hypophosphataemia.
- Primary hypoparathyroidism is due to inadequate PTH secretion (usually as a result of thyroid surgery). This results in low plasma calcium, high plasma phosphate, and tetany.
- Secondary hyperparathyroidism is caused by a fall in serum calcium (e.g. in vitamin D deficiency). PTH levels rise leading to excess loss of phosphate in the urine.
- Secondary hypoparathyroidism is caused by an increase in plasma calcium levels (e.g. excessive vitamin D intake). The biochemical profile will show raised plasma calcium, depressed PTH levels, and raised plasma phosphate.
- Vitamin D (cholecalciferol) is mainly synthesized in the skin under the action of UV light or sunlight. It is then transported to the liver where it is hydroxylated to 25-(OH)-vitamin D, the main circulating form, and again in the kidney to 1,25-dihydroxycholcalciferol, the biologically active form of vitamin D (Figure 6.10).

113

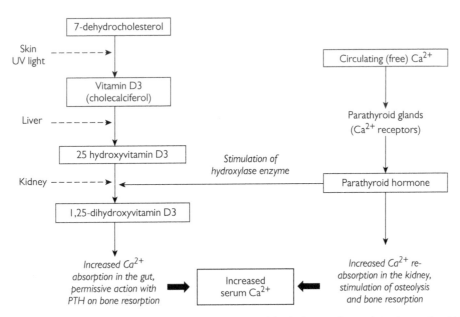

Figure 6.10 Synthesis of vitamin D (cholecalciferol) and the regulation of 'free' calcium in the circulation by parathyroid hormone (PTH) and di-hydroxy cholecalciferol. Cells of the parathyroid gland detect the levels of Ca^{2+} in the circulation by a unique calcium sensing receptor.

- During pregnancy there is an increased synthesis of maternal vitamin D, which helps to meet the increased demands for calcium.
- Its main actions include increased calcium reabsorption from the small intestine, and a permissive effect on the action of PTH on bone. PTH increases the action of the 1α-hydroxylase enzyme in the kidney. Vitamin D deficiency causes hypocalcaemia and osteomalacia (rickets in children).
- At very high levels vitamin D increases bone resorption.

Calcitonin

- Calcitonin is a water-soluble peptide hormone, which is released from the parafollicular C-cells of the thyroid gland.
- The C-cells are independent of the thyroid gland and are indeed of different embryological origin, arriving in the thyroid gland by cell migration.

- The main signal for the secretion of calcitonin is raised free calcium concentration.
- Calcitonin lowers plasma calcium by suppressing the bone resorption activity of osteoclasts.
- It is not a major regulator of calcium homeostasis in humans and Ca^{2+} levels are unaffected in the absence of calcitonin, e.g. after thyroidectomy.

Effect of gravity and weight bearing

- Weight bearing stress increases bone mineralization, and inactivity and absence of weight bearing stress promotes bone demineralization.
- With loss of gravity, plasma calcium and urinary excretion of calcium rise whilst PTH levels fall.
- Excess bone demineralization and remodelling is associated with a rise in serum alkaline phosphatase level, and increased urinary excretion of hydroxyproline (breakdown product of collagen).

Hormones of the hypothalamic-pituitary gonadal axes

The steroid hormones of both the testes and ovaries are controlled by gonadotrophin-releasing hormone (GnRH), which stimulates the release of LH and FSH from the gonadotrophs of the anterior pituitary gland (Figure 6.11). These hormones control steroid synthesis of the testes and ovaries. The major hormones include testosterone secreted by Leydig (interstitial) cells of the testes, and oestradiol and progesterone secreted by developing ovarian follicles and the corpus luteum (Figure 6.11).

The functional cells of the testis are:

1. The seminiferous tubules—comprised of spermatogonia, spermatocytes at various stages of development, and the Sertoli cells, which form tight junctions with each other and form the blood-testis barrier.
2. The Leydig cells, which synthesize and secrete testosterone.

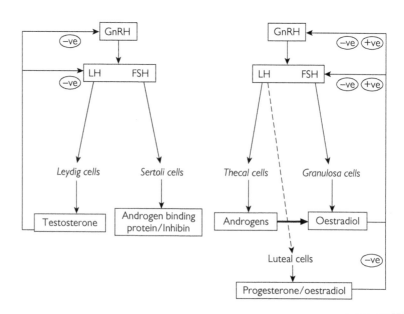

Figure 6.11 Control of hormone secretions in the gonads and their feedback effects on the hypothalmo-pituitary axis. Oestradiol exerts a positive feedback effect at mid-cycle to stimulate the pre-ovulatory surge.

The functional cells of the ovary are:

1. The follicles in the cortex of the gland, which synthesize and secrete mainly oestradiol and progesterone.
2. The corpus luteum, which secretes progesterone and oestradiol and is important in maintaining pregnancy in the first trimester.

Steroid synthesis and development of mature sperm and oocytes are controlled by LH and FSH.

Testicular function

Spermatogonia (46XY) are the precursors of spermatocytes and they divide mitotically to maintain a source of cells for spermatogenesis. Spermatognoia push their way through the tight junctions between adjacent Sertoli cells and undergo two meiotic divisions to become secondary spermatocytes. By a process known as spermiogenesis (loss of cytoplasm, chromatin condensation, formation of a cuff of mitochondria in the mid-piece, and flagellum formation) they become spermatids and then mature sperm. During this entire process, which takes about 9–10 weeks, they are moving towards the lumen of the seminiferous tubule (Figure 6.12).

Spermatogenesis is 'nurtured' by the Sertoli cells, which organize waves of spermatogenesis.

- Sertoli cells synthesize and secrete androgen-binding protein into the seminiferous tubules, which binds up testosterone to about 50-fold the concentration found in plasma. The target cell of FSH in the adult male is the Sertoli cell, which is absolutely essential for sperm development.
- Sertoli cells possess aromatase activity and therefore convert androgens to oestrogens, and also transport sperm into the lumen of the seminiferous tubules and produce inhibin, which exerts a negative feedback effect on FSH secretion at the level of the pituitary gland.
- Normal spermatogenesis requires the synergistic actions of testosterone and FSH on Sertoli cell function.

Testosterone is synthesized and secreted by the Leydig cells in response to LH. Up to 95% of circulating testosterone is derived from the testis, and the rest from peripheral conversion of adrenal androgens.

- Only 2% of circulating testosterone is in the free form; the rest is either bound to albumin (~40%) or SHBG (~60%).
- Under normal conditions, testosterone exerts negative feedback effects on LH secretion (not on FSH) and testosterone is important in the development and maintenance of the reproductive tract.
- Injection of exogenous testosterone (e.g. methyltestosterone) suppresses LH secretion, thus removing the stimulus for testosterone production by the Leydig cells. The Leydig cells undergo atrophy in the long term, and produce less testosterone for the nourishment of the Sertoli cells, which results in diminished sperm production. A very high level of methyltestosterone also exerts a modest negative feedback on FSH levels.

- The actions of testosterone on the penis, scrotum, and prostate and other peripheral tissues are dependent on its conversion to the more active form dihydrotestosterone (DHT) by the enzyme 5α-reductase in target cells.
- Testosterone is mainly metabolized to androsterone and etiocholanolone, and excreted as water-soluble glucuronides and to a lesser extent sulphates. DHT is excreted as 3α- and β-androstanediols.

Ovarian function

The maximum complement of primordial follicles in the ovary is achieved at 20 weeks' gestation when it is approximately 7 million, and decreases progressively from this point such that at birth each ovary contains about 2 million primordial follicles and 300 000 by menarche. Primordial follicles consist of a single oocyte halfway through its first meiotic division and surrounded by a flattened layer of granulosa cells.

Folliculogenesis

- Cohorts of follicles begin to develop into primary and then secondary follicles. The oocyte enlarges, becomes surrounded by the zona pellucida, granluosa cells divide forming several layers, and fibroblasts of the ovarian stromal cells differentiate into the inner thecal cells.
- This process is considered to be independent of gonadotophins, although there is increasing evidence that this initial growth is dependent on hormones and growth factors.
- The initiation of follicular growth to a preantral follicle (~0.2 mm) takes place over well in excess of 120 days. Further, and final, maturation takes about 65 days, and over two menstrual cycles cohorts of preantral follicles and antral follicles and the oocyte become surrounded by the cumulus oophorous.
- They become recruitable follicles and during the luteal phase of the second menstrual cycle follicles that have not undergone atresia may be 'selected' for further development.
- Over a period of 5 days, only one of these follicles is selected and becomes the dominant follicle. Then, over 10 days, this grows from about 2 mm to 20 mm, secreting increasing amounts of oestradiol and becoming a mature Graafian follicle.
- The later stages of follicular development (preantral to dominant) are controlled by gonadotrophins, particularly FSH, and throughout this process there is continued follicular atresia.

Endocrinology of the menstrual cycle
Follicular phase

- This begins with the first day of menstruation and is associated with a rise in FSH secretion that stimulates the growth and differentiation of cohorts of preantral and antral follicles. As a result oestrogen synthesis and

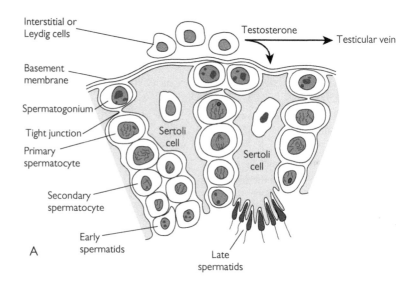

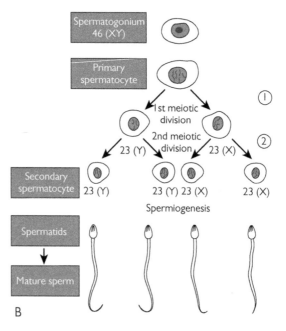

Figure 6.12 Cross-section of a seminiferous tubule (A) and the process of spermatogenesis (B). Reproduced from SS Nussey & SA Whitehead, *Endocrinology, an integrated approach*, Taylor and Francis, with permission. Copyright 2001.

secretion rises, reaching a peak at mid-cycle, whilst LH and FSH secretions decline (negative feedback) (Figure 6.13).

- When oestrogen levels reach a peak concentration (>750 pmol/l) sustained for 24–48 h, oestrogen no longer provides negative feedback but switches to a positive feedback effect on GnRH/gonadotrophin secretion, resulting in a pre-ovulatory surge of LH and a smaller surge of FSH (Figure 6.13). This induces completion of the first meiotic division of the oocyte (to give a mature oocyte and polar body) and initiation of the second meiotic division.

Ovulation occurs 9–12 hours after the LH surge. Only the LH surge is required for ovulation.

- The circulating oestrogen stimulates the female sex accessories.

Luteal phase

- The granulosa and thecal cells of the empty follicle rapidly proliferate and form the corpus luteum. The corpus luteum synthesizes progesterone and to a lesser extent oestradiol (Figure 6.13).

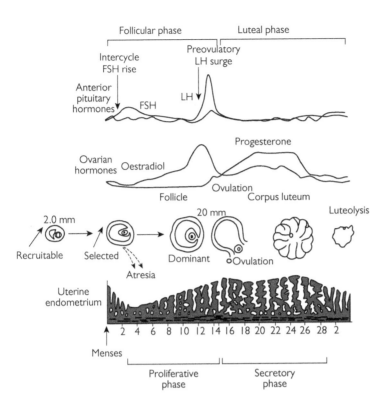

Figure 6.13 Hormonal profile during a typical menstrual cycle in relation to final stages of folliculogenesis, ovulation, formation of the corpus luteum, and changes in the endometrium.

- During the luteal phase, progesterone provides the major feedback to LH secretion.
- Small amounts of gonadotrophins, particularly LH, are required to maintain the secretory activity of the corpus luteum but, in the absence of conception, the corpus luteum undergoes luteolysis (a process not well defined but believed to be apoptotic) about 14 days after ovulation.
- The loss of negative feedback from oestradiol and progesterone induces the intercycle rise in FSH secretion and another cycle begins.
- If conception occurs the corpus luteum does not undergo luteolysis but is maintained by human chorionic gonadotrophin (HCG) secreted by the developing placenta.

Endometrial changes during the menstrual cycle

- **Proliferative phase:** Oestradiol increases the rate of mitotic division of endometrial glandular cells leading to proliferation (Figure 6.13).
- **The secretory phase:** Under the action of oestradiol and progesterone further proliferation and secretory activity occur during the luteal phase.

Ovarian steroidogenesis

- Progesterone and androgen production in thecal cells is stimulated by LH.
- The androgens diffuse across the basement membrane into the granulosa cell layer where, under the influence of FSH, the androgens are converted to oestrogens under the action of aromatase.
- Just prior to ovulation, granulosa cells develop LH receptors and can respond to the pre-ovulatory surge of LH. Steroid secretions of the corpus luteum are mainly stimulated by LH.
- Oestradiol and progesterone are transported in the circulation bound to sex hormone-binding globulin (SHBG) and albumin, with progesterone having a low affinity for SHBG but a higher affinity for cortisol-binding globulin. About 2% of these hormones exist in free form in the circulation.
- Because oestradiol and progesterone are lipid-soluble and bound to plasma proteins, they cannot be easily filtered or excreted by the kidneys. Oestradiol is excreted as a conjugate but is mostly converted to oestrone and oestriol.
- Progesterone is metabolized to pregnanediol and oestradiol to estrone and then oestriol or catecholoestrogens in the liver. This is then conjugated with glucuronide or sulphate prior to excretion in the urine.

Endocrinology of pregnancy

Throughout pregnancy the fetoplacental unit secretes hormones into the maternal bloodstream and these alter the function of all maternal endocrine glands (Figure 6.14).

The placenta can synthesize and secrete proteins but cannot synthesize steroids de novo and therefore requires steroid precursors of fetal or maternal origin.

The following maternal serum hormone changes occur during pregnancy:

- Placental proteins: HCG peaks at 10 weeks and decreases to a lower plateau. Human placental lactogen (hPL) rises with placental weight, coinciding with the period of maximal fetal growth. It induces insulin resistance and has been used as an index of placental wellbeing.
- Oestrogens are synthesized in the placenta from DHEA (a weak androgen) produced by the fetus, and oestradiol,

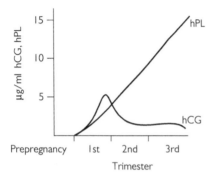

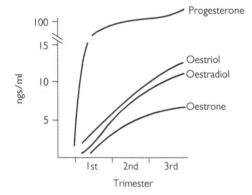

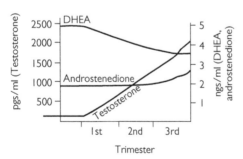

Figure 6.14 Hormonal changes during the three trimesters of pregnancy. hCG, human chorionic gonadotrophin; hPL, human placental lactogen; DHEA, dehydroepiandrosterone.

oestriol, and oestrone steadily increase to term. The high oestrogen output drives an increase in the expression of oxytocin receptors in the myometrium as pregnancy progresses.

- Androgens are derived from the fetoplacental unit and testosterone levels rise 10-fold compared to prepregnancy levels, DHEA falls, and there is a small rise in androstenedione.
- Progesterone is synthesized mainly by the corpus luteum in the first 2–3 months of pregnancy, and by the placenta afterwards. Placental production of progesterone depends on the availability of substrates (maternal cholesterol) and the size of the placenta, and appears to be uncontrolled. Progesterone rises steadily until term. 17-hydroxyprogesterone peaks at 5 weeks and then declines.
- Pituitary hormones: LH and FSH secretions decline, while prolactin rises to term.
- Thyroid hormones: Total T_4 and T_3 rise during the first trimester, then plateau. TBG increases so free T_4 and T_3 are unchanged.
- Adrenal steroids: Cortisol increases steadily to three times prepregnancy values and aldosterone plateaus at 34 weeks.

Fetal pituitary gland

- This secretes ACTH, which stimulates the fetal adrenal glands to secrete large quantities of very weak and water-soluble androgens.
- They pass to the liver where their structures are modified before they are delivered to the placenta. Here placental aromatase converts them to oestriol, the main oestrogen produced in the last 6 months of pregnancy.
- Oestriol and progesterone exert the massive increase in the myometrial mass, and all the uterine glands and stromal elements.

Hormonal changes in puberty

The endocrinology of puberty consists of two phases:

1. Adrenarche: the rise in adrenal androgens between the ages of about 6–8 years.
2. Gonadarche: activation of gonadal sex steroid production occurring several years later.
   - The onset of puberty is characterized by an increase in frequency and amplitude of GnRH pulses, which stimulates LH and FSH secretion and hence gonadal steroidogenesis.
   - Several theories have been put forward to account for the increased GnRH pulsatility and these include a relative reduction of melatonin secretion and attainment of adequate body fat. Adipose tissue secretes hormones, including leptin, and leptin appears to play a permissive role in puberty. Kisspeptin, released from hypothalamic neurons, stimulates GPR54 receptors on GnRH neurosecretory cells and increases GnRH secretion. Both leptin and kisspeptin are essential for puberty and attainment of fertility.

Hormone changes in the menopause

Menopause is defined as the cessation of menstruation because the ovary no longer contains follicles responsive to FSH. It results in an oestrogen and progesterone-deficient state with an increase in the secretion of LH and FSH. The decline of oestrogens during the perimenopause is associated with vasomotor symptoms in the short term, including hot flushes, night sweats, vaginal dryness, and depressive episodes. Longer-term effects in the post-menopause include osteoporosis, increased incidence of cardiovascular disease, and changes in lipid metabolism and profile.

Pineal gland

- Situated between the two cerebral hemispheres, the pineal gland secretes melatonin during the dark phase of the light/dark cycle.

- It receives an input from the suprachiasmatic nucleus (SCN) via the superior cervical ganglion. The SCN itself receives a direct input from the retina and is thought to be responsible for driving numerous physiological functions that show a daily rhythm, including the circadian rhythm of ACTH/cortisol secretion and melatonin.

- Melatonin is synthesized from tryptophan and melatonin treatment in humans reduces GH and LH secretion. It may be used beneficially to improve sleep patterns and can be used to treat sleep disturbances associated with jet lag.

ADDITIONAL FACTS AND REVISION MATERIAL

Hypothalamic-pituitary hormones

- Usually released in pulses to prevent down-regulation of the end organ receptors.

Steroid and thyroid hormones

- Cortisol increases blood glucose by inhibiting peripheral glucose uptake and increasing hepatic gluconeogenesis. Cortisol is catabolic to muscles and therefore delivers the resultant amino acids to the liver for gluconeogenesis. Cortisol does not break down liver glycogen.

- Glucagon requires cortisol to work and if cortisol is absent, fasting hypoglycaemia develops rapidly. Cortisol is also required for the vasoconstrictive actions of catecholamines and if absent (as in Addison's disease) hypotension develops.

- Steroid and thyroid hormones are transported in plasma attached to carrier proteins, except for adrenal androgens, which are conjugated with sulphate moieties in the liver. This renders them water-soluble such that they can be transported dissolved in plasma.

Extragonadal effects of androgens during puberty

- Androgens increase GH secretion, which in turn increases IGF-1.

- IGF-1 stimulates cell division in cartilage and epiphyseal plates of long bones.

- Testosterone in males (and adrenal androgens in females) exerts the mineralization of the epiphyseal plates of the long bones at the end of puberty.

- Androgens therefore initiate and terminate the growth spurt. Oestrogens can also cause plate closure.

- Administration of testosterone in puberty may lead to a short stature and conversely excessive growth during puberty may be terminated by testosterone administration.

Miscellaneous

- Recall that Sertoli cells possess aromatase activity, therefore Sertoli cell tumours are associated with elevated oestrogens.

CHAPTER 7

General and Systemic Pathology

General pathology

Cellular injury

Cellular injury involves the disruption and failure of critical cellular functions, which if persistent may lead to cell death. Cellular injury may be reversible or irreversible. The cell may respond by adaptation or death, depending on the type, duration, and severity of the injury, and also on the cell type and its metabolic state.

Causes of cellular injury

1. Hypoxia: With oxygen deprivation there is reduced or absent ATP production leading to the failure of Na⁺-K⁺ pumps, protein production, and anaerobic metabolism, in which glycolysis is the only source of ATP and is associated with high production of lactate. Hypoxia may be caused by ischaemia, cardiopulmonary failure, or anaemia.
2. Infection: Micro-organisms can damage cells directly, or via their toxins, or as a result of host response.
3. Immunologic damage
4. Genetic diseases
5. Physical injury (burns or trauma)
6. Chemical injuries
7. Nutritional injury: Examples of nutritional injury include marasmus (total deficiency of calories) and kwashiokor, which is selective protein deficiency.

Mechanism of cellular injury

- Reduced ATP production leads to failure of critical cell functions including the Na⁺-K⁺ pump with loss of membrane integrity, increased membrane permeability, and influx of calcium ions. Calcium is a secondary messenger that activates a spectrum of intracellular enzymes including lipases, proteases, ATPases, and endonucleases, which break down cellular components.
- Mitochondrial dysfunction from the formation of non-selective mitochondrial permeability transition (MPT) channels within the inner membrane of the mitochondria results in the loss of electron gradient, which is important for electrical transport chains.
- Oxygen-derived free radicals break down strands of DNA.

Important cellular systems susceptible to cellular injury

1. Cell membrane and its barrier function
2. ATP production from mitochondrial damage
3. Genome—DNA disruption
4. Protein synthesis

Reversible changes following cell injury

- With reduced ATP production, Na⁺-K⁺ ATPase shuts down, K⁺ rushes out of the cell, and Na⁺ rushes in accompanied by water. This leads to cellular oedema, swelling of the endoplasmic reticulum, formation of membrane blebs, and loss of specialized cell structures such as the microvilli.
- Reduced ATP production leads to the detachment of ribosomes from the endoplasmic reticulum and reduced protein synthesis.
- There is a switch from aerobic to anaerobic metabolism for cellular energy. Glycogen is used up in fuelling glycolysis with resultant lactate production and a fall in pH as lactic acid accumulates, with adverse effects for cellular enzyme function.

Irreversible changes following cell injury

- Membrane damage and the resultant calcium influx, which activates all intracellular enzymes including lactate dehydrogenase, troponins, and creatinine phosphokinase (all of which may leak out of the cell following a myocardial infarction), or aspartate and alanine transaminases (AST, ALT), which may also leak out of hepatocytes from cell death and oedema during hepatitis B virus infection.
- Marked mitochondrial dysfunction suggested by mitochondrial swelling or increased density, loss of ATP production, and the formation of mitochondrial permeability transition channels.
- Lysosomal rupture with release of lysosomal enzymes and autolysis.
- Nuclear death suggested by pyknosis and karyorrhexis.

Cellular death

There are two mechanisms of cell death:

1. necrosis
2. apoptosis.

Necrosis

- Coagulative necrosis—usually due to protein denaturation but with the shape of the organ maintained by the proteins sticking together, although the nuclei and other organelles are disrupted, dislocated, and dead.
- Liquefactive necrosis—due to the action of tissue digestive enzymes, classically seen in the brain and the pancreas.
- Caseous necrosis—features are between coagulative and liquefactive necrosis. The organ is semi-solid and semi-liquid with granulomas, multi-nucleated giant Langerhans cells, and epitheloid cells evident under the microscope.
- Fat necrosis—caused by the action of lipases and seen in the breast, pancreas, omentum, and skin. It has a chalky white appearance. When fat cells die, they liberate negatively-charged free fatty acids from triglycerides, which attract positive calcium ions leading to calcium deposition in fat or saponification.
- Fibrinoid necrosis, which appears pink on hematoxylin and eosin (H & E) staining due to protein deposition.
- Gangrenous necrosis—a gross descriptive term for dead, necrotic, jet-black tissue. There are two forms of gangrenous necrosis:
  1. wet gangrene where the tissues are undergoing liquefying necrosis
  2. dry gangrene (coagulative necrosis).

Apoptosis

- This is programmed cell death, which usually affects single cells or a small group of cells, in contrast to necrosis, which affects many different cells. Apoptosis is executed by a cascade of enzymes, known CASPASE.
- The nucleus is pyknotic, the cell cytoplasm is shrunken and becomes more pink, and fragments of apoptotic (dead) cells are phagocytosed by adjacent macrophages and epithelial cells.
- Characteristically there is no inflammation, unlike necrosis.
- Stimuli for apoptosis include cell injury and DNA damage, which result in p53 gene expression; this prevents damaged cells from entering the cell cycle. Other stimuli for apoptosis include hormone or growth factor deficiency, death signals from T cells, and tumour necrosis factor (TNF) binding to TNF receptor-1.
- Anti-apoptotic genes include the bcl-2 gene, which immortalizes cells such as cancer cells.
- Physiologic examples of apoptosis include the removal of tails and webs for formation of fingers during embryogenesis, corpus luteolysis and the menstrual cycle, and breast involution post-lactation.

Cellular adaptation

In general cellular adaptation follows a prolonged and persistent cellular stress. All forms of cellular adaption are potentially reversible if the stress is removed, although some forms of adaptation are premalignant.

- Hypertrophy—there is an increase in cellular organelles and structural proteins, often secondary to increased demands on the organ.
- Atrophy—the cell decreases in size and functional ability due to a reduced blood supply, nutrition, hormone stimulation, or aging.
- Hyperplasia—there is an increased number of cells (for example endometrial hyperplasia, ductal atypical hyperplasia of the breast, and benign prostatic hypertrophy, which is more of a hyperplasia than hypertrophy).
- Metaplasia—a change from one cell type to another, e.g. from columnar epithelium to squamous epithelium in the bronchus, and the transition from squamous epithelium of the oesophagus to columnar cell type (so-called Barrett's epithelium due to reflux disease). This is a premalignant state.
- Dysplasia—the sequence of changes leading to neoplasia; the cells are disorganized but not malignant, e.g. dysplastic cervical cells.

Other types of cellular injury

- Accumulation of products such as: proteins, e.g. in the proximal convoluted tubule (hyaline droplets) or plasma cells (Russell bodies); fat or lipids leading to atherosclerotic plaques; and pigments deposited in the brain, heart, or liver, e.g. hemosiderin (accumulation of iron), hemosiderosis (iron accumulation and overload present within the Kuppfer cells and macrophages), and hemochromatosis (organ damage from hemosiderosis).
- Hyaline disease—accumulation of pink protein material on H & E stain.
- Calcification could be dystrophic, that is calcium deposition in dead or dying tissue, or metastatic, which usually occurs in areas of high blood flow such as the kidneys and the lungs.

Inflammation

Acute inflammation

This is the immediate response of the body to any form of injury. It is of short duration and is characterized by the cardinal signs of redness (rubor), pain (dolor), heat (calor), swelling (tumour), and loss of function. There are three main aspects of acute inflammation:

1. haemodynamic changes
2. cellular (inflammatory cells) response
3. chemical mediators.

1. Haemodynamic changes

There is an initial transient vasoconstriction, which is followed by a massive vasodilatation (mediated by histamine, bradykinin, and some prostaglandins). The vasodilatation is associated with increased vascular permeability (mediated by histamine, bradykinin, serotonin, and leukotrienes), resulting in the leakage of proteins, immunoglobulins, and polymorphs. The intravascular fluid becomes more concentrated and slows down, allowing the inflammatory cells (polymorphs) to marginate and leave the blood vessel.

2. Cellular response

- During inflammation, soluble mediators initiate cellular activation of leukocytes and endothelial cells, whereas adhesion molecules allow the interaction of leukocytes with the vessel wall and all subsequent adhesive interactions that are required for emigration into the tissue (Figure 7.1).
- Polymorphs contain a large number of digestive enzymes for killing micro-organisms, including myeloperoxidases, which are oxygen-dependent killing enzymes. They are bactericidal by increasing the permeability of bacterial membranes. There are also secondary granules including phospholipases, lysosomes, collagenases, and lactoferrin, which bind iron and thus deny the bacteria iron. Polymorphs appear first followed by macrophages.

Steps in neutrophil migration

1. Release of pro-inflammatory mediators, e.g. by tissue macrophages.
2. Expression of adhesion molecules and secretion of pro-inflammatory mediators by the endothelial cell.
3. The neutrophils marginate and adhere to the vessel wall with the aid of adhesion molecules including selectins (expressed by the endothelial cells as E-selectin and L-selectin on the leukocytes; selectin is also expressed on platelets as P-selectin). Other adhesion molecules include integrins, which mediate the firm adhesion of leukocytes by binding members of the immunoglobulin family of adhesion molecules expressed on endothelial cells. The most important adhesion molecules that serve as ligands for the integrins during leukocyte-endothelial cell interactions are the intercellular adhesion molecules ICAM-1 (expressed on the surface of inflamed endothelium recruiting leukocytes to sites of inflammation), ICAM-2 (constitutively expressed on endothelial cells but unaffected by inflammatory mediators), ICAM-3 (which binds LFA-1 and mediates leukocyte interactions; it is highly expressed on leukocytes but absent on endothelial cells), and vascular cell adhesion molecule (VCAM-1), which is expressed primarily on endothelial cells, up-regulated by inflammatory mediators, and plays a role in mediating leukocyte-endothelial interactions.
4. Capture
5. Rolling
6. Activation and adhesion
7. Spreading
8. Diapedesis
9. Migration

10. Ingestion of foreign particles, bacteria, etc.
11. Apoptosis of the polymorphs
12. Elimination of the polymorphs by phagocytosis.

Histamine up-regulates the expression of E-selectin on the endothelial cell. IL-1 and TNF up-regulate E-selectin, ICAM, and VCAM.

Neutrophil molecules are up-regulated by chemotactic factors.

Disorders of the inflammatory steps

1. Cellular adhesions may be impaired by diabetes mellitus, steroid administration, acute alcohol intoxication, leukocyte adhesions defect (an autosomal recessive disorder), and integrin subunit deficiency, which leads to recurrent bacterial infections.
2. Emigration with pseudopods, which go through endothelial cells to the basement membrane where they release enzymes such as collagenases to facilitate passage.
3. Chemotaxis: Polymorphs always follow a chemotactic trail including bacterial products containing N-formyl methionine at the end, leukotriene B4 molecules, C5a complement, and Il-8 produced by macrophages.
4. Phagocytosis and degranulation aided by opsonization: Any of the three major opsonins, Fc portion of IgG, C3b, and mannose-binding protein, may have defects.
5. Phagolysosomes for intracellular killing due to respiratory bursts including oxygen-free radicals and hydrogen peroxide.

Diseases associated with inflammatory steps

1. *Chronic granulomatous disease of childhood:*
   - an autosomal recessive or X-linked condition
   - there is a deficiency of NADPH oxidase
   - there is no respiratory burst, no superoxide, and no hydrogen peroxide (H_2O_2), so there is no killing of catalase-positive organisms such as *Staph. aureus* and salmonella
   - therefore there are recurrent bacterial infections.
2. *Myeloperoxidase deficiency*
   - an autosomal recessive disorder
   - causes recurrent usually candidal infection.

Chemical mediators of inflammation

Vasoactive amines

- Histamine and serotonin, which are produced by various cells such as basophils, platelets, and mass cells.
- They cause vasodilatation and increased vascular permeability.
- They are triggers for the release of IgE mediating disease, physical injury, and anaphylaxis.
- Serotonin from platelets increases vasodilatation and vascular permeability.

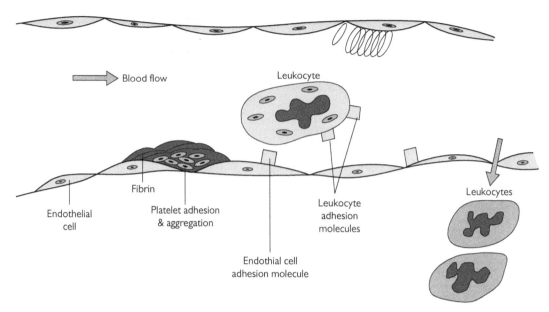

Figure 7.1 Cellular response in inflammation. Neutrophil margination brings these inflammatory cells into contact with the endothelium. They line the endothelium in a tightly packed formation (pavement) mediated by adhesion molecules activated by inflammatory mediators released by other cells, including platelets, red blood cells, and other leukocytes.

The kinin system

- The end product of bradykinin is formed by factor XII, which activates pre-kallikrein, which cleaves kininogen.
- Bradykinin mediates pain and increases vascular permeability.

Arachidonic acid pathway and products of the cyclo-oxygenase pathway

- Thromboxane released by platelets causes vasoconstriction and platelet aggregation.
- Prostacyclins released by endothelial cells cause vasodilatation and inhibit platelet aggregation.
- Prostaglandin E_2 mediates pain and fever and keeps the ductus arteriosus patent *in utero*.
- Lipoxygenase pathway; leukotriene B4 is chemotactic for neutrophils. Leukotrienes C4, D4, and E4 are vasodilators and increase vascular permeability.

Complement system

- Membrane attack complex C5b–C9, which punch holes in bacteria.
- C3b is an opsonin.
- C5a is a neutrophil chemotactic factor.
- C3a and C5a are anaphylactic toxins and stimulate the release of histamine.

Cytokines

- IL-1 and TNF exert a broad range of effects including fever, enhancement of adhesion molecules, increase of acute phase reactants, and stimulation of other cells: endothelium, neutrophils, and fibroblasts.

Outcomes of acute inflammation

1. Resolution and regeneration of normal tissue.
2. Resolution and tissue destruction leading to healing and scarring.
3. Persistence of the bacteria with abscess formation such that there is ongoing acute inflammation and the walling off of that area by the body.
4. Chronic inflammation.

Chronic inflammation

Causes

1. Recurrent bouts of acute inflammation
2. Persistent infection
3. Infection with mycobacterium, fungi, viruses, and parasites
4. Response to foreign bodies or tumours
5. Autoimmune disease

Important cellular mediators of chronic inflammation

These include macrophages, lymphocytes, eosinophils, and basophils.

Macrophages

- Come from the bone marrow and travel within the bloodstream as monocytes.

- Settle in tissues and become tissue macrophages where they are given different names depending on the tissue or organ in which they are found, e.g. Kupffer cells in the liver and microglia in the brain.
- Produce a wide spectrum of cytokines that contribute to granuloma formation.

Lymphocytes

- Include B and T helper and suppressor cells.
- They release lymphotoxins, a chemotactic factor.

Eosinophils

- Have an important role in parasitic infections and allergies.
- They contain important major toxins for killing parasites.
- They are attracted by eotoxins.

Basophils (or mast cells)

- Positioned around blood vessels especially in the skin and lungs.
- They are important in IgE-mediated reactions.

Chronic granulomatous inflammation

- A collection of modified macrophages or epitheliod cells.
- Contain giant cells, which are multi-nucleated cells with a rim of lymphocytes and plasma cells.
- The presence of caseation suggests TB.
- Typical examples of chronic granulomatous diseases include TB, leprosy, syphilis, cat scratch fever, viral and fungal infections, foreign bodies, sarcoidosis, and Crohn's disease.

Host response to organisms

Although there are hundreds of thousands of organisms that can infect the body, the body has only five ways of responding to these organisms, namely:

1. Exudative inflammation: Response to bacterial infection characterized by exudate—inflammatory fluid dominated by proteins and inflammatory cells, especially polymorphs. Commonly seen in bacterial pneumonia and meningitis.
2. Necrotizing inflammation: Caused by a very virulent organism, which causes far more tissue destruction and death than just the inflammation or response to it.
3. Granulomatous inflammation: Response to slow-growing organism, for example tuberculosis.
4. Interstitial inflammation: Response to viruses, for example viral myocarditis.
5. Cytopathic inflammation:
   - affected cell is altered in some demonstrable way under the microscope

- common with viruses and may be evident as viral inclusions
- examples include rabies, CMV inclusions within the nucleus, and herpes.

Wound healing and repair

a. Regeneration

The damaged tissue is replaced with cells of the same type, depending on the cell type injured. These cells can be classified into:

1. *Labile cells*—epithelial cells of the skin, bowel epithelium—cells with the ability to proliferate throughout life.
2. *Stabile cells*—low level replication capacity over time, e.g. liver may regenerate slowly after resection.
3. *Permanent cells*—cells with limited ability to replicate, for example cardiac myocyte and neurons.

b. Tissue repair

The tissue architecture is destroyed and the tissue is replaced with scar (granulation tissue). Granulation tissue contains fibroblasts, which are synthetically active and lay down type 3 collagen initially and subsequently type 1 collagen, which is strong collagen. Wounds healed by secondary intention may contract down because of myofibroblasts. The granular red appearance of granulation tissue is because of capillaries.

c. Aberrations in wound healing

Delay in wound healing may be caused by:

1. infection
2. foreign body
3. diabetes mellitus
4. vitamin deficiency
5. ischaemia.

d. Excessive wound healing

1. *Hypertrophic scar:*
   - Excessive production of granulation tissue leading to a protuberant and raised scar.
   - This is a genetically determined event.
2. *Keloid:*
   - Also has genetic predisposition.
   - Commoner in the earlobes, face, neck, and forearms.
   - The scar is made up of pink bundles of type 3 collagen.
   - Normal wound starts with type 3 and matures to type 1 collagen over time.
   - In keloids the type 3 collagen remains indefinitely.

Types of collagen

1. Type 1 is the most common, has the highest tensile strength, and is found everywhere in the body including bones, skin, tendons, and in most organs.

2. Type 2 collagen is found in cartilage and vitreous humour only.
3. Type 3 is found in granulation tissue, embryonic tissue, the uterus, and in keloids.
4. Type 4 collagen is found in basement membranes.

Pathology of circulation

Oedema

This is defined as excessive fluid in the intercellular or interstitial space.

Causes

1. *Increased hydrostatic pressures*, e.g. congestive cardiac failure (CCF), portal hypertension, renal problems, and venous thrombosis.
2. *Decreased colloid osmotic pressure*, e.g. liver disease, nephrotic syndrome, and kwashiorkor.
3. *Lymphatic obstruction*, e.g. following surgery.
4. *Increased vascular permeability* from drugs or chemicals, e.g. bleomycin hyaline damage of the lung epithelium.

Related terminologies

- *Anasarca*—generalized total body oedema
- *Effusion*—fluid in body cavities, e.g. peritoneal, pleural, or pericardial
- *Transudate*—oedema fluid of low protein content, specific gravity <1.02.
- *Exudate*—oedema fluid with a high protein content and polymorphs, specific gravity >1.02. It is described as fibrinous exudate or eosinophilic exudate, depending on what constitutes the exudate.
- *Hyperaemia*—this is an active process of vasodilatation (e.g. in blushing) due to neurogenic factors and histamine.
- *Congestion*—a passive process, e.g. CCF.

Haemostasis

The goal of haemostasis is to form a fibrin platelet plug to stop bleeding. Three key factors are required to achieve this, namely: vascular wall, platelets, and the coagulation cascade.

Vascular wall

- Vascular injury elicits transient vasoconstriction mediated by the endothelium, resulting in blood flow changes with turbulence and stasis, which are factors that favour fibrin clot formation.
- Then there is release of tissue factors from the injured cells, activating the extrinsic coagulation pathway.
- Exposure of the subendothelial collagen, which is highly thrombogenic, stimulates/activates the intrinsic coagulation pathway. Endothelial release of von Willebrand factor (vWF) aids platelet aggregation.

Platelets

- Made in the bone marrow and carried in the bloodstream to the injury site.
- At the injury site platelets adhere to the vascular wall collagen with the aid of vWF.
- Platelets cannot adhere directly to collagen, so the vWF does the adherence and the platelets adhere to the vWF via a receptor, glycoprotein-1b (GP1b).
- Platelet activation follows, with a change in shape and degranulation.
- ADP released with activation and degranulation of platelets recruits more platelets to add to the clot through GP2b3a.
- A defect in GP2b3a leads to Glanzmann thromboaesthenia.
- Platelet disorders will present with bruising, ecchymosis, petechial haemorrhages including nose bleeds, and heavy periods.
- Investigations would include platelet count and bleeding time tests, which detects qualitative platelet problems.

Immune thrombocytopenic purpura (ITP)

- Autoantibodies produced against own platelets, which coat the platelets.
- The IgG-coated platelets are destroyed in the spleen leading to thrombocytopenia.
- Two forms of ITP are recognized:
  1. *Acute form*, usually a self-limiting illness seen in children after a viral illness.
  2. *Chronic form*, usually in women of reproductive age and commonly associated with lupus. May present with nose bleeds, menorrhagia, and ecchymosis.
- Findings include thrombocytopenia, prolonged bleeding time, normal coagulation tests, reduced platelets on peripheral film, large mega-thrombocytes, and proliferating megakaryocytes on bone marrow biopsy.
- Treatment includes immunoglobulin (this floods the Fc receptors in the spleen and prevents platelet phagocytosis), steroids (reduce antibody production), and splenectomy.

Thrombotic thrombocytopenic purpura (TTP)

- Due to generalized and widespread platelet thrombi formation (not true thrombi but fibrin and platelets stuck together).
- Characteristically there is no activation of the coagulation system.
- Usually affects adult females.
- There is a clinical pentad of fever, thrombocytopenia, microangiopathic haemolytic anaemia, neurological symptoms, and renal failure.
- Lab findings include thrombocytopenia, prolonged bleeding time, normal coagulation (PT and PTT) test, fragmented red blood cells, and schistocytes on blood film.

Haemolytic uraemic syndrome (HUS)

- On the opposite end of the disease spectrum to TTP.
- The same pentad of signs and symptoms is involved.
- TTP has more neurologic symptoms; HUS has more renal problems.
- TTP is usually found in adults, HUS usually in children, and they are associated with bloody diarrhoea after infection from *E. coli*, 0157H$_7$.

Coagulopathies

- Most clotting factors are produced by the liver, except factor VIII (FVIII).
- They circulate as pro-enzymes and need conversion or activation with calcium.
- Intrinsic pathway requires activation by contact factors, such as contact with collagen, high molecular weight kininogen, and kallikein.
- Extrinsic pathway activated by tissue factors (aka tissue thromboplastin).
- Coagulation problems tend to present with deep bleeding, e.g. haematomas, haemarthrosis, and delayed post-traumatic bleeding.
- Prothrombin time, which measures extrinsic and common coagulation pathways, is prolonged.
- PTT, which measures the intrinsic and common coagulation pathways, is increased.
- Thrombin time tests for adequate levels of fibrinogen, fibrinogen degradation products (FDP), and D-dimers.

Haemophilia A (FVIII deficiency)

- An X-linked recessive disorder and therefore affects males.
- Haemarthrosis, easy bleeding following trauma.
- Single abnormality is raised PTT.
- Treatment is FVIII replacement.

Thrombophilia B (FIX deficiency)

- Also an X-linked disorder.
- Clinically identical to haemophilia A.
- Distinction made by FVIII and FIX assays.

Acquired coagulopathies

1. *Vitamin K deficiency:*
   - Associated with deficiency of clotting factors II, VII, IX, and X.
   - May occur with prolonged broad spectrum antibiotic therapy because vitamin K is produced by gut flora, which may be reduced or eliminated by long-term antibiotic therapy.
   - PT elevated and later PTT also elevated.
   - Treatment is vitamin K first, and if that is adequate the diagnosis is made.

2. *Liver disease:*
   - All factors except FVII are reduced.
   - PT elevated earlier on.
   - PTT elevated later.
3. *von Willebrand disease (vWD):*
   - An inherited bleeding disorder.
   - Characterized by either a deficiency or a qualitative defect of vWF.
   - vWF is produced by endothelial cells for attachment to collagen and provides a surface for platelets to attach themselves.
   - Clinical features, like with other platelet problems, include nose bleeds and petechial haemorrhages; platelet count is normal but the bleeding time is prolonged.
   - PT is normal and PTT may or may not be normal. Occasionally it is increased because FVIII circulates in the body attached to vWF, which stabilizes it, and therefore a defect in vWF leads to a rapid degradation of FVIII leading to prolonged PTT.
   - Diagnosis is made by platelet aggregometry.
   - Treatment is by desmoprossin (an ADH analogue), which causes more release of vWF from the endothelial cells.

Disseminated intravascular coagulopathy (DIC)

- Always secondary to another disease, e.g. abruption, malignancy, leukaemia, or infection (particularly Gram-negative sepsis).
- There is generalized formation of thrombi, which uses up all the platelets, coagulation factors, and fibrinogen in a consumptive coagulopathy leading to excessive bleeding.
- Diagnosis requires the presence of four conditions:
  1. reduced platelet count
  2. increased PT and PTT
  3. reduced fibrinogen
  4. increased fibrinogen degradation products (or D-dimers).
- Treatment—treat the underlying cause and correct the coagulopathy.

Thrombosis

Thrombosis is usually due to the violation of the Virchow triad of vessel wall integrity, disturbances of blood flow, and changes in the constituents of blood. Thrombosis may therefore be due to:

1. endothelial injury
2. alteration of laminar flow, e.g. aneurysms, polycythemia, immobility
3. hypercoagulable state, e.g. tissue injury, nephrotic syndrome, pregnancy, oral contraceptive use.

Differences between a thrombus and a clot

- Thrombus occurs within the vasculature, unlike blood clot.

- Thrombus contains fibrin, platelets, and white and red blood cells (RBCs).
- Thrombus has a shape and contains lines of Zahn (pale lines of platelet and fibrin alternating with red lines composed of RBCs) unlike blood clot.
- Thrombus lead to occlusion or embolization.

Pulmonary embolism (PE)

- Over 95% of cases of PE are from deep vein thrombosis (DVT) in the deep leg veins or pelvic iliac veins on the right side of the heart.

Outcomes of DVT

1. *No sequelae:*
   - Asymptomatic—most common presentation; there may be dyspnoea and tachypnoea but with no infarction and therefore no sequelae.
2. *Infarction:*
   - Approximately 15% of PE, usually in patients with pre-existing lung or heart disease.
   - There may be shortness of breath, haemoptysis, chest pain, and pleural effusion.
   - In fatal cases post-mortem may show the classic wedge form with the apex pointing towards the pathology.
3. *Sudden death:*
   - Approximately 5% of PE, particularly with saddle emboli.
4. *Chronic pulmonary hypertension:*
   - Occurs in about 3% of PE.
   - Usually from longstanding showering type, which is followed by sclerosis of the pulmonary vessels.

Systemic emboli

- Majority will lead to infarction.
- Usually from the heart after a myocardial infarction, atrial fibrillation, or infectious endocarditis.
- Emboli may lodge in the legs, spleen, gastrointestinal tract, or brain.
- Paradoxical emboli—embolus that starts from the venous side of the circulation and ends up in the arterial side, usually through a heart defect.

Infarction

- A localized area of necrosis secondary to ischaemia.
- Usually due to an embolus or thrombi.
- Torsion and vasospasm are other causes, especially in the ovary and testes.
- In most body tissues infarctions lead to coagulative necrosis, except in the brain where there is liquefactive necrosis. The dead tissue provokes an inflammatory response and the inflammatory cells remove the dead tissue leaving behind a scar.

- Predisposing factors to infarction:
  - tissue vulnerability to infarction, e.g. the brain or heart because of their requirement for high blood flow compared to tendons or fat
  - presence or absence of collateral circulations; organs with a single blood supply tend to have a pale infarct, whereas organs with dual or more sources of blood supply tend to have haemorrhagic infarction.

Shock

- Widespread hypoperfusion of cells and tissues from vascular collapse/reduction in cardiac output, leading initially to reversible injury but if prolonged may lead to irreversible cell injury.

Causes

1. Hypovolaemic shock, e.g. trauma, postpartum haemorrhage.
2. Cardiogenic shock, e.g. myocardial infarction.
3. Septic shock, e.g. from Gram-negative endotoxaemia, which releases IL-1, IL-6, TNF, and IL-8, resulting in massive vasodilatation, adult respiratory distress syndrome (ARDS), DIC, and multi-organ dysfunction; mortality from septic shock is ≥50%.
4. Neurogenic shock from brain or spinal cord injury.
5. Anaphylactic shock from type 1 hypersensitivity reaction.

Three major stages of shock

1. Compensatory stage—perfusion to the vital organs is maintained by reflex mechanisms including catecholamine release and activation of the sympathetic and renin-angiotensin systems (RAS).
2. Decompensated stage—reduced tissue perfusion resulting in reversible cellular injury, metabolic acidosis, and electrolyte disturbances.
3. Irreversible stage—organ failure and death even if the original injury is removed.

Selected individual organ injury in shock

- Lungs—ARDS or diffuse alveolar damage (DAD).
- Kidneys—acute tubular necrosis (ATN); the proximal convoluted tubular cells are very susceptible to hypoxia and die quickly in the process and fall off into the tubular lumen.
- Adrenals—bilateral adrenal infarction (Waterhouse-Friderichsen syndrome) commonly associated with Gram-negative endotoxaemia due to meningococcal meningitis.
- Intestines—ischaemic necrosis and haemorrhage.
- Liver—centrilobular necrosis (aka shocked liver).

Genetic syndromes

- *Down syndrome:*
  - trisomy 21

- 95% secondary to non-disjunction, 4% Robertsonian translocation
- features include flat face, low nasal bridge, wide-set eyes, short broad neck, low-set ears, speckled appearance of the iris (brush field spots), single simian crease in the hand, cardiac defects including ASD, VSD, duodenal atresia (double bubble sign on ultrasound scan), and Hirschsprung's disease
- 15 to 25% have increased risk of leukaemia, particularly acute lymphocytic leukaemia
- Alzheimer's disease (amyloid protein deposition in the brain from the extra chromosome 21) by ≥40 years of age.

- *Edward syndrome:*
  - trisomy 18, 46 XX/XY + 18
  - features include severe mental retardation, low-set ears, overlapping flexed fingers, micrognathia, rocker-bottom feet (from excessive connective tissue at the base of the foot), and death soon after birth (severe malformations).

- *Patau syndrome:*
  - trisomy 13, 47 XX/XY + 13 non-disjunction
  - features include severe mental retardation, microcephaly, extra digits, cleft lip and palate, chromosomal deletions (e.g. 46 XY/XY 5p–), and VSD.

Sex chromosome disorders

- *Klinefelter's syndrome:*
  - 47 XXY/48XXXY
  - a meiotic chromosomal non-disjunction disorder
  - results in male hypogonadism, atrophic, fibrotic testes, no production of testosterone, infertility, high-pitched voice, gynaecomastia.

- *Turner's syndrome:*
  - 45 X0
  - female hypogonadism (two X chromosomes required for normal ovarian development), the ovaries are streaked (by the fibrous tissue bands)
  - primary amenorrhoea, reduced oestrogen, short stature, failure of secondary sex characteristics, cystic hygromas (dilated lymphatic channels underneath the skin, which eventually leave redundant skin around the neck), aortic coarctation, hydrops fetalis, may be stillborn.

Sexual determination

Can be considered at four levels:

1. karyotype—presence or absence of the Y chromosome
2. gonadal sex—presence of testicular or ovarian tissue
3. ductal sex—presence of Wolffian or Mullerian duct
4. phenotype—external sexual characteristics.

True hermaphrodite
- Presence of ovotestis; extremely rare.
- Ambiguous genitalia.

Female pseudo-hermaphrodite
- Genetically female, phenotypically male.
- Caused by exposure of a female fetus to androgens, e.g. congenital adrenal hyperplasia.

Male pseudo-hermaphrodite
- Genetically male, phenotypically female
- Caused by testicular feminization.
- There is a defect in the androgen receptor.
- Undescended testes.

Inheritance patterns

1. Autosomal recessive
2. Autosomal dominant
3. X-linked disorders
4. Genetic imprinting—genetic defect in which the symptoms differ depending on whether the gene was inherited from paternal or maternal chromosomes.

1. Autosomal recessive disorders

- General characteristics:
  - early in onset, presenting early in infancy or childhood
  - complete penetrance (i.e. likely to express if inherited)
  - tends to involve enzyme proteins, e.g. cystic fibrosis, alkaptonuria, albinism, glycogen storage disease
  - mutation of both alleles required.

- Phenylketonuria (PKU):
  - autosomal recessive disorder
  - defect in the enzyme phenylalanine hydroxylase leading to accumulation of toxic levels of phenylalanine in the brain
  - light-coloured skin and hair
  - treatment is dietary restriction of phenylalanine.

- Cystic fibrosis (CF):
  - the defect is in the CF transmembrane conductance regulator, a chloride channel protein responsible for anion transport
  - the gene is on chromosome 7 and the deletion is at position 508 in 70% of cases
  - there is production of viscid mucus, which blocks the ducts in organs, e.g. in the lung leading to pneumonia and bronchiectasis, and in the gut leading to meconium ileus. Other features include pancreatic atrophy and fibrosis, and congenital absence of the vas deferens.

2. *Autosomal dominant disorders*

- General characteristics:
  - variable in onset; some may represent in adulthood
  - incomplete penetrance (variable expression in time and degree)
  - mutations in structural or regulatory proteins, e.g. receptors
  - mutation is only required on one allele.

- Familial hypercholesterolaemia:
  - most common inherited disorder (affecting 1 in 500)
  - defect is a mutation in the LDL receptor gene
  - no functional LDL receptors in the liver, therefore LDL-cholesterol levels increase, and the liver responds by producing even more cholesterol, because of lack of negative feedback
  - no inhibition of HMG-CoA reductase, which exacerbates the process
  - may be heterozygous or homozygous
  - xanthomas (lipid-laden macrophages) and premature artherosclerosis.

- Marfan's syndrome:
  - defect is in the fibrillin gene (a glycoprotein that functions as a scaffold protein and helps to align elastin fibres)
  - affects skeletal systems
  - affected individuals are tall with long arms, legs, bones, and fingers
  - hyperextensible joints and chest wall deformities
  - bilateral subluxation of the lens, aortic dissection from cystic medial necrosis leading to aneurysms, aortic insufficiency and mitral valve prolapse.

- Ehlers–Danlos syndrome:
  - there are 10 different variants: type 3 is the most common; type 4 results from a defect in type 3 collagen, and patients usually die of ruptured aorta or colon
  - hyperflexible and hyperextensible joints, and lax skin
  - there may be poor wound healing and dislocations.

- Neurofibromatosis (Von Recklinghausen's disease) Types 1 and 2:
  - approximately 90% of cases are Type 1
  - mutation is in neurofibroma NF1 tumour suppressor gene on chromosome 17, responsible for producing neurofibromin
  - patient presents with café-au-lait spots, nerve bundle, and branch lesions
  - increased risk of pheochromocytoma and meningiomas
  - pigmented iris
  - Type 2—10% of cases
  - mutation in tumour suppressor gene type 2 on chromosome 22
  - gene product is merlin but its function is unknown.

3. *X-linked diseases*

- Fragile X syndrome:
  - a triplet nucleotide (GCC) repeat mutation
  - mental retardation and large jaws, ears, and testes
  - more common in males than females
  - diagnosis is with gene probe analysis.

- Huntington's disease:
  - triplet repeat (CAG) in Huntington gene resulting in defective Huntington's protein
  - patients make purposeless movements (aka Huntington's chorea)
  - early onset dementia
  - atrophy of the caudate nucleus of the brain.

- Prader-Willi syndrome:
  - defect on chromosome 15, inherited from paternal chromosomes
  - there is hypogonadism, mental retardation, obesity, and hypotonia.

- Engelman syndrome (Happy Puppet syndrome):
  - defect also on chromosome 15, but inherited under maternal chromosomes
  - mental retardation, seizures, ataxia, and inappropriate laughter.

Immunopathology

Hypersensitivity reactions

There are four types. Three require antibodies; the other is completely cell mediated.

Type 1 hypersensitivity reaction

This anaphylactic type is characterized by plasma cell production of IgE antibodies on exposure to antigen, and the IgE antibodies circulate and attach to mast cells. Next time there is exposure to the antigen, the antigen causes cross-linkage of the IgE on the mast cells, which degranulate leading to release of histamine, leukotrienes, and prostaglandins. There is influx of eosinophils to amplify and sustain the reaction. Clinical examples include anaphylactic reactions, food allergies, atopy, and asthma.

Type 2 hypersensitivity reaction

This involves the production of cytotoxic IgG or IgM antibodies directed against specific tissues, cells, or cell receptors. This leads to: autoimmune haemolytic anaemia if the target cell is the red blood cell; Grave's disease in the case of antibodies against the TSH receptor; myasthenia gravis when antibodies are produced against the acetylcholine (Ach) receptor; or Goodpasture's disease with production of antibodies against type 4 collagen in the basement membrane, leading to acute glomerulonephritis. Attachment of the antibodies leads to inflammation, which activates compliment for cytotoxicity or antibody-dependent cell-mediated phagocytosis.

Type 3 hypersensitivity reaction

This is due to the deposition of circulating antigen-antibody immune complexes in tissues where they cause inflammation and disease, e.g. skin in lupus, joints in rheumatoid arthritis, blood vessels in vasculitis or polyarteritis nodosa, and kidney in glomerulonephritis.

Type 4 hypersensitivity reaction

This is a completely cell-mediated hypersensitivity reaction with no antibody involvement. The reaction is delayed and mediated by Th1 cells. Two types of T-cell mediated hypersensitivity reaction exist, namely delayed hypersensitivity reaction, which is responsible for granuloma formation, and cytotoxic T-cell mediated reaction, which is responsible for fighting tumours and viruses and for graft rejection.

Autoimmune diseases

- Systemic lupus erythematosus (SLE):
  - a chronic autoimmune disease characterized by loss of self-tolerance and production of lots of autoantibodies
  - affects women more than men, usually reproductive-age women, and Africans more than Caucasians
  - due to autoantibodies against nuclear proteins including histones, DNA, and other RNA proteins
  - antinuclear antibodies (ANA) are commonly raised, but they are not specific. Specific antibodies for SLE are anti-dsDNA (double-stranded DNA), and anti-SM antibodies (aka anti-Smith); anti-dsDNA is the more sensitive of the two
  - tissue injury in SLE is usually a combination of types 2 and 3 hypersensitivity reaction; that is antibody targeted against specific tissue and deposition of immune complexes
  - diseases include anaemia, thrombocytopenia, arthritis, neutropenia, lymphopenia, malar skin rash, diffuse glomerulonephritis and membranous glomerulonephritis leading to nephrotic syndrome, endocarditis, and pericarditis
  - treatment is with steroids and immunosuppressants.

- Sjögren's syndrome:
  - an autoimmune disease characterized by the destruction of the salivary and lacrimal glands leading to dry mouth and dry eyes respectively
  - often associated with other autoimmune diseases, usually rheumatoid arthritis
  - characteristic antibodies include anti-ribonuclear protein antibodies SSA and SSB
  - increased risk of lymphoma, particularly non-Hodgkin's lymphoma.

- Scleroderma (progressive systemic sclerosis):
  - characterized by the stimulation of fibroblasts by IL-1 and platelet-derived growth factor (PDGF)
  - the stimulated fibroblasts lay down excess amounts of collagen in different organs
  - affects reproductive-age women mostly
  - two types of scleroderma are described, diffused and localized
  - *diffused scleroderma* is associated with anti-DNA topoisomerase-1 antibodies and affects approximately 70% of cases; there is widespread involvement of the hands and face leading to thick and fibrotic claw-like fingers, and also involvement of the internal organs including the oesophagus (dysphagia), gastrointestinal tract (malabsorption), lungs (fibrosis, dyspnoea), heart (arrhythmias), and kidneys (renal failure)
  - *localized (form) scleroderma (aka the CREST syndrome):* C—calcinosis, R—Raynaud's phenomenon, E—oesophageal dysmotility, S—sclerodactyly, T—telangiectasia. It is associated with anti-centromere antibodies involving the skin, hands, and face, leading to clawed hands and smooth, tight face; it may also involve the internal organs later in its course. The localized form has a more benign prognosis compared to the systemic form.

Immunodeficiency syndromes

- X-linked agammaglobulinemia (Bruton's tyrosine kinase (BTK) mutation): An inherited disorder characterized by failure to produce mature B cells (i.e. plasma cells and therefore immunoglobulins). There are recurrent bacterial infections, usually from 6 months of age when maternal antibodies wane from the infant's circulation: staphylococcal infections, strep pneumonia, haemophilus, and influenza. The mutation is in B cell protein Bruton's tyrosine kinase.
- Common variable immunodeficiency: A B-cell maturation disorder. There is reduced immunoglobulin production affecting one class usually. The patient suffers recurrent infections with parasites such as *Giardia lamblia* and bacteria. There is increased risk of developmental lymphomas and gastric carcinoma; both sexes are equally affected. There is also association with other autoimmune diseases.
- Di George syndrome: Failure of development of the third and fourth pharyngeal pouches; that is, the parathyroid and thymus glands. Classically, the patient presents with hypocalcaemia and tetany; there are recurrent fungal and viral infections because of the absence of T cells.
- Severe combined immunodeficiency syndrome (SCID): Affects cell-mediated and humoral immunity. There are two modes of inheritance, autosomal recessive or X-linked. In the autosomal recessive type there is absence of adenosine deaminase, which leads to accumulation of deoxyadenosine, which is toxic to stem cells and lymphoid cells. As a result there is death and loss of stem cells. Affected children suffer all types of infections with viruses, bacteria, fungi, parasites, and protozoa. They should not be given any live attenuated vaccines. They suffer from unusual infections including *Pneumocystis carinii*. Treatment is bone marrow transplant and gene therapy.
- Wiskott-Aldrich syndrome: An X-linked disorder. The mutation is in the gene for the Wiskott-Aldrich syndrome protein (WASP). Patients present with a classic clinical triad of recurrent infections, severe thrombocytopenia,

and skin rash. There is an increased risk of lymphomas and treatment is with bone marrow transplant.

Secondary immune deficiency syndromes

Disease conditions that may cause secondary impairment of the immune system include diabetes mellitus, collagen vascular diseases, alcoholism, organ transplant and immunosuppressant therapy, and AIDS.

Types of organ rejection

1. Hyperacute rejection

This is caused by preformed antibodies, which attach to the vessels of the new organ once reconnected *in situ* and cause thrombosis and infarction of the organ, usually within minutes.

2. Acute rejection

Takes weeks to months after transplantation and the onset is abrupt as the patient is weaned off immunosuppressant therapy. There is renal failure, oliguria, and azothemia. Microscopically there is vasculitis, interstitial lymphocytes, and neutrophil vasculitis. Treatment is to increase the dose of immunosuppressants.

3. Chronic rejection

This takes months to years after transplantation to develop. There is gradual onset of renal failure with increased blood pressure. Microscopy shows intimal fibrosis with the vessels progressively narrowing until the organ becomes ischaemic and infarcts, which is irreversible.

Amyloidosis

This is a group of diseases characterized by the deposition of extracellular protein (amyloid protein) with very specific properties around small blood vessels. Principally it affects the liver, spleen, and kidneys. There is no known treatment for amyloidosis.

Common and characteristic features of amyloid

- Amyloid is deposited in a very specific configuration called a 'β-pleated sheet'.
- It is eosinophilic pink under the microscope.
- It gives a bright red/pink colour when stained with Congo red and because of its β-pleated sheet the Congo red also produces another effect when placed under polarized light—'apple green birefringence' (i.e. some areas will have green and others yellowish colouration).

Three major components of amyloid

1. Fibrillar protein, which is specific for each disease.
2. Amyloid component.
3. Glycosaminoglycan (heparin sulphate).

Systemic forms of amyloidosis

Primary amyloidosis

- Usually caused by plasma cell malignancy including multiple myloma and B-cell lymphoma.

- The protein deposited as amyloid is the light chain called AL type (amyloid-light chain).

Reactive systemic amyloidosis (secondary amyloidosis)

- The fibrillar protein is called serum amyloid A (SAA), which is an acute phase reactant protein produced by the liver.
- This type of amyloidosis occurs in inflammatory states such as tuberculosis, rheumatoid arthritis, SLE, Crohn's disease, ulcerative colitis, and longstanding osteomyelitis, and it is the underlying inflammatory disease that stimulates the liver production of SAA.

Familial Mediterranean fever (inherited amyloidosis)

- Autosomal recessive disorder.
- Also produced by SAA protein.
- Characterized by recurrent bouts of infections, fever, and neutrophil dysfunction.

Haemodialysis-associated amyloidosis

- Usually diagnosed on dialysed patients; the dialysing membrane is not very good at handling and filtering proteins, especially $β_2$ macroglobulin, which accumulates and deposits in tissues, especially in the wrists where it may cause carpal tunnel syndrome.
- The amyloid protein is called $Aβ_2$ macroglobulin.
- The protein accumulated is $β_2$ macroglobulin.

Localized forms of amyloidosis

Senile cerebral amyloidosis (Alzheimer's disease)

- The amyloid protein is Aβ.
- The fibrillar protein is called β-amyloid precursor protein (BAPP).
- The gene for BAPP is located on chromosome 21, which is why Down syndrome patients with an extra chromosome 21 get Alzheimer's disease.
- The amyloid is found in the centre of all amyloid plaques and also within the cerebral vessels.

Senile cardiac amyloidosis

- Usually in older men over 70 years of age and may result in heart failure.
- Restrictive cardiomyopathy.

Endocrine organs and tumour amyloidosis

- For example, medullary carcinoma of the thyroid, which is a C-cell tumour producing calcitonin.
- The tumour is surrounded by deposits of pro-calcitonin, which forms β-pleated sheets resulting in amyloid.
- Prognosis is very poor.

Neoplasia—basic principles

- 90% of neoplasias are of epithelial origin (cells are proliferating at a higher rate and exposed to environmental carcinogens).

- 10% are of mesenchymal tissue origin.
- Age is a factor, e.g. seminomas are commoner in men of 15–35 years of age compared to yolk sac tumour or teratoma, which are commoner in young children.
- Hereditary predisposition, e.g. familial retinoblastoma, multiple endocrine neoplasia syndrome (MENS), and familial polyposis coli are of autosomal dominant inheritance.

Acquired pre-neoplastic dysplasias

- Cervical dysplasia
- Endometrial hyperplasia
- Chronic atrophic gastritis
- Liver cirrhosis
- Ulcerative colitis

Causes

Chemical carcinogens

Carcinogenesis is a multi-step process involving mutagens and promoters. Mutagens cause mutation in the DNA. Promoters cause cell proliferation. Chemical carcinogens include:

- nitrosamines for gastric cancer
- asbestos
- arsenic foreskin cancers and liver angiosarcomas
- alklating agents
- benzene compounds.

Radiation

- Ultraviolet radiation from the sun produces pyridine dimers in DNA, which increases the risk of cancers, especially in patients with scleroderma pigmentosa (an autosomal recessive condition with defective DNA repair).
- Ionizing radiations including X-rays, γ-rays, α- and β-particles, protons, and neutrons damage cells and may lead to carcinoma, e.g. thyroid, and leukaemia.

Oncogenic viruses

1. Human T cell leukaemia virus and RNA virus (HTLV I)—responsible for human T cell leukaemia and lymphoma.
2. Hepatitis B virus—hepatocellular carcinoma.
3. Epstein–Barr virus—Burkitt's lymphoma, B cell lymphoma, and nasopharyngeal carcinomas and tumours.
4. HPV—benign squamous papillomas, increased risk of CA cervix.
5. Kaposi's sarcoma-associated herpes virus 8.

Smoking

There are over 4000 components in cigarettes, 40 of which are known human carcinogens, including carbon monoxide, arsenic, and cyanide. The addictive component is nicotine, a causative agent of cancer of the lung, oral cavity, stomach, oesophagus, cervix, pancreas, kidney, ureter, and bladder. It is a major risk factor for endothelial injury with increased risk of coronary disease from vasospasm, chronic obstructive airways disease, chronic bronchitis, early menopause, increased risk of miscarriage, and fetal growth restriction.

Carcinogenesis

Carcinogenesis requires the accumulation of multiple mutations acquired either as inherited germ-line mutations or over a lifetime's acquisition, in: growth promoting genes, i.e. proto-oncogenes (over-expressed by tumours); tumour suppressor genes (growth inhibitor genes); and apoptotic genes.

Proto-oncogenic

- Activated proto-oncogenes lack regulatory capacity and tend to over-express.
- Clinically important oncogenes include: erb1, squamous cell carcinoma of the lung (EGF receptor is over-expressed); erb2, ovarian or breast cancer (EGF receptor amplified); erb3; bcl; c-myc; I-myc; and N-myc.

Tumour suppressive genes

- Inhibit cells from entering the cell cycle.
- p53 gene is expressed whenever the cell DNA is damaged and this is most commonly mutated in tumours.
- BRCA genes and NF-1 and -2 for neurofibromatosis.

Apoptosis-regulating genes

- bcl_2 prevents apoptosis and is amplified by some tumours, such that the tumour cells become immortalized, e.g. follicular lymphomas.
- p53 prevents the mutated cells from proliferating and promotes apoptosis of the damaged cells.

Benign neoplasia

These are small, slow-growing, and encapsulated with well-defined borders; they are well differentiated and look like the original tissue under the microscope. They are non-invasive and never metastasize.

Serum tumour markers

These are normal cellular components that are over-expressed in disease/tumours and have three major applications:

1. Useful in screening, e.g. prostate specific antigen (PSA) for prostatic cancer.
2. Monitoring treatment efficacy.
3. Detection of disease recurrence, e.g. carcino-embryonic antigen (CEA).

Tumour markers include:
- α-feto protein (AFP)—hepatomas and yolk sac tumours
- β-hCG—trophoblastic tumours and choriocarcinomas
- calcitonin—thyroid C-cells
- carcino-embryonic antigen (CEA)—lung, pancreas, breast, and colon
- CA 125—epithelial ovarian tumours
- CA$^{19-9}$—important for pancreatic cancers
- Placental alkaline phosphatase—seminomas
- PSA and prostatic acid phosphotase—prostate cancer

Vasculitides

This is a group of diseases characterized by acute immu-nologic damage and fibrinoid necrosis of affected vessels, usually medium-sized arteries.

- Polyarthritis nodosa:
  - due to segmental necrotizing vasculitis
  - there are acute lesions in the form of arteries undergo-ing fibrinoid necrosis, surrounded by polymorphonu-clear cell infiltration alongside healing lesions made up of proliferating fibroblasts, and healed lesions, which are nodular areas of fibrosis
  - sequelae include thrombosis, weakened vessels, and aneurysms
  - any organ may be involved except the lungs
  - medium-sized arteries are usually involved, including kidneys, heart, gastrointestinal system, and muscles
  - there is a low-grade fever, malaise, and weight loss
  - 30% of cases are associated with infection, e.g. hepatitis B virus
  - autoantibodies against own neutrophils (specifically against neutrophil peroxidise) are present in 75% of cases
  - a variant of polyarthritis nodosa displays vasculitis with granulomas and eosinophilia.

- Wegener's granulomatosis:
  - a rare necrotizing vasculitis with granuloma formation
  - usually in the age group of 40–60 years
  - affects the nose, lungs, sinuses, and kidneys resulting in pneumonia, sinusitis, nasal ulceration, and dominant renal disease, with cause of death usually acute glom-erulonephritis nephritis
  - microscopy reveals fibrinoid necrosis and granulomas
  - autoantibodies against neutrophils present in 93% of cases
  - if untreated (usually with cyclophosphamide) mortality is 80% within a year.

- Temporal (giant cell) arteritis:
  - this is the most common form of arteritis and usually occurs in the elderly
  - associated with HLA DR4

- small and medium-sized arteries involved, particularly the facial artery; the aortic arch may be involved includ-ing the cranial branches
  - patients present with throbbing headaches, visual dis-turbances, facial pains, fever, malaise, weight loss, and nodularity of arteries
  - the ESR is raised and there is formation of granulomas with segmental multi-nucleated giant cells
  - treatment is with steroid with typically a good response.

- Takayasu arteritis (pulseless disease):
  - a granulomatous arteritis with loss of the pulse from the thickening intima of the vessels
  - affects the aortic arch and its branches
  - usually involves young Asian women
  - response to steroid is variable.

- Thromboangitis obliterans (Buerger's disease):
  - affects young male smokers
  - involves the extremities
  - vessel lumen obliterated by inflammatory thrombi
  - patient may present with gangrene or claudication
  - treatment is to stop smoking.

- Kawasaki disease:
  - affects children <4 years of age
  - common in Hawaii and Japan
  - there is an acute febrile illness, conjunctivitis, lymph-adenopathy, fever, maculopapular skin rash, and coronary artery involvement in 70% of cases with thrombosis or aneurysm in 1 to 2% of patients
  - disease is self-limiting and is thought to be due to a virus.

- Raynaud's disease:
  - usually affects young women
  - precipitated by exposure to cold temperatures or stress
  - there is painful blanching of the fingers, leading to cya-nosis, when the fingers may become blue
  - when the vessel spasm is relieved they turn red
  - Raynaud's disease is an entity of its own, whereas Raynaud's phenomenon is a feature of another disease, e.g. scleroderma.

Systemic pathology

Selected respiratory pathology

Sarcoidosis

- Idiopathic condition commoner in people of African an-cestry.
- Affects women more than men in their middle ages.
- May be asymptomatic or patients may present with fa-tigue, malaise, shortness of breath, fever, and night sweats.

- Chest X-ray may show bilateral hilar lymphadenopathy, which is diagnostic.
- Affects the lungs, lymph nodes, skin, heart, central ner-vous system, eyes, and bone marrow, especially of the fingers and toes.
- Angiotensin-converting enzyme may be raised.
- Tissue biopsy may show non-caseating granulomas.

Adult respiratory distress syndrome (ARDS, shock lungs)

- Diffuse damage to the alveoli and alveolar capillaries, resulting in progressive respiratory failure; unresponsive to oxygen therapy.
- Causes include shock, sepsis, burns, radiation, pulmonary infections, drugs, oxygen toxicity, gastric aspiration, and trauma.
- Patient may present with dyspnoea, tachypnoea, hypoxemia, cyanosis, and use of accessory muscles of respiration.
- Chest X-ray may show bilateral lung field opacities; stiff, leathery, heavy, non-compliant, and solid lungs on gross examination.
- Microscopy shows interstitial space oedema, infiltration by inflammatory cells (usually chronic), loss of type I pneumocytes, which are replaced by pink hyaline membranes comparable to newborn respiratory distress syndrome.
- Underlying cause should be treated; the patient will be mechanically ventilated with oxygen supplementation.
- Mortality is 50%.

Newborn respiratory distress syndrome (RDS, hyaline membrane disease)

- Associated with prematurity.
- 60% of neonates <28 weeks will suffer from RDS.
- Associated with elective caesarean section, diabetes mellitus, and multiple births.
- Due to the deficiency of pulmonary surfactant.
- The infants are usually normal at birth, followed by rapid onset of respiratory insufficiency.
- Chest X-ray reveals ground glass appearance.
- Microscopic findings are identical to ARDS.
- Treatment is with surfactant, oxygen, and ventilation.
- Mortality is as high as 30%.
- Long-term sequelae include bronchopulmonary dysplasia, pulmonary hypertension, and increased pulmonary arterial pressure.

Selected renal pathology

Acute glomerulonephritis (AGN)

- More common in children after group A, β-haemolytic streptococcal throat or skin infection. Other bacteria, viruses, parasites, and systemic diseases can also cause AGN.
- Anti-streptolysin O antibody titres are raised, there are RBC casts in the renal tubules, and electron microscopy shows epithelial humps (immune complexes) underneath the podocytes of the kidney.
- Specific immunofluorescent tests will reveal granular deposits of IgG, IgM, and complement (C3) throughout the glomeruli.
- 95% of children will recover fully compared to 60% of adults.

Goodpasture's syndrome

- This is an autoimmune disease characterized by the production of autoantibodies directed against type IV collagen in the basement membrane of the glomerulus and the lungs.
- It is a type 2 hypersensitivity reaction.
- It usually affects young males and is rapidly progressive with poor prognosis.
- The treatment is plasmapheresis, steroids, and cytotoxic drugs.

IgA nephropathy (Berger's disease)

- Usually affects children and young adults and is the most common nephritic disease worldwide.
- It may follow an upper respiratory tract infection and may be associated with other immune diseases.
- Microscopy shows mesengial proliferation due to IgA deposition.
- There may be renal failure within 20–25 years.

Polycystic disease of the kidney (adult type)

- Autosomal dominant inheritance.
- The mutation is in the polycystic kidney disease (PKD) gene, which is located on chromosome 16 and produces polycystin-1.
- Onset is in adulthood, usually in the 40s and 50s, and presents with hypertension, renal insufficiency, and grossly enlarged kidneys.
- There are extra-renal manifestations including pancreatic and hepatic cysts, Berry aneurysms, and an increased risk of mitral valve prolapse.
- The child type of PKD is rare and of autosomal recessive inheritance. It presents in infancy with progressive renal failure.

Selected gastrointestinal tract pathology

Hirschsprung's disease (congenital aganglionic megacolon)

- Congenital absence of ganglionic cells, usually affecting the rectum and sigmoid colon.
- The patient presents with constipation, abdominal distension, and vomiting.
- Affects 1–2% of Down syndrome babies.
- Affects boys more commonly than girls.
- Microscopy of colonic biopsy reveals absence of ganglionic cells.

Malabsorption syndromes

Coeliac sprue

- This is an IgA disease associated with HLA, B8, DR3, and DQ.
- It is due to hypersensitivity reaction to gluten and gliadin (IgA or IgG antibodies to gliadin in 90% of cases).

- There is malabsorption, flatulence, diarrhoea, and fatty stools.
- Microscopy of biopsy shows loss of microvilli, increased lymphocytes within the epithelium, and increased plasma cells within the lamina propria.
- It is associated with other IgA diseases including Berger's nephropathy and dermatitis herpetiformes.
- Treatment is with dietary restriction.

Tropical sprue

- This is a malabsorption syndrome of unknown aetiology.
- Microscopic findings are identical to coeliac disease but there is usually a history of travel.

Inflammatory bowel disease

Crohn's disease (regional enteritis)

- Usually affects Caucasian women, peak age 10–30 years and 50–60 years.
- Less common than ulcerative colitis.
- There is usually fever, peritoneal fistulas, and malabsorption if the terminal ileum is involved.
- May affect any part of the gastrointestinal system from the mouth to the anus, but the terminal ileum is the more common site.
- Diagnosis is made by endoscopy, which shows skip areas (lesions) and strictures, and by biopsy, which shows transmural inflammation, non-caseating granulomas, and strictures.
- Unlike ulcerative colitis there are not many extra-intestinal manifestations.
- About 1–3% may progress to carcinoma.

Ulcerative colitis

- Associated with HLA B27.
- Always involves the rectum from where it spreads proximally, usually to the large intestine, and rarely to the ileum.
- There is extensive mucosal ulceration and formation of pseudopolyps (areas that have not ulcerated and therefore stand out like polyps); there are no strictures.
- Microscopy shows inflammation limited to the mucosal and the submucosal layers, and crypt abscesses.
- Complications include toxic megacolon and a 5–25% risk of colonic cancer.
- Extra-intestinal manifestations—primary sclerosing cholangitis.

Pseudomembranous colitis (antibiotic-associated colitis)

- Usually associated with a course of broad spectrum antibiotic therapy. Although the condition is frequently quoted to be due to clindamycin therapy, it may follow treatment with any broad spectrum antibiotic. It is also mainly associated with *Clostridium difficile* but may be caused by other organisms.
- There is acute colitis characterized by formation of pseudo-membranes, composed of neutrophils, mucin,

fibrin, and necrotic cellular debris in a mushroom-shaped appearance.
- Treatment is with metronidazole, or vancomycin as a last resort and to avoid development of resistant strains.

Familial adenomatous polyposis syndrome

- This is an autosomal dominant disorder.
- The defect is in the APC gene on chromosome 5q.
- The patients have hundreds or thousands of adenomatous polyps, and before the age of 40 the majority of them would develop colonic cancer.
- The treatment is prophylactic total colectomy by the age of 40.

Hereditary non-polyposis colorectal cancer (HNPCC)

- An autosomal dominant inherited disorder.
- There are no polyps but there is an increased risk of other cancers, including endometrial and ovarian cancers.

Peutz-Jegher's syndrome

- An autosomal dominant disorder.
- There are multiple hamartomatous polyps, usually in the small intestine.
- Other features include melanin pigmentation on the lips and oral cavity.
- There is increased risk of carcinoma of the lungs, pancreas, breasts, and uterus.

Carcinoid tumours

- These are serotonin-producing neuroendocrine tumours.
- They occur most commonly in the appendix where they are usually benign.
- They may occur in the terminal ileum where they are malignant.
- If metastasis to the liver occurs then the serotonin produced may be secreted directly into the hepatic vein, which empties into the inferior vena cava and right side of the heart to cause the *carcinoid heart syndrome*, including fibrosis of the endocardial surface of the right atrium, right ventricle, tricuspid valve, and pulmonary vessels. The serotonin is metabolized and destroyed when it reaches the lungs.
- Carcinoid syndrome is due to the systemic effects of serotonin and includes diarrhoea, flushing, bronchospasm, wheezing, and fibrosis.
- The diagnosis is made by the presence of breakdown products of serotonin in urine, 5-hydroxyindoleacetic acid (5HIAA).

Haemochromatosis

- Due to the accumulation of iron in tissues, leading to tissue damage. It usually affects northern Europeans and there is a predilection for men.
- The primary form is an autosomal recessive hereditary disorder associated with HLA-HG on chromosome 6p.

There is excessive intestinal absorption of iron, which accumulates in tissues.

- The secondary form is associated with multiple blood transfusions for chronic anaemia.
- There is micronodular cirrhosis of the liver, pancreatic damage from iron deposition leading to diabetes mellitus, and iron deposition in the skin, which makes the skin bronze-coloured, produces the so-called bronze diabetes. Iron accumulation in the heart leads to congestive cardiac failure and cardiac arrhythmias, and hypogonadism if iron is deposited in the gonads.
- The diagnosis can be made by the finding of raised serum iron levels, raised ferritin, and tissue biopsy with Persian blue stain, which demonstrates iron staining.

Alpha-1-antitrypsin deficiency

- An autosomal recessive disorder characterized by the production of defective α-1-antitrypsin, which accumulates in the hepatocytes and causes liver damage.
- The α-1-antitrypsin fails to reach the circulation and perform its normal function of preventing damage to the lung parenchyma, such that there is destruction leading to the development of emphysema.
- Alpha-1-antitrypsin is produced by the protease inhibitor (PI) gene on chromosome 14, and although there are over 70 PI genes described, the most common one accounts for 90% of cases. The most severe form is the homozygous state, which produces very severe disease with 15% or lower antitrypsin levels available.
- In the liver there is micronodular cirrhosis and an increased risk of hepatocellular carcinoma, and panacinar emphysema in the lungs.

Selected red blood cell pathology
Anaemias: microcytic anaemia
1. *Iron deficiency anaemia*

- Causes of iron deficiency anaemia:
  1. Reduced dietary intake—common in the elderly and in children.
  2. Reduced absorption, e.g. after gastrectomy or in malabsorptive states.
  3. Increased demand in pregnancy.
  4. Increased blood loss, e.g. in menorrhagia and GI pathology.
- Iron is found in haemoglobin, myoglobin, enzymes, and cytochromes and is stored as ferritin in the reticuloendothelial system and within macrophages. Serum ferritin is in equilibrium with macrophage ferritin, and is a good indicator for total body iron storage. Transferrin is a transport protein for iron and is associated with total iron binding capacity (TIBC).
- In iron deficiency anaemia, storage iron (i.e. ferritin) is reduced in the first instance, and then bone marrow iron is diminished within the macrophages. This is followed

by reduced circulating iron, partly because of increased output of the transport protein from the liver, so TIBC is increased and then there are small red blood cells with reduced MCV and MCHC.

2. *Thalassaemia*

This is characterized by a defect in the α- or β-globin chain of the haemoglobin.

a. α-thalassaemia:
- There are four α-globin chain genes on chromosome 16 and normal individuals have all four chains.
- α-thalassaemia is due to gene deletion, so there are four clinical disease states, the first three of which are: *silent carrier*—one gene deleted, so 75% of globin chains are produced with normal clinical functioning; *α-thalassaemia trait*—two genes deleted, so 50% α-chain production; *haemoglobin H disease*—three α-genes deleted, so only 25% α-chain production. Because of the deficiency of α-chains in this disease state, the abundant β-chains pair up to make haemoglobin H (β_4), which easily denatures and forms Heinz bodies detected on crystal blue stain. The final and most severe form is *hydrops fetalis*, when no α-chains are produced at all, with increased γ_4 (Bart's) haemoglobin resulting in hydrops fetalis and intra-uterine death.

b. β-thalassaemia:
- Two genes located on chromosome 11 make the two β-globin chains, and point mutation in either of them results in reduced or no β-chain production.
- The clinical states include *β-thalassaemia minor*, where one gene is knocked out. These patients are usually asymptomatic unless stressed either by infection or hypoxia. Haemoglobin electrophoresis will show raised haemoglobin A_2 and F. In *β-thalassaemia major*, where both genes are knocked out, the individuals are normal at birth as they are protected by haemoglobin F, but from 6 months of age, as haemoglobin F begins to decline, symptoms will emerge.
- There is usually severe haemolytic anaemia, jaundice, and gall stones. These patients will need repeated blood transfusions to survive. The majority will die in late teenage years from haemochromatosis. There may be erythroid hyperplasia with bony deformities. Haemoglobin electrophoresis will show reduced haemoglobin A and increased haemoglobin A_2 and F.

3. *Anaemia of chronic disease*

- This is characterized by macrophages holding down the iron and not releasing it to the bone marrow for red cell production. This happens because the chronic inflammation releases inflammatory cytokines, particularly IL-1, which increases lactoferrin, and lactoferrin in turn binds iron in macrophages. Iron studies in these patients show a reduction in iron indices except for a raised serum ferritin.

Anaemias: Macrocytic anaemia

Megaloblastic anaemia

- There is impaired DNA synthesis as a result of vitamin B_{12} and folate deficiency.
- Vitamin B_{12} is stored in the liver, and because liver storage may last for more than a year, deficiency states from dietary insufficiency are rare; however, they can occur in strict vegans.
- Other causes of B_{12} deficiency include reduced absorption from diseased or damaged stomach (parietal cells or intrinsic factor) and damage to the pancreas or the terminal ileum (where intrinsic factor-B_{12} complex is absorbed).
- The clinical signs include large, sore tongue, anaemia, and subacute combined degeneration of the spinal cord with loss of vibration and position sense.
- Diagnosis is made by the measurement of B_{12} in serum.
- Schilling test is used to exclude pernicious anaemia (antibodies against intrinsic factor, or B_{12}). A loading dose of B_{12} is injected to saturate the body sites first, and then radioactive B_{12} is given orally. If there is no intrinsic factor, the patient will not absorb the radioactive B_{12}, so cannot secrete radioactive B_{12} into the urine. In the second part of the test, B_{12} is given together with intrinsic factor to test whether the terminal ileum is working (corrected Schilling test).
- Treatment of B_{12} deficiency is with intramuscular injection of serum B_{12} and reticulocytosis may be expected within 5 to 7 days.
- Body storage of folic acid lasts for about one month only. Folate deficiency is common in elderly patients, alcoholics, malabsorption syndromes, increased requirements as in pregnancy, and decreased utilization, e.g. with methotrexate treatment. There are no neurological signs, but homocysteine level is increased. Treatment is with folate replacement.

Sickle cell anaemia

- Results from a single nucleotide change in the β-globin chain at position 6, where glutamic acid is replaced by valine.
- The heterozygous form (AS or SC trait) is usually asymptomatic until stress, such as high altitude or hypoxia, and this variant protects against malaria.
- The homozygous form (SS) is a severe condition in which the abnormal haemoglobin agglutinates when it becomes deoxygenated and changes the shape of the red blood cell. The red blood cells can no longer pass through the capillaries with ease, leading to infarction of tissues from microthrombi.
- Sickling is promoted by infection, dehydration, hypoxia, and low pH.
- Sickled RBCs are destroyed in the reticuloendothelial system leading to haemolytic anaemia, bone marrow hyperplasia, raised bilirubin, jaundice, and gall stones.

- Haemoglobin F and C improve the disease, so some treatment approaches include the administration of hydroxyuria, which increases the concentration of haemoglobin F.
- Vaso-occlusive crises occur as a result of hypoxia, dehydration, infection, or acidosis. The pains typically affect the bones and joints.
- Splenic infarction from repeated infarctions makes these patients highly susceptible to capsulated organisms including strep pneumonia and *Haemophilus influenzae*, and these patients need pneumovax and HIB vaccines.
- Acute chest syndrome is an emergency in which the sickled red cells get stuck in the pulmonary vasculature, presenting as shortness of breath.

Haemoglobin C disease

This is also a β-globin chain abnormality, with a point mutation also at position 6 in which glutamic acid is replaced by lysine. The patient presents with mild normochromic, normocytic anaemia and target cells in the peripheral blood.

Microangiopathic haemolytic anaemia (DIC, TTP, HUS)

- Haemolysis is due to traumatic fragmentation of RBCs in the vascular beds with intravascular thrombi formed as part of the DIC.
- Peripheral blood film will show schistocytes.
- In TTP-HUS there is formation of hyaline thrombi within the vasculature (platelets and fibrin stuck together without the activation of the coagulation cascade). If the coagulation cascade is activated, DIC would occur.

Glucose-6-phosphate dehydrogenase (G6PD) deficiency

- G6PD is the rate-limiting enzyme in the hexose monophosphate (HMP) shunt and this deficiency is the most common human enzyme defect.
- G6PD produces NADPH, which keeps glutathione in its reduced state (the antioxidant form), without which there would be oxidative stress from oxidant drugs, foods, or infection. Reduced-state glutathione breaks down H_2O_2.
- With G6PD deficiency there is a low level of reduced glutathione.
- The pathology involves an abnormality of the folding of the enzyme protein rather than a deficiency in the quantity of the enzyme G6PD produced.
- There are well over a hundred variants of G6PD including the very common A-type found in people of African origin, which usually presents with a mild and self-limiting acute haemolysis. The Mediterranean type is associated with acute and potentially fatal haemolysis, pallor, and jaundice, classically following ingestion of fava beans.

Hereditary spherocytosis

- This is an autosomal dominant disorder characterized by a defect in the cytoskeleton protein *spectrin*, which is responsible for keeping the RBC in its normal biconcave shape.
- Without spectrin the RBC becomes spherical, loses its central pallor, and is not as easily deformable. It is unstable in this state and unable to negotiate its way through capillaries.
- There is chronic haemolysis.
- The diagnosis is made with increased osmotic fragility.

Selected endocrine pathology

Multiple endocrine neoplasia syndrome (MENS)

- Autosomal dominant disorder characterized by hyperplasia and neoplasia of endocrine organs. There are three types: MENS 1, 2, and 3.
- In MENS 1, there is a genetic mutation in the MEN 1 gene, and the features include pituitary adenomas, parathyroid adenoma, pancreatic adenoma (usually an islet cell gastrin-producing tumour—gastrinoma), and peptic ulcer: the so-called 4Ps. The gastrinoma produces the Zollinger Ellison syndrome.
- In MENS 2, the genetic mutation is in the *RET proto-oncogene*. Features include medullary carcinoma of the thyroid (originating in the C-cells producing calcitonin, with raised calcium levels), parathyroid adenoma or hyperplasia, and pheochromocytomas.
- MENS 3 shares medullary carcinoma of the thyroid and pheochromocytoma with MENS 2 and in addition is characterized by neurofibromas or neuromas.

Selected bone and muscle pathology

Ankylosing spondylitis (AS)

- This is a seronegative (rheumatoid factor negative) arthropathy associated with HLA B27 (90% of cases) and usually affects young men.
- It affects the sacroiliac joints and the spine with fusion of the vertebrae.
- AS is associated with ulcerative colitis and other inflammatory bowel diseases.

Reiter's disease

- Classic triad of conjunctivitis, urethritis, and arthritis of the ankles and knees, often triggered by bacillary dysentery or sexually transmitted infections.
- Young men (age range 20–30 years) are more affected than women.

Duchenne's muscular dystrophy (most common and most severe muscular dystrophy)

- An X-linked inherited disorder, so affects males.
- The defect is in the dystrophin gene on the X chromosome, which makes dystrophin, an important structural protein of muscle.
- Mutation results in the absence of dystrophin.
- Affected individuals are normal at birth but there is progressive muscular weakness from about age 5, ascending in pattern, starting from the ankles and calves upwards.
- Once the diaphragm becomes involved there is respiratory insufficiency; recurrent infections ensue and subsequently death.

CHAPTER 8

Medical Microbiology

Classification of pathogenic micro-organisms

There are thousands of named species of micro-organisms but only a small fraction of these commonly cause human disease. These pathogens include bacteria, fungi, parasites, and viruses. A general classification of major pathogenic bacteria, fungi, viruses, and parasites are given in Tables 8.1–8.4, but simply:

- Bacteria are classified according to their shape and Gram-stain appearance, although some bacteria do not take up stain.

- Viruses are classified according to whether they are RNA or DNA viruses, and whether they are enveloped or non-enveloped.

- Fungi can be classified into yeasts (single-celled) and moulds (which form hyphae), although some pathogenic species can display different forms at different temperatures—the dimorphic fungi.

- Parasites include single-celled eukaryotic organisms (protozoa) and multi-celled higher animals (worms and flukes).

Bacteria

Morphology and structure of bacteria

Bacteria are free-living, single-celled, self-replicating micro-organisms. There are two major groups of bacteria:

- the Eubacteria, which include almost all known bacterial pathogens
- the Archaebacteria, which are often adapted to extreme environments (e.g. the bottoms of lakes, or hot springs) but do not seem to play a pathogenic role.

They are classified as prokayotes—that is, they have a relatively simple intracellular structure, with no mitochondria, plastids, Golgi apparatus, or intracellular membrane system, and no separate nucleus.

Bacteria are generally either spherical (cocci) or elongated and rod-like (bacilli); bacilli may be curved or spiral. They are usually one to several microns in length and so are visible by light microscopy, unlike viruses. Bacterial cytoplasm contains a single chromosome, several thousand ribosomes, and possibly storage granules of glycogen or other compounds. Many bacteria also have free circular elements of DNA known as plasmids.

- The bacterial cell envelope consists of a cell membrane, as in eukaryotes, surrounded by a cell wall, which eukaryotes lack. The cell membrane consists of a phospholipid bilayer, with many embedded membrane proteins (Figure 8.1).

- The membrane is relatively impermeable, even to hydrogen ions, and the membrane proteins control transport of nutrients, waste products, and other molecules into and out of the cell. The energy for these processes, when they occur against a concentration gradient, is derived from a hydrogen ion (or proton) gradient across the membrane; this proton gradient is in turn maintained by the breakdown of high-energy substrates such as glucose or (in photosynthetic bacteria) by utilization of sunlight.

- The cell wall gives rigidity to the bacterium and enables it to withstand the osmotic pressure generated by the active transport of various molecules into the cell (this pressure can be considerable, estimated as several times atmospheric pressure).

- There are two main groups of bacteria, based on the composition of the underlying cell wall structure: the Gram-positive and Gram-negative bacteria. The name derives from a common stain used for diagnostic microscopy: the Gram stain or Gram reaction (Figure 8.2). Gram-positive organisms retain violet dye stain because of their thick (20–80 nm peptidoglycan), less permeable external layer. Gram-negative organisms lose the violet dye and take up a red counter-stain applied after washing with alcohol because of their thinner (5–10 nm peptidoglycan) layer, which is overlaid by an outer membrane of lipopolysaccharide and lipoproteins. A few bacterial

Table 8.1 Simple classification of medically important bacteria

Gram stain	Shape	Major groups (Genera)	Clinically important species
Gram positive	Rod	Bacillus	B. cereus
			B. anthracis
		Listeria	L. monocytogenes
		Corynebacteria	C. diphtheriae
		Clostridium	Clostridium perfringens
			C. tetani
			C. botulinum
	Coccus—in clusters	Staphylococcus	Staphylococcus aureus
			S. epidermidis
	Coccus—in chains or pairs	Streptococcus	Streptococcus pyogenes
			S. agalactiae
			S. milleri
			S. pneumoniae
		Enterococcus	Enterococcus faecalis
			E. faecium
Gram negative	Rod	Enterobacteriaceae	Escherischia coli
			Proteus spp.
			Klebsiella spp.
			Enterobacter spp.
			Serratia spp.
		Pseudomonas	Pseudomonas aeruginosa
			P. cepacia
		Haemophilus	Haemophilus influenzae
			H. ducreyi
		Brucella	Brucella abortus
			B. melitensis
	Coccus	Neisseria	N. meningitides
			N. gonorrhoea
Not seen by Gram stain		Mycobacteria	M. tuberculosis
			M. bovis
			M. leprae
			M. avium-intracellulare
		Mycoplasma	Mycoplasma pneumoniae
			M. hominis
		Ureaplasma	Ureaplasma urealyticum
		Chlamydia	Chlamydia trachomatis
			C. pneumoniae
		Treponema	Treponema pallidum

species are 'Gram-variable' and show a mixture of the two types of cell.

- Both types of cell wall are predominately composed of peptidoglycan, a polymer of sugar (glycan) chains, cross-linked by amino acids (peptides). Peptidoglycan is the principal molecular target of the beta-lactam group of antibiotics (penicillins and cephalosporins).

- The Gram-positive cell wall is relatively thick, with poly-saccharides known as teichoic acids attached to the outer surface.

- The Gram-negative cell wall is much thinner, and is in turn surrounded by a second membrane—the outer membrane or lipopolysaccharide layer. This is composed of a phospholipid bilayer, like the inner membrane, but it also contains lipoproteins and lipopolysaccharides anchored to the membrane.

- The lipopolysaccharides of the Gram-negative outer membrane in particular are toxic to humans and animals, and constitute the 'endotoxin' of Gram-negative organisms. The outer membrane also contains porins—proteins that control the passage of molecules into and out of the cell.

- Many bacteria (especially bacilli and spiral organisms) are motile, due to the presence of flagella—spiral whip-like structures formed of a single type of protein, flagellin, which are anchored on the (inner) membrane, and

Table 8.2 Simplified classification of pathogenic viruses

Nucleic acid	Envelope present	Subgroups	Clinically important species
DNA viruses	Enveloped	Pox viruses	Smallpox virus Vaccinia virus
		Herpes viruses	Herpes simplex virus I & II Varicella-zoster virus Cytomegalovirus Epstein-Barr virus
	Non-enveloped	Hepadnaviridae	Hepatitis B virus
		Adenoviruses	Human adenovirus
		Papovaviruses	Human papillomavirus BK & JC virus
		Parvovirus	Parvovirus B19
RNA viruses	Enveloped	Togaviridae	Rubella virus
		Flaviviridae	Yellow fever virus
		Coronavirus	Human coronavirus
		Paramyxoviruses	Mumps virus Parainfluenza virus Measles virus Respiratory syncytial virus (RSV)
		Rhabdoviruses	Rabies virus
		Orthomyxoviruses	Influenza virus (A, B, & C)
		Bunyaviruses	Hantavirus
		Retroviruses	HIV I & II HTLV I & 2
	Non-enveloped	Picornaviruses	Enteroviruses (including coxsackie & polio viruses) Hepatitis A virus Rhinovirus
		Caliciviruses	Norovirus

extend outside the cell. The membrane anchor, or basal body, functions as a turbine motor powered by the membrane proton gradient; this spins the flagellum like a propeller and generates movement.

- Flagella can be arranged in a number of ways; some bacteria have a single unipolar flagellum, some are covered in flagella (peritrichous), and some have a tuft of flagella at one end (lophotrichous).
- Gram-negative bacteria also have other hair-like structures known as fimbriae, composed of protein, which are shorter than flagella but much more numerous. They are involved in adhesion to inert surfaces and other cells, and many play an important role in virulence.
- Many bacteria are surrounded by a capsule or slime layer, also known as the glycocalyx. This is composed of different sugar polymers and it is thought to assist in binding to host tissues, confer resistance to phagocytosis, and possibly prevent drying out.

Growth and metabolism of bacteria

Bacteria multiply by binary fission, and when nutrients are plentiful some species can divide extremely rapidly—every 10 minutes for *Clostridium pefringens*, and every 30 minutes for *E. coli*. Some bacteria, especially the *Mycobacteria*, grow much more slowly, with a generation time of 15–20 hours.

Experiments where bacteria are inoculated into liquid nutrient media show four phases of growth:

1. an initial *lag phase*, where the bacteria prepare for replication and growth
2. a *logarithmic* or *exponential growth phase*
3. when the supply of nutrients and other requirements of metabolism such as oxygen becomes limited and waste products accumulate, the organisms enter the *static phase*, where growth is limited and balanced by the death of some cells
4. finally, when the nutrient supply is exhausted and deaths exceed growth, the number of viable cells declines—the *death phase*.

The potential for rapid exponential growth allows bacteria to quickly colonize any available ecological niche, but for most bacteria in their natural state, nutrients are limited and they exist in a static phase of growth.

Table 8.3 Simplified classification of pathogenic fungi

Major groups	Subgroups/genera	Pathogenic species	Typical disease
Yeasts & yeast-like fungi (always or predominately single-celled)	Candida	Candida albicans C. tropicalis C. glabrata	Vaginal or oral thrush Invasive candidiasis Candida endophthalmitis
	Cryptococcus	Cryptococcus neoformans	Meningitis in the immunocompromised
	Pneumocystis	Pneumocystis carinii (recently renamed P. jiroveci)	Pneumonia in the immunocompromised
Moulds (always or predominately form a mycelium)	Aspergillus	Aspergillus fumigatus A. flavus A. niger	Invasive aspergillosis
	Mucorales	Rhizopus spp. Rhizomucor spp. Mucor spp.	Mucormycosis/zygomycosis
	Dermatophytes: Trichophyton, Epidermophyton, & Microsporum	Trichophyton rubrum Epidermophyton floccosum Microsporum canis	Tinea pedis (athlete's foot) Tinea capitis (scalp ringworm) Tinea corporis (body ringworm) Onychomycosis (fungal nail infection)
Dimorphic fungi (yeast or mould form, according to temperature and conditions of growth)	Histoplasma	Histoplasma capsulatum	Pulmonary and systemic infections
	Coccidioides	Coccidioides immitis	
	Paracoccidioides	Paracoccidioides brasiliensis	
	Blastomyces	Blastomyces dermatitidis	
	Sporothrix	Sporothrix schenkii	Sporotrichosis

- Some bacteria can suspend growth and metabolism entirely when faced with adverse conditions, and form an extremely tough and resistant spore. Such spore-formers include *Bacillus* (e.g. *B. anthracis*, the cause of anthrax) and *Clostridia* (e.g. *C. difficile*, a cause of antibiotic-associated diarrhoea). Bacterial spores can withstand boiling at 100°C, and can survive for many months or even years.

- Bacterial growth requirements vary for each species: all require sources of carbon, iron (an essential component of cytochromes, catalase, and other enzymes), nitrogen, sulphur, phosphate, magnesium, sodium, and potassium ions, as well as trace elements.

- Each species has an optimum growth temperature range; most pathogenic bacteria are adapted to grow in or on animal hosts, and thus have optimum growth temperatures between 20°C and 40°C (mesophiles). A small number of pathogens are normally environmental organisms adapted to lower temperatures (psychrophiles)—these organisms, for example *Listeria monocytogenes*, can grow on refrigerated food.

Bacteria vary in their need for, and ability to deal with, oxygen. This element, with its high electron affinity, has the potential to form toxic radicals ($\bullet OH$, O_2^-) but is also needed as a final electron acceptor in oxidative phosphorylation (or respiration), which is the most efficient way to obtain usable energy from sugar substrates. The enzymes catalase and superoxide dismutase convert the superoxide radical into harmless H_2O and O_2. Thus, four groups of bacteria can be considered, according to their use of oxygen:

1. Obligate anaerobes: Do not use oxygen in respiration and lack the means to deal with toxic oxygen radicals; only thrive where oxygen is very low or absent. Examples include Actinomyces, Bacteroides, and Clostridium. Many gut and oral organisms are anaerobes and play a role in infections of these sites.

2. Microaerophilic organisms: Possess *superoxide dismutase* but not *catalase*, and so can handle low levels of oxygen but do not carry out respiration. Includes gut pathogens such as *Campylobacter*, and oral *Streptococci*.

3. Facultative anaerobes: Possess *catalase* and *superoxide dismutase*, and thus tolerate oxygen. Can carry out respiration if oxygen is present but can still generate energy by fermentation in the absence of oxygen. This group includes *Staphylococci* and the gut-dwelling Enterobacteriaceae.

4. Obligate aerobes: Need oxygen and carry out respiration. They cannot carry out any energy-generating reactions in the absence of oxygen and so need oxygen for growth. Examples include *Pseudomonas* and the *Mycobacteria*.

Bacteria have a diverse range of biochemical pathways to allow a variety of substrates to be used as energy sources, including sugars, amino acids, and lipids. These pathways can be broadly divided into:

1. *Fermentation*—exemplified by the breakdown of glucose by the Embden-Meyerhof pathway, which provides a low yield of ATP and NADH, and can lead (via pyruvate) to

Table 8.4 Simplified classification of common pathogenic parasites

Major groups	Subgroups	Examples of pathogenic species (common name in parentheses if appropriate)	Typical disease
Protozoa (single-celled)	Intestinal protozoa	*Entamoeba histolytica* *Giardia lamblia* *Balantidium coli* *Cryptosporidium parvum*	Dysentery Gastroenteritis
	Blood or tissue protozoa	*Plasmodium* spp. *(falciparum, vivax, ovale, malariae)* *Trypanosoma* spp. *Leishmania* spp. *Toxoplasma*	Malaria Sleeping sickness Chaga's disease Kala-Azar Cutaneous leishmaniasis Toxoplasmosis
	Urogenital protozoa	*Trichomonas vaginalis*	Vaginitis
	Other protozoa	*Naegleria fowleri* *Acanthamoeba*	Meningitis Keratitis
Helminths (worms etc.)	Cestodes (tapeworms)	*Taenia sagatina* (beef tapeworm) *Taenia solium* (pork tapeworm) *Diphyllobothrium latum* (fish tapeworm) *Echinococcus granulosus* (hydatid tapeworm)	Intestinal tapeworm infestation Hydatid disease
	Trematodes (Flukes)	*Fasciola hepatica* (liver fluke) *Paragonimus westermanii* (lung fluke) *Schistosoma* spp. *(mansoni, haematobium, japonicum)* (blood flukes)	Liver/Lung fluke infestation Schistosomiasis
	Nematodes (roundworms)	*Trichinella spiralis* *Trichuris trichura* (whipworm) *Ascaris lumbricoides* *Necator americanus* & *Ancylostoma duodenale* (hookworms) *Enterobius vermicularis* (pinworm or threadworm) *Strongyloides stercoralis* *Wuchereria bancrofti* *Onchocerca volvulus* *Dracunculus medinensis* (Guinea worm)	Intestinal roundworm infestation Tissue roundworm infestation
Ectoparasites (external parasites, living on or in skin)	Lice	*Pediculus humanus var corposis* (human body louse) *Pediculus humanus var capitis* (human head louse) *Phthirus pubis* (pubic/crab louse)	Infestation of the body/ head/pubic area Body louse may also spread other bacterial infections such as typhus
	Fleas	*Pulex irritans* (human flea)	Bites (plague etc. spread by other species of flea)
	Mites	*Sarcoptes scabei*	Scabies

the typical fermentation products of ethanol, lactic acid, or acetic acid.

2. *Respiration*—which involves the further breakdown of pyruvate by the Krebs cycle, generating CO_2 and NADH. High-energy electrons from NADH are then transferred along a series of carrier molecules, which are embedded in the cell membrane. The energy from these transfers is coupled to the generation of a proton gradient across the cell membrane. This proton gradient is then used to generate ATP, as well as to drive active transport across the membrane. The final electron acceptor is usually oxygen but in some cases it is another compound such as nitrate or sulphate.

Bacterial genetics

The bacterial chromosome is circular, usually contains one to several million base pairs, and is elaborately folded and coiled to fit inside the cell.

● Plasmids (separate DNA molecules) typically carry genes for features that allow the organism to exploit a specific environment, such as resistance to antibiotics or other

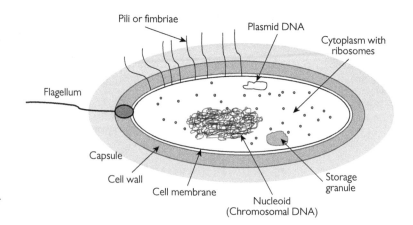

Figure 8.1 Typical bacterial cell. Adapted from an image by Dr Peter Riley with permission.

toxic substances, a colonization or virulence factor, or the ability to use an unusual substrate. They seldom code for essential functions of the organism.

- Bacteria can exchange DNA and acquire (or lose) genes by varied means:
  1. **Transformation:** Many bacteria can take up free DNA (released by dying organisms, not necessarily of the same species) from the extracellular environment.
  2. **Transduction:** DNA can also be transferred from one bacterium to another by means of viruses that infect bacteria (bacteriophages).

3. **Conjugation:** Bacteria can exchange DNA directly (usually plasmids) by forming a long protein structure, the sex pilus, which binds two cells and allows a conjugal bridge to form, through which DNA can pass. This occurs most frequently with Gram-negative organisms and allows genes coding for antibiotic resistance (for example) to spread rapidly.

Bacterial pathogenesis

The first step in causing disease is to reach and gain entry to the host. Bacteria are rarely able to penetrate intact skin and usually enter by a mucosal surface (respiratory

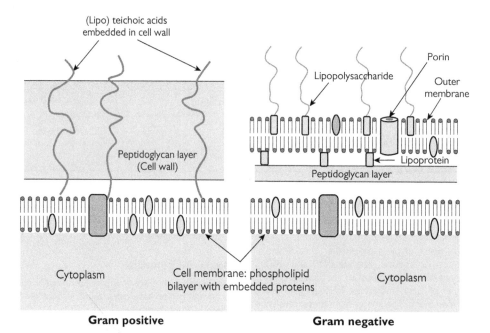

Figure 8.2 Comparison of Gram-positive and Gram-negative bacterial cell walls. Adapted from an image by Dr Peter Riley with permission.

or genital), are ingested, or are inoculated as a result of surgery, injection, or trauma.

- Slime capsules and fimbriae can function as bacterial virulence factors, assisting colonization of the host or immune evasion.
- Many bacteria secrete compounds (usually proteins) that have toxic effects on the host, such as staphylococcal toxic shock toxin, diphtheria toxin, tetanus toxin, and the cholera enterotoxin. These are known as exotoxins to make the distinction from Gram-negative endotoxins, which are the lipopolysaccharide portion of the outer membrane, and are not actively secreted but released when the organism dies.

Host defences against infection

Host defences can be considered in terms of immune and non-immune defences; immune defences can then be further divided into innate immunity and acquired immunity. Non-immune defences are often overlooked and include physical and chemical factors, summarized in Table 8.5.

Normal flora and pathogens

Most skin and mucosal surfaces have resident bacteria, which can range from a few thousand organisms per cm^2 of skin to 10^{11} organisms per gram of faeces. These bacteria are generally harmless and they play an important role in resisting colonization of the skin and mucosa by other, potentially pathogenic micro-organisms. Removal or alteration of the microflora, for example by antibiotic use, may render the host vulnerable to infection by low-virulence organisms such as *Candida* or enterococci, or by *Clostridium difficile*.

Diagnosis of bacterial infection

Bacteria are visible by light microscopy. Shape and Gram-staining characteristics can be easily determined, and they can be grown on solid agar-based media, forming visible

Table 8.5 Non-immune factors contributing to defence against infection

Physical	Chemical
Integrity of skin	Lysozyme (tears, sweat, urine)
Ciliary action in airways	Gastric acid
Cough and gag reflexes	Fatty acids from sebaceous glands
Flow of urine and tears	

colonies from a single organism after overnight culture (in most cases—*Mycobacteria* being the notable exception). These properties are the mainstay of initial diagnostic techniques, but different combinations of tests are used for different sample types.

- For samples from sites with a heavy normal flora (for example faeces, or mouth swabs) microscopy may not be useful, as one would find bacteria in any case. Exceptions are cases where there is obvious clinical infection and plentiful pus or infected materiel—microscopy may then suggest the likely pathogen or disease, for example a urethral discharge that reveals numerous Gram-negative diplococci is likely to be gonorrhoea, or a vaginal swab that contains many bacteria-studded epithelial cells ('clue cells') suggests bacterial vaginosis.
- Microscopy is more useful in samples that are normally sterile, such as CSF or joint fluid—any bacteria seen are likely to be significant.
- Culture of bacteria can be on agar or in liquid (broth) media. Liquid culture is more sensitive, and is appropriate for samples that are normally sterile, or where infecting bacteria may be scanty, for example blood cultures. Liquid culture is, however, more prone to contamination.
- Agar-based media can be broadly categorized as:
  - enriched/unenriched
  - selective/unselective
  - differential/undifferential.
- Enriched media, for example chocolate agar (which contains red blood cells heated until they lyse and release their nutrients; it does *not* contain any chocolate), are suitable for growing fastidious organisms (i.e. bacteria that grow only in specially fortified artificial culture media) such as *Haemophilus* or *Neisseria*.
- Selective media contain compounds that inhibit the growth of some (non-pathogenic) bacteria, increasing the chance that the pathogens of interest will be recognized. Such media are often used for faeces and genital samples to help distinguish pathogens from the normal flora.
- Differential media contain colour indicators so that different types of bacteria produce different coloured colonies, aiding early recognition. Many of the media used in faeces culture are both selective and differential.

Once grown, pathogenic bacteria are usually further identified to genus or species level by simple biochemical or serological tests, and antibiotic susceptibilities can also be determined (usually by agar disc methods).

Common pathogenic bacteria

Staphylococci

These are Gram-positive cocci, which grow in clumps or clusters.

- They include the potential pathogen *S. aureus* (which is carried harmlessly in the noses of 30% of the population) and less virulent skin *Staphylococci*, including *S. epidermidis*.

- They are distinguished in the lab by the fact that *S. aureus* produces a coagulase enzyme, causing serum to clot; thus, other *Staphylococci* are sometimes referred to as 'coagulase-negative *Staphylococci*'.
- *S. aureus* causes skin and soft tissue infections such as cellulitis, boils, and surgical wound infection, and it can also cause bacteraemia, endocarditis, and osteomyelitis.
- *S. aureus* produces exotoxins, which can cause food poisoning, and also staphylococcal toxic shock syndrome, seen in tampon-users, where the vagina gets infected with *S. aureus* and the toxin is absorbed systemically.
- Most *S. aureus* (>90%) are resistant to penicillin by means of beta-lactamase production, but can still be treated with flucloxacillin, which is not degraded by the beta-lactamase. Some *S. aureus* have a mutant penicillin-binding protein in the cell wall (pbp 2a), which renders it resistant to all beta-lactam antibiotics. This is referred to as methicillin-resistant *S. aureus*, or MRSA. These organisms can still be treated with several other antibiotics, including vancomycin.

Streptococci and *Enterococci*

Streptococci and *Enterococci* are Gram-positive cocci that normally grow in chains, or sometimes pairs. Classification of these organisms often confuses the student. Each has its own proper species name, but they are also categorized first by their appearance when grown on blood agar; thus there are:

- Beta-haemolytic *Streptococci* (which cause complete haemolysis of the red cells in the agar), alpha-haemolytic *Streptococci* (which cause partial lysis and thus green/brown discoloration of the agar), and gamma-haemolytic *Streptococci* (which cause no lysis at all). The alpha-haemolytic *Streptococci* are also known as viridans *Streptococci*.
- Beta-haemolytic *Streptococci* are further categorized according to the particular sugar-compounds on their outer cell surface—the Lancefield Group. Lancefield Groups are often used interchangeably with species names. Thus, Group A beta-haemolytic *Streptococci* are equivalent to *S. pyogenes*, and Group B beta-haemolytic *Streptococci* equate to *S. agalactiae* (a significant cause of neonatal sepsis).
- *Enterococci* were formerly known as 'faecal streps', being found in the gut, but they are genetically a separate group and belong to Lancefield Group D. The *Streptococci* are generally susceptible to penicillin or amoxicillin; *Enterococci* tend to be more resistant, and some may even be resistant to vancomycin.

Nocardia and *Actinomyces*

These are both branching Gram-positive rods, which may cause spreading or disseminated infection.

- *Nocardia* is aerobic, and is also (weakly) acid-fast (see '*Mycobacteria*' section below). It is normally an environmental organism and tends to infect the immunocompromised or those with chronic lung disease. Typical diseases are brain abscess and persisting suppurative lung infection. The most common species is *N. asteroides*.
- *Actinomyces* (commonest species: *A. israelii*) are anaerobic, not acid-fast, and may colonize and infect the mouths of those with poor dentition. Infections are usually secondary to oral colonization and include cervicofacial abscesses, and aspiration or swallowing of organisms leading to thoracic, abdominal, and disseminated disease. There is no strong association with immunosuppression. Pus from these lesions often contains 'sulphur granules', which consist of a mycelial mass and may be up to a few mm in size.

Aerobic Gram-positive bacilli

Corynebacteria are aerobic, and include *C. diphtheriae*. This often carries a bacteriophage that codes for a potent exotoxin, which causes the illness diphtheria.

- The toxin is a classic subunit toxin: the beta-unit binds to host cells and the alpha-unit is released into the cytoplasm, where it switches off protein production leading to cell death.
- The illness begins as pharyngitis and the effects of the toxin are first seen in local upper airway tissues, and later in the heart and nervous tissue.
- A potent vaccine made from inactivated toxin means this illness is now very rare in the developed world.

Other *Corynebacteria* are less virulent and typically live on the skin; they are frequent contaminants of blood cultures. *Listeria monocytogenes* is widely distributed in the environment and is mainly a soil-dwelling aerobe, which can also be carried asymptomatically in the gastrointestinal tract of humans and many animal species.

- It can contaminate processed meats, dairy foods, and salads during preparation.
- It can grow at wide ranges of pH (5.6–9.6) and temperature (1–45°C), and thus can multiply in refrigerated food.
- The infection is usually harmless to healthy adults but it can cause meningitis in the immunocompromised and the elderly.
- In pregnancy it can cross the placenta to infect the fetus, resulting in miscarriage, preterm delivery, or term delivery of a baby with septicaemia or meningitis. Pregnant women are advised to avoid certain high-risk foods, pâté and soft cheeses in particular.
- Ampicillin is considered the drug of choice for treatment.

Bacillus spp. are a large group of aerobic spore-forming environmental organisms, mostly harmless. Exceptions are *B. cereus*, which can cause food poisoning (typically associated with reheated rice), and *B. anthracis*, the cause of anthrax.

Enterobacteriaceae and *Pseudomonas*

The Enterobacteriaceae are a large group of related Gram-negative rods that typically live in the gut. The most commonly encountered member is *Escherischia coli*; other examples are given in Table 8.1.

- They cause a similar range of infections, from uncomplicated urinary tract infections (rarely, with associated septicaemia) and hospital-acquired pneumonia, to post-operative pelvic and abdominal infections.
- They are all facultative anaerobes and are distinguished from each other by a range of biochemical tests, the simplest of which is lactose fermentation (*E. coli* ferments lactose; most of the remainder don't).
- All are penicillin resistant; many are resistant to ampicillin, and some carry genes for 'extended-spectrum beta-lactamases' (ESBLs), which confer resistance to a wide range of antibiotics.
- *Pseudomonas* cause similar infections to Enterobacteriaceae but are more antibiotic-resistant, and more likely to be found in hospitals than the community. They are obligate aerobes and can be distinguished from the Enterobacteriaceae by producing a positive oxidase test.

Neisseriae

Neisseriae are aerobic Gram-negative cocci, typically found in pairs; they grow best with added CO_2 and are oxidase positive. There are several species, distinguished by their use of different sugars; the two pathogenic species are *N. meningitidis* and *N. gonorrhoeae*.

- *N. meningitidis* causes meningococcal sepsis and meningitis; it is spread by respiratory droplets and saliva.
- There are several serogroups based on capsular polysaccharide; A, B, and C are the most common, and a vaccine against Serogroup C is now widely used in the UK. The organism remains penicillin sensitive and this is the agent of choice.
- *N. gonorrhoeae* causes gonorrhoea, acute pelvic inflammatory disease, rarely septicaemia and septic arthritis, and ophthalmia neonatorum in babies born to mothers with active genital disease.
- The organism is fastidious, susceptible to drying out or cooling, and has complex nutritional requirements, needing special enriched media to grow.
- Spread is sexual, and the usual site of infections in females is the endocervix, and the urethra in males.
- Antibiotic resistance, particularly to penicillin and also quinolones, is common.

Haemophilus

- The main pathogenic species, *Haemophilus influenzae*, is a small Gram-negative rod. It is nutritionally fastidious, needing haemin (X-factor) and nicotinamide (V-factor) for growth; this is the basis of laboratory identification.

- *H. influenzae* causes chest infections, especially in smokers, and capsulate Type b strains can cause serious invasive disease in non-immunized young children, including meningitis and epiglottitis. There is a non-typeable *H. influenzae* (NTHI), which has no capsule.
- The other important *Haemophilus* is *H. ducreyi*, the causative agent of chancroid (soft ulcer).

Anaerobic organisms

Anaerobes are a diverse group of organisms, most of which are Gram-negative rods living in the gut or oral cavity.

- The most common anaerobes encountered clinically are *Bacteroides fragilis* (commonest organism in the colon) and related species, *Prevotella*, *Porphyromonas*, *Fusobacteria* (which have a characteristic fusiform shape) and the *Clostridia*.
- The *Clostridia* are distinguished by being spore-forming Gram-positive rods, often soil-dwelling.
- Some *Clostridia* give rise to specific clinical syndromes—toxin-related in the case of tetanus (from *C. tetani*) and botulism (*C. botulinum*), and also gas gangrene caused by *C. perfringens* infection of damaged tissue.
- The other anaerobes are typically found as part of mixed bowel bacteria in intra-abdominal infections, and occasionally in lung, brain, and liver abscesses. Apart from the *Clostridia*, the other anaerobes are difficult to identify, and most general diagnostic laboratories only identify them as unspecified anaerobes by their inability to grow in air and susceptibility to metronidazole.

Mycobacteria

These are related to the Gram-positive bacteria, but the presence of waxy lipid compounds in their cell walls means they do not take up the Gram stain. They need to be heated to allow stain to penetrate, and the stain is retained despite washing with alcohol or acid—the origin of the acid-fast stain. Two common forms of this stain are the Ziehl-Neilsen stain and the Auramine stain.

- *Mycobacteria* grow very slowly compared to other bacteria, and thus diagnostic cultures may take several weeks. Traditionally Lowenstein-Jensen media was used, but many laboratories have now switched to using automated broth culture systems.
- Important species include *M. tuberculosis*, *M. bovis* (the cause of bovine tuberculosis), *Bacille-Calmette-Guerin* (the BCG vaccine strain), *M. leprae* (the cause of leprosy, and non-cultivable), and also *Mycobacterium avium-intracellulare*, which causes opportunistic infections in patients with advanced HIV.

Treponema and other spiral bacteria

Treponema pallidum is a long, slender, coiled bacterium, the cause of syphilis. Related treponemal strains cause endemic non-venereal syphilis, yaws (*T. pallidum pertenue*), and pinta (*T. carateum*).

- The organism cannot be cultured (except using animals, which is not practicable in a routine laboratory) and so serological tests are used for diagnosis.
- The serological tests are divided into those that detect antibodies to specific treponemal antigens, and those that detect non-specific antigens ('lipoidal', 'reagin', or 'non-treponemal'). The specific tests are useful to detect evidence of treponemal infection at some time, and specific IgM assays can point to recent infection. However, these specific tests cannot distinguish old but still active disease from inactive disease, which is where the reagin tests are useful—the level of reagin antibody correlates with disease activity. The classic reagin test is the 'Venereal Disease Reference Laboratory' test—the VDRL.
- Treponemes can sometimes be visualized directly, in lesions of primary and secondary syphilis (see below), using phase-contrast or dark-ground microscopy.
- Venereal syphilis has three stages:
  1. *Primary syphilis* is marked by a painless ulcer (chancre) at the site of inoculation (usually genital); this then heals.
  2. Some weeks later there is a generalized fever and rash, associated with systemic dissemination of the treponemes throughout the body (*secondary syphilis*). This resolves, but some patients go on to develop latent syphilis.
  3. After several years this latent syphilis presents as progressive vascular or neurological disease (*tertiary syphilis*).
- Mothers with primary or latent infection may spread the infection haematogenously through the placenta to their babies, resulting in *congenital syphilis*. Affected babies may be stillborn, or survive but are born with the systemic (i.e. secondary) phase of syphilis.

Borrelia

- This is another group of spiral bacteria.
- *B. burgdorferi* is carried by *Ixodes* ticks, which usually infect deer.
- Infection results in Lyme disease, characterized by an initial rash at the site of the tick bite (erythema chronicum migrans) followed by chronic neurological or bone/joint problems; a common manifestation is isolated Bell's palsy.
- Culture of the organism is difficult and serology is used for diagnosis.

Leptospira interrogans

- This is another pathogenic spiral organism.
- It is excreted in rodent urine, and thus often contaminates drains, canals, sewers etc.
- Humans with occupational or recreational contact with such water may become infected and develop leptospirosis.

- This varies in severity; the most severe form (Weil's disease) is characterized by fever and liver and renal failure. There may also be meningitis and myocarditis.

Mycoplasma, Rickettsia, and related organisms

Mycoplasma

- These organisms are unusual among bacteria in having no cell wall. Therefore, antibiotics that inhibit cell wall synthesis, e.g. penicillin and cephalosporin, will be ineffective in *Mycoplasma* infections.
- Mycoplasmas grow slowly on routine media; colonies are small and easily missed. Colonies are often glassy in appearance and may have an opaque central zone, giving rise to a 'fried egg' appearance.
- *M. pneumoniae* causes 'atypical' pneumonia, generally less severe and less acute than pneumococcal disease. It is the most common cause of pneumonia in young adults.
- *Ureaplasma urealyticum* (characterized by the presence of a urease enzyme, allowing it to metabolize urea) has been implicated in respiratory and other infections of neonates. However, its exact role is unproven, as is the role of *Ureaplasma* and other mycoplasmas such as *M. hominis* and *M. genitalium* in a variety of urogenital infections.

Rickettsia

- These organisms are obligate intracellular parasitic bacteria.
- They generally have an arthropod vector (ticks, mites, fleas, or lice) to aid spread between hosts, and include the agents of typhus and spotted fevers.
- Multiplication occurs in capillaries, leading to vasculitis.
- Because they cannot grow outside a host cell, diagnosis is by serology.
- They are resistant to the penicillins and treatment is usually with a tetracycline.

Q-fever

- This is due to infection with another intracellular bacterium, *Coxiella burnetti*.
- Livestock animals are often the source, and infections are seen in farmers and abattoir workers. There may be a risk of adverse outcome in pregnancy, though this is probably low.

Chlamydia

- These are obligate intracellular bacteria—they cannot generate their own ATP and must obtain this from their host.
- They exist in two forms: the elementary body is the small infective form taken up by a host cell; this then reorganizes into the reticulate body, which replicates and eventually fills the cell (giving rise to the inclusion body seen on microscopy). These then convert into elementary bodies and are released (or the cell lyses).

- There are three main species: *C. psittaci* causes severe pneumonia—psittacosis—and is usually acquired from pet birds. *C. pneumoniae* is a purely human pathogen and causes a milder pneumonia. *C. trachomatis* has different biotypes or strains: LGV causes lymphogranuloma venereum, spread sexually, while the 'trachoma' group, comprising several serovars or subgroups, cause ocular and genital infections. Ocular infections include trachoma, found in tropical areas and spread by flies, and inclusion conjunctivitis, which can affect the newborn (direct spread from an infected mother) or occasionally adults (autoinoculation from genital lesions). Genital infections are spread sexually and are frequently asymptomatic, which facilitates onward transmission. They include urethritis (men), cervicitis, and occasionally pelvic inflammatory disease, which can lead to scarring of the uterus or Fallopian tubes, with risk of infertility, miscarriage, or ectopic pregnancy (women).
- *Chlamydia* cannot be grown on solid media. Cell culture is possible but difficult, and diagnosis is usually by enzyme immunoassay detection of antigen, or (more recently) by amplification of nucleic acid, which has the advantage of being able to use urine rather than cervical or urethral swabs.

Viruses

Viruses are much smaller and biochemically simpler than bacteria; they range from approximately 20 to 250 nm in size. They lack the cellular machinery for independent growth and replication outside a host cell. All animals, plants, protozoa, and even bacteria can be infected by different viruses.

Viral structure

Typically, a virus consists of nucleic acid (either DNA or RNA, but not both) surrounded by a protein coat (capsid). This capsid is composed of repeating protein subunits called capsomeres. The virus particle consisting of nuclear materiel and capsid is sometimes referred to as the nucleocapsid.

- The nucleic acid may be single- or double-stranded.
- There is no cytoplasm.
- There may be other proteins within the capsid that are associated with DNA/RNA replication.
- In most viruses (except the large poxviruses) the capsid has a strict geometric arrangement, either *icosahedral*, with 20 sides formed of equilateral triangles, or *helical*, with the capsomeres attached to the coiled nucleic acid.
- Viruses consisting only of the viral genome and capsid are classified as *naked* or *non-enveloped*. If there is an additional outer covering of lipid and/or protein membrane surrounding the genome and protein coat, then the virus is classified as an *enveloped* virus (Figure 8.3).
- Enveloped viruses are susceptible to environmental conditions because the lipids in the envelope are targets for agents such as detergents. Naked viruses, on the other hand, are less susceptible and more resistant.

Virus replication and other consequences of virus infection of cells

Viruses must enter (or at least their DNA/RNA must enter) the host cell in order to initiate their own replication. In the case of viruses infecting animal cells, the virus first adheres to the target cell, perhaps by binding to a specific receptor molecule (adsorption). It then enters the cell by endocytosis

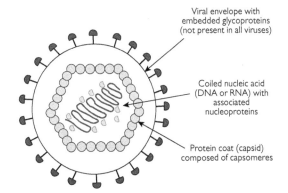

Viral envelope with embedded glycoproteins (not present in all viruses)

Coiled nucleic acid (DNA or RNA) with associated nucleoproteins

Protein coat (capsid) composed of capsomeres

Figure 8.3 Structure of a typical virus. Many viruses lack the lipid membrane or envelope. Adapted from an image by Dr Peter Riley with permission.

(penetration), and the envelope (if present) and capsid are removed to release the viral genome. What happens next depends on the particular virus, and especially on whether it contains RNA or DNA.

- RNA may be 'ready-to-use' as messenger RNA, in which case it can be used directly for translation into viral proteins and synthesis of more RNA (as happens with the polio virus). Alternatively it may be necessary to transcribe the RNA into DNA, which can then be inserted into the host genome before being used as a template for viral protein production and synthesis of more viral RNA (as happens with the retroviruses, including HIV).
- Nucleic acid from DNA viruses is translated into viral proteins via mRNA, and used as a template for synthesis of further viral DNA.
- Nucleocapsids undergo self-assembly. They then leave the cell, either by causing cell death and lysis or by passing through the cell membrane. In the latter case, they may acquire a membrane coating upon exit, which contains incorporated viral proteins—this is the origin of the viral envelope.

Virus infection of cells can have consequences other than immediate cell death. Some viruses can cause latent infection, remaining in the host cell for many years in a dormant state. Occasionally, such viruses are triggered to resume replication, which may result in a clinical relapse. Examples are herpes simplex and varicella-zoster viruses, which enter dormancy in nerve ganglia and cause cold sores and shingles respectively when they are reactivated. Other viruses may cause a persistent infection, with continued virus replication over months or years, without cell death. Hepatitis B and C viruses are examples of such chronic viral infections. Still other viruses (oncogenic viruses) have the ability to 'transform' the host cell in some way, usually by inducing uncontrolled growth and thus tumours or lymphoma. To do this, some or all of the virus DNA needs to become incorporated into the host genome. Examples of virus-associated tumours are given in Table 8.6.

Diagnosis of viral infection

The small size of viruses means that they cannot be seen by light microscopy, and their inability to reproduce outside a host cell means they cannot be cultured on solid media like bacteria, so other techniques must be employed. Common diagnostic techniques are summarized in Table 8.7.

In general, most infections are diagnosed by immunoassay, with PCR increasing in use and popularity. Most laboratories do not have an electron microscope and do not have facilities for cell culture.

Table 8.6 Virus-associated malignancies

Virus	Type of malignancy
EBV	Burkitt's lymphoma & B-cell lymphoma (in association with HIV) Nasopharyngeal carcinoma
Papovavirus	Cervical cancer
Hepatitis B virus	Hepatocellular cancer
Human herpes virus 8	Kaposi's sarcoma (in association with HIV)
HTLV-I	Adult T-cell leukaemia

Table 8.7 Common methods for detecting viral infection

Technique	Advantages	Disadvantages
Electron microscopy	'Catch-all' method—can see any virus present	Expensive, complex machinery needed Time-consuming to operate
Tissue (cell) culture	'Catch-all' method Virus obtained for further analysis	Slow (several days to get result) Expensive Difficulty in maintaining cell lines
Enzyme immunoassay (for viral antigens or host antibodies)	Quick Can be automated IgM assays can distinguish recent infection	Not appropriate for all viral species
Fluorescence microscopy for viral antigens expressed by host cells	Suitable for investigating respiratory infections	Expensive
Polymerase chain reaction (PCR)	Highly sensitive Increasingly quick Can be automated	DNA extraction can be difficult Expensive

Common pathogenic viruses

Herpes viruses

These enveloped DNA viruses are marked by latency after the initial infection, with further illness possible after months or years.

- The site of latency can be nerve ganglia (herpes simplex, varicella-zoster) or lymphocytes (cytomegalovirus, Epstein-Barr virus).
- Replication inside a host cell involves both host-encoded and virus-encoded enzymes; one of the latter, thymidine kinase, is the target for the antiviral agent acyclovir.

Herpes simplex I and II

These are similar viruses with some antigenic differences. HSV-I usually affects the mouth or face and is spread by oral or salivary contact; most people have a primary infection in childhood. Latent infection can re-emerge as cold sores of the lips, sometimes triggered by various stimuli: cold, sunlight, and other infections. HSV-I is also the most common cause of viral encephalitis.

HSV-II affects the genital area and is spread by sexual contact. It can also lead to recurring painful genital lesions. Childbirth during a primary HSV-II infection can lead to severe generalized neonatal infection. With increasing oro-genital sexual contacts both HSV-I and II cause oral and genital lesions.

Varicella-zoster virus (VZV)

This causes chickenpox in the non-immune. Latent infection can re-emerge as shingles (localized vesicular skin lesions, in the region of a single dermatome). Nearly all adults are immune. Infection in pregnancy may be associated with severe disease and pneumonitis; rarely, the fetus may be infected *in utero* and suffer reactivation leading to scarring and limb hypoplasia.

Cytomegalovirus (CMV)

This causes an acute illness with fever, malaise, headache, and sometimes mild hepatitis. Latency occurs in blood mononuclear cells and can re-emerge in immunocompromised patients (including HIV) to cause a variety of syndromes, including retinitis and colitis. The virus is found in blood and body fluids, and spread occurs at birth, from breast milk, from direct contact with other children, and later on through sexual contact. Primary infection of a pregnant mother may lead to severe congenital infection of the infant, with growth restriction, fever, jaundice, pneumonitis, and thrombocytopenia.

Hepatitis viruses

Hepatitis A virus

This is related to the enteroviruses and is spread via the faeco-oral route. After a relatively short incubation period of around a month jaundice develops in most patients; children are often asymptomatic. There is no chronic infection or carriage of the virus, and infection confers lifelong immunity. Effective vaccines are available; they can also be used after exposure, for example during outbreaks. Diagnosis is by detection of IgM in serum.

Hepatitis B virus (HBV)

This differs from other hepatitis viruses in being an enveloped DNA virus (the rest are RNA viruses). Blood and body fluids contain the virus (not faeces) and spread is via blood and sexual contact, or vertically during childbirth. The incubation is longer, usually 2–3 months; many infections are subclinical, and about 5–10% of infected individuals develop persistent infection, associated with ongoing infectivity. This may lead to chronic hepatitis, cirrhosis, and hepatocellular cancer.

Hepatitis B virus has different components, which are the basis of different serological tests:

- Surface antigen (HBsAg) refers to envelope proteins; HBsAg in the blood suggests an active infection but does not indicate whether the virus can be passed to others. Sometimes this antigen is produced in abundance and can be found in the bloodstream without being attached to virus particles. Modified HBsAg is the main vaccine component. Antibodies to HBsAg indicate previous exposure to hepatitis B virus, but the virus is no longer present and

the person cannot pass on the virus to others. This antibody provides lifelong immunity from HBV infection unless the individual develops immune impairment from HIV infection, renal failure, or treatment with immunosuppressants. Vaccination also causes the production of antibodies to HBV surface antigen.

- Core antigen (HBcAg) is the capsid protein but disappears early in the course of infection. Antibodies to the core antigen are produced during an acute HBV infection and afterwards. They are present in chronic HBV carriers as well as in those who have cleared the virus, and usually persist for life. Their presence implies a past infection at some time, as this antigen is absent from the vaccine.

- The e-antigen is a protein contained within the capsid; its presence in the blood implies that a large number of infectious virus particles are present, and thus a high level of infectivity. Conversely, the presence of antibody to the e-antigen, even in the presence of HBsAg, implies low-level infectivity. Some strains of HBV common in the Middle East and Asia do not make the e-antigen and in these areas testing for HBeAg is not very useful.

- Hepatitis B vaccine should be given to those at high risk of infection, for example family or sexual contacts of cases, healthcare workers, and babies born to carrier-status and infectious mothers (these babies should also be given hepatitis B immune globulin). Some countries practise universal HBV vaccination.

Hepatitis C virus

This is an enveloped RNA virus; like HBV it is present in blood and other fluids. It is very common among IV drug users and can be spread by unsterile injection equipment.

- The link with sexual spread is less clear than with HBV.

- There are six genotypes, which determine the response to therapy.

- Most infections are asymptomatic but the incidence of chronicity is very high. Most cases present many years after initial infection with chronic liver disease.

- There is no vaccine but interferon combined with ribavirin given for prolonged courses (6–12 months depending on genotype) can halt the progression of chronic hepatitis.

Parvovirus

Parvovirus B19 is the only human pathogenic parvovirus; it causes erythema infectiousum in children (also known as 'fifth disease', or 'slapped-cheeks disease').

- It is the only single-stranded DNA virus.

- It is spread by the respiratory route.

- Infections are often asymptomatic or mild but may result in classic 'slapped-cheek disease', with redness of the cheeks followed by a generalized rash.

- Adults more often present with pain and swelling of the joints.

- The virus infects red cell precursors, and may precipitate an aplastic crisis in patients who already have chronic haemolytic anaemia.
- Infection in pregnancy may result in fetal infection, with anaemia and hydrops—but most infections in pregnancy have no ill effect on the fetus.

Measles, mumps, and rubella

Rubella

Rubella virus—an enveloped RNA virus of the Togavirus group—causes rubella or German measles.

- It is characterized by an incubation period of 2–3 weeks, with a coryzal prodrome and lymphadenopathy preceding a maculopapular rash.
- The illness in childhood is usually mild; adults more often present with arthritis or arthralgia.
- The most serious consequences follow infection during pregnancy, with a high chance of serious birth defects, especially early in gestation.
- The congenital rubella syndrome includes deafness, cataracts or retinopathy, mental retardation, microcephaly, and cardiac abnormalities. The illness is prevented by the MMR vaccine, but cases are still seen in the unvaccinated.

Mumps

Measles and **mumps** are both members of the Paramyxoviridae, with a tube-shaped or helical RNA-containing nucleocapsid, coiled within a lipid envelope.

- As with rubella, they are spread by respiratory droplets, affect mainly children (in unvaccinated populations) and can be effectively prevented by the MMR vaccine.
- Mumps has an incubation of 2–4 weeks and presents with unilateral parotitis, and possibly meningitis or encephalitis.
- Adult cases in the male may develop epididymo-orchitis, which may then lead to testicular atrophy; as this is usually unilateral, sterility is very rare.

Measles (rubeola)

- This is the most infectious of the exanthems.
- After an incubation of 10–14 days, a prodromal coryzal illness develops; the virus is shed from the respiratory mucosa from this time.
- Late in the prodrome, Koplik's spots may develop on the oral mucosa—these resemble grains of salt or sand.
- The rash is erythematous and maculopapular, and spreads from face to trunk to extremities.
- Pneumonia is common and accounts for most of the deaths. Acute encephalitis is rare, and very rarely childhood infection is followed by subacute sclerosing panencephalitis (SSPE), which leads to progressive and irreversible dementia.

Respiratory viruses

Influenza virus

This consists of a coiled RNA nucleocapsid within a lipid envelope containing neuraminidase (N) and haemaglutinin (H) glycoproteins. There are three types: influenza A is found in humans and animals (including pigs and birds), whereas B and C infect humans only and cause milder illness. Incidence is seasonal, with winter epidemics.

- Continual mutations of the influenza A genome lead to gradual changes in the surface antigens (antigenic drift), allowing a degree of immune evasion and contributing to the yearly epidemics.
- More dramatic antigenic changes (antigenic shift) occur rarely, leading to effectively new viruses; this can result in global pandemics. Antigenic shift is thought to occur by combination of animal and human strains. The clinical features are of a sudden onset severe fever, with generalized aches, headache, chills, cough, and prostration. Pneumonia, which can involve bacterial superinfection, may complicate the illness. A vaccine is available, but because of antigenic drift it needs to be reformulated and re-administered yearly to be effective.

Adenovirus

This is an un-enveloped (or naked) DNA virus. It can cause respiratory tract infections, and more rarely epidemic conjunctivitis, or gastroenteritis.

Others

- **Respiratory syncytial virus** (RSV) is the major cause of bronchiolitis in young children.
- **Parainfluenza virus** causes laryngotracheobronchitis (croup).
- **Rhinovirus**, which is related to the enteroviruses, is the main cause of the common cold.

Enteroviruses, norovirus, and rotavirus

Enteroviruses are a large group of small, un-enveloped RNA viruses, which are spread by the faeco-oral route. They cause a viraemia with a range of illnesses, which can involve the nervous system (viral meningitis, polio), cardiac system (viral myocarditis), or can present as a fever or exanthema. Polio virus, echo viruses, and coxsackie viruses are all members of this group.

Norovirus causes gastroenteritis with predominant vomiting, tending to cause institutional outbreaks (winter vomiting disease). Rotavirus is an RNA virus with a double-layered capsid, giving it a characteristic wheel-like appearance on electron microscopy. It is the commonest cause of gastroenteritis in infants and young children.

HIV

Human immunodeficiency virus (HIV) is a retrovirus, possessing reverse transcriptase, and causes acquired immune deficiency syndrome (AIDS).

- The virus binds via an envelope glycoprotein, gp41, to the CD4 molecule on the surface of T lymphocytes.
- The viral RNA enters the cell and is transcribed into DNA by the reverse transcriptase. The viral DNA is then incorporated into the host genome, and serves as a template for further virus production. The cell produces numerous viruses and sheds these into the bloodstream, until it dies some days later.
- Spread is either sexual, by infected blood, during childbirth, or by breastfeeding.
- Infection is followed by a seroconversion illness some weeks later, with fever and a rash, and then a long period of latency, during which the number of CD4+ lymphocytes gradually declines. Eventually the immune system fails and the patient begins to succumb to a variety of infections, many with low-virulence opportunistic pathogens, and some associated with malignancy.

HIV can be controlled, but not eradicated, by different antiviral drugs, which are usually given in combination. These include nucleoside-, nucleotide-, and non-nucleotide-reverse-transcriptase inhibitors, and protease inhibitors, which block the action of viral protease enzyme.

The risk of transmission from mother to baby can be reduced by suppression of maternal viraemia using combination anti-HIV drugs (highly active anti-retroviral therapy), avoidance of breastfeeding, and elective caesarean section if appropriate. This necessitates recognition of infected mothers, and in the UK and most other developed countries routine antenatal screening for HIV is recommended.

Papillomaviruses

Human papillomaviruses (HPV—wart viruses) are DNA viruses that specifically infect skin and mucous membrane cells.

- There are over 70 described types, each with a tendency to infect certain anatomical sites. Types 1, 2, 3, and 4 cause warts of the hands and feet; Type 7 causes Butcher's warts (common warts in people who regularly handle raw meat, poultry, and fish), and Types 6, 11, 16, and 18 cause anogenital warts.
- They are spread by direct or indirect contact—in the case of anogenital warts, by sexual contact. They usually resolve after 1–2 years.
- Female genital warts, which may be hidden in the cervix, may be premalignant, leading eventually to cervical cancer. Vaccines against genital HPV types have recently become available, which should be able to prevent the associated cancers.

Fungi

Fungi are a large and diverse group of eukaryotic organisms, with over 100 000 species. They range from poisonous toadstools to brewer's yeast—but only a few of these cause infection. They have chitin-containing cell walls, and most live in or on decaying organic matter. Some species exist mainly in a single-celled form (yeasts), but most grow in branching filaments (hyphae) forming a mycelium (moulds). Some can exist in both forms—the dimorphic fungi. Fungal taxonomy is complex and ever-changing, and a pragmatic division into yeasts, moulds, and dimorphic fungi is more helpful to the clinician.

Most fungal infections are of an opportunistic nature, caused by an organism whose normal habitat is the environment, but some species are adapted to animal hosts. Opportunistic infections are seen in the immunocompromised and chronically ill or debilitated, and can range from mucosal candidiasis to life-threatening invasive aspergillosis.

Superficial fungal infections are generally diagnosed by microscopy and culture of swabs (or skin scrapings, for dermatophytes). However, many of the invasive fungi, apart from yeasts, do not grow easily in the lab, and diagnosis may therefore need histology, serology, or molecular tests such as antigen detection or PCR.

Candida

These yeasts, of which the commonest species is *Candida albicans*, are a common cause of both superficial and invasive disease.

- *Candida albicans* is typically distinguished in the laboratory by its ability to form a 'germ tube'—a single hypha—when cultured in serum.
- Oral *Candida* infection (oral thrush) can occur in otherwise healthy adults, but may be a marker for immunosuppression; HIV patients may get severe oral and oesophageal *Candida* infections.
- *Candida* is a common cause of vaginal infection and discharge (which is typically creamy-white); this is more common in diabetes, in pregnancy, and following antibiotic use, but many infections occur without any of these factors.
- Recurrent vulvovaginal candidiasis is usually due to subtle shifts and dysregulation of local vaginal cell-mediated immunity rather than repeated episodes of new infections.
- Invasive *Candida* infections are seen in the setting of hospital patients (typically seriously ill, in intensive care) and intravenous drug users—in both cases, the yeasts gain entry via the intravenous route, and may spread to the heart, bones, eyes, or other organs.

Dermatophytes

Dermatophytes cause a variety of skin, nail, and hair infections, and are named for their anatomical site (Table 8.3). There are many species, and some have an animal origin.

- The fungi use keratin for growth, and the infection remains in the upper layer of the skin, typically spreading outwards with central healing—classic ringworm.

- Most infections respond to topical antifungal agents, for example azoles such as ketoconazole or miconazole (and basic hygiene and ventilation in the case of athlete's foot), but some fungal nail infections persist despite treatment, necessitating nail removal.

Invasive moulds and dimorphic fungi

Except for the dimorphic fungi, these are usually seen in immunocompromised hosts. The most common infection encountered is invasive pulmonary disease caused by *Aspergillus fumigatus*, usually occurring in haematology/

oncology patients. Fungi of the *Mucor/Rhizopus* group can cause invasive infection of the facial sinuses and tissues—rhinocerebral mucormycosis.

The dimorphic fungi (Table 8.3) are generally not found in the UK or Europe, being native to the New World or tropical regions, but should be suspected in travellers from those areas with typical illnesses. Because of their potential to cause serious disease in healthy people, and to spread by airborne spores, they are classed as dangerous pathogens, and laboratory staff should be alerted if they are suspected in a sample.

Parasites

These include both single-celled protozoa and larger parasitic animals—all eukaryotes.

Protozoa are distinguished from bacteria by their larger size (from 5 microns to 1 mm), motility (in many species), and lack of a cell wall. Many of the parasitic protozoa have complex life-cycles, which may include hardy cysts that can survive in the environment and trophozoite forms that infect the host. In addition, several hosts may be infected; the host where sexual reproduction takes place is known as the definitive host, and the other(s) are known as intermediate hosts.

Intestinal parasitic protozoa

These are common in overcrowded areas with poor hygiene. They are generally diagnosed by visualization of the cysts in stool samples; cyst excretion may be low or intermittent, and so several samples may need to be examined.

Entamoeba histolytica

- This is an intestinal amoeba, the cause of amoebic dysentery.
- It has a cyst form that is spherical with four nuclei, averaging 10–15 microns in diameter, and a motile amoeboid trophozoite form that is larger (up to 40 microns) with a single nucleus.
- The cyst size is important to allow other non-pathogenic amoebae to be distinguished, but it is now recognized that 'E. histolytica' is really two species, one highly pathogenic (E. histolytica) and the other non-pathogenic (E. dispar). These are indistinguishable microscopically and can only be separated by molecular or serologic methods.
- E. histolytica may spread via the portal veins and cause an amoebic liver abscess, which can present months or years after the episode of dysentery.
- Diagnosis depends on the clinical presentation; acute dysentery is best diagnosed by examining a fresh sample (a 'hot stool') for trophozoites, which may contain ingested red cells. Older samples rarely contain visible trophozoites, but cysts may be seen.
- In amoebic liver abscess, cysts may be absent from the faeces, and serology is more definitive in the diagnosis.

Aspiration of the cyst should be avoided, for fear of peritoneal seeding of amoebae.
- Treatment of both amoebic dysentery and liver abscess is with metronidazole, followed by diloxanide furoate to eradicate organisms within the gut.

Giardia lamblia

This is a binucleate flagellate protozoan. It may cause low-grade but chronic diarrhoea, or persisting asymptomatic carriage. Cysts are oval, typically 10–12 microns in length, thin-walled, with up to four nuclei visible. Metronidazole is generally an effective treatment.

Cryptosporidium parvum

- This is the commonest parasitic infection reported in the UK; it may arise from livestock animals or other humans.
- Like *Giardia*, it may be spread via contaminated drinking water.
- The cysts are small (2.5 microns) and easily overlooked—they can be detected using modified acid-fast stains.
- Paromomycin was formerly used to treat severe infections seen in AIDS patients; more recently nitazoxanide has been licensed in the USA (but not yet in the UK) for treatment.

Tissue and blood protozoa

Plasmodium

Malaria is caused by four species of *Plasmodium*—*P. falciparum*, *P. vivax*, *P. ovale*, and *P. malariae*.

- The infection is spread by the bite of the female anopheline mosquito, and only exists where these mosquitoes are found—tropical and some subtropical areas.
- The infectious sporozoites are injected into the bloodstream along with mosquito saliva and pass into liver cells, where they multiply. They then re-emerge into the bloodstream as merozoites. The merozoites invade and multiply in red cells; most produce more merozoites, leading to more red cell infection, but a small number form male and female gametes.

- The gametes, when taken up by a biting mosquito, complete sexual reproduction in the insect's stomach, and migrate as sporozoites to the salivary glands.
- Diagnosis is usually by visualizing parasites within red cells on a blood film.
- There are important differences between the four species:
  1. *P. vivax* and *ovale* can enter a dormant phase in liver cells (hypnozoite) leading to relapsing infection.
  2. *P. falciparum* infection can be very severe, with infected red cells blocking and damaging capillaries in the brain, kidneys, and other organs. *P malariae* is milder but may persist for many years.
- Patients with sickle cell trait have relative resistance to the harmful effects of malaria infection, which is probably why this haemoglobinopathy has persisted in Africans.
- Chloroquine is the preferred treatment, but in many areas *P. falciparum* is resistant, and so other agents such as quinine or artemether will be needed.

Leishmania

This refers to a group of flagellate parasites that can cause a range of illnesses, divided into visceral, cutaneous, and mucosal infections. There are many species, of which the best known is *L. donovanii*, but species and syndromes often overlap. They are spread by the female sandfly, which is found in many tropical and subtropical areas (including the Mediterranean); animals may act as a reservoir for some species.

- There is a biphasic lifecycle, with a motile flagellate form—the kinetoplast—existing in the sandfly, and the non-motile amastigote found within human cells, mainly of the reticuloendothelial system.
- Visceral leishmaniasis (Kala-Azar) involves enlargement of the liver and spleen, with fever and wasting; the organism can be seen in cells aspirated from liver, spleen, bone marrow, or lymph nodes.
- Cutaneous leishmaniasis (Oriental sore) involves infection of dermal macrophages in the site of the original sandfly bite, leading to a chronic ulcer. In South America, cutaneous lesions may heal only to be followed by secondary lesions in the oropharyngeal area—mucocutaneous leishmaniasis.

Trypanosoma

Trypanosoma brucei is spread by the bite of the tsetse fly and is confined to tropical Africa, causing African trypanosomiasis (sleeping sickness). The parasites first enter red cells and then spread to the nervous system, reticuloendothelial system, and possibly other organs such as skin and myocardium. Clinical features include fever, hepatosplenomegaly, and progressive drowsiness and coma.

Trypanosoma cruzii is found in South America, is spread by the faeces of reduviid bugs, and causes Chagas disease. A generalized chronic tissue infection, with a possible autoimmune component, results in typical features of cardiomyopathy and

dilatation of the gastrointestinal tract, with oesophageal reflux and constipation.

Toxoplasma gondii

Toxoplasma gondii causes toxoplasmosis, a common infection with particular consequences in pregnancy and immunodeficiency.

- The trophozoites undergo sexual reproduction in the gastrointestinal tract of cats, which are the definitive host.
- Oocysts are passed out in the faeces and ingested by other animals, where trophozoites exist and migrate throughout the body, forming tissue cysts. The natural cycle is maintained by cats ingesting the tissue cysts in prey animals such as mice.
- Humans can be infected either by handling soil contaminated with cat faeces, or by ingesting raw/undercooked meat containing tissue cysts. Acute infection in humans is usually subclinical, or may present as a glandular fever-like illness.
- Tissue cysts persist in humans as in other animals, and in immunosuppression (e.g. HIV) these cysts can activate. This is most often seen as toxoplasma encephalitis, from dormant brain cysts.
- Chronic latent infection is common (90% seroprevalence in some countries in Europe) and poses no risk in pregnancy, but acute or re-activated infection during pregnancy may lead to congenital infection of the infant, with choroidoretinitis or brain damage.

Genital protozoa

Trichomonas vaginalis

- This is a motile, flagellate, pear-shaped protozoan, 10 × 7 microns in size. It is a common cause of vaginal and urethral infections.
- It is usually spread sexually, and the vaginal infection is characterized by an elevated vaginal pH (>4.5), an intense and disproportionate vulvovaginal irritation and soreness, and a green or yellow frothy discharge with a fishy odour.
- Male patients are usually asymptomatic.
- Metronidazole is the usual treatment, although resistant strains occur.

Helminths

These include Platyhelminths (flat) and Nematodes (round); the former are divided into Trematodes (flukes) and Cestodes (tapeworms). Flukes are leaf-shaped, up to a few centimetres in length, with one or two suckers to aid attachment to the host and a blind-ending gut. They all have freshwater snails as intermediate hosts, and some have a second intermediate host—fish or crustaceans. They may reside mainly in the blood and bladder (schistosomiasis), liver (e.g. *Clonorchis sinensis*—Chinese lever fluke), intestine, or lung (e.g. *Paragonimus westermanii*).

Tapeworms

The tapeworms are multi-segmented flattened worms, sometimes up to 10 metres in length, with a scolex (head) attached to the intestinal wall by hooks or suckers, and the worm residing in the intestinal cavity. Each segment, a proglottid, is hermaphrodite and produces eggs. The worm has no intestine, nutrients being absorbed directly from the host intestinal contents. As it grows, proglottids break off the end; eggs or whole proglottids may be passed in the stool. With some species (e.g. *Echinococcus granulosus*), ingested ova migrate from the gut to tissues where they form larval cysts, which may enlarge sufficiently to cause illness (hydatid disease).

Roundworms

Roundworms include intestinal species and those that invade tissues. The commonest intestinal nematode outside tropical areas is probably the common pinworm or thread-worm, *Enterobius vermicularis*, a small worm (approximately 1 cm long). The female emerges from the anus at night to lay eggs on the perineum; this leads to the main symptom of nocturnal anal itch.

The larvae of the roundworm *Ascaris lumbricoides* have a curious cycle of migration from the gut through the lung before being coughed up and swallowed again. The hookworms (*Ankylostoma duodenale* and *Necator americanus*) enter the body via penetration of the skin (usually of the feet in barefoot people) and are a common cause of chronic anaemia in tropical areas. *Strongyloides stercoralis*, a small worm (2 mm) can cause a chronic gut infection, maintained by emerging larvae penetrating the anal skin and migrating back to the intestine. Ongoing infection has been found in ex-prisoners of war 50 years after their return to the UK.

Control of infection

Mechanisms of action of antibiotics

The sites of action of the major groups of antibiotics are shown in Figure 8.4.

Sterilization and disinfection

- Sterilization implies eradication of all organisms on an object, whereas disinfection means 'removing pathogens' or 'making safe'—a less precise concept. Sterilization is necessary for pharmaceutical compounds and any medical equipment that goes into a 'sterile area'—wound dressings, syringes and needles, and surgical devices.
- Surgical devices are sterilized by steam autoclaving at 135°C for 3 minutes (or 125°C for 15 minutes); these high temperatures are necessary to kill spores. Steam autoclaves are used as the steam penetrates fabrics and instrument packs, unlike dry heat. Autoclaving must be preceded by manual cleaning to be effective—this is particularly important with hollow-bore instruments, as steam penetration may be blocked by debris.
- Single-use items such as needles and syringes are usually sterilized by irradiation at the site of manufacture.

Delicate instruments such as endoscopes will not survive autoclaving, so must be washed and disinfected between patients. Gluteraldehyde was formerly the main disinfectant used but was withdrawn due to safety concerns; peracetic acid and superoxidized water are now preferred.

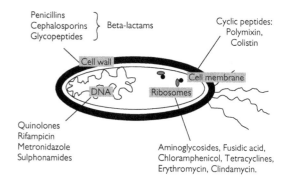

Figure 8.4 Bacterial cellular targets of antibiotic action. Adapted from an image by Dr Peter Riley with permission.

ADDITIONAL FACTS AND REVISION MATERIAL

Selected bacterial toxins, their target tissues and modes of action

- In general, exotoxins are released by live bacteria, whereas endotoxin ('lipid A' within Gram-negative lipopolysaccharide cell walls) is released when the organism dies.

- *Clostridium botulinum* toxin inhibits the release of acetyl choline at nerve terminals leading to flaccid paralysis, whilst the tetanus toxin (from *C. tetani*) inhibits the release of glycine and GABA, which are inhibitory neurotransmitters, thus resulting in spastic paralysis.

- α-toxins produced by *C. perfringes* and *Staph. aureus* are cytotoxic and cause cell death and destruction.
- The botulinum, diphtheria, and strep erythrogenic toxins are not encoded on the bacterial chromosomes but on bacteriophages.
- Diphtheria toxin inhibits elongation of protein during synthesis.
- Enterotoxigenic *E. coli* (ETEC) and *Vibrio cholera* produce toxins that activate the cAMP pathway leading to water secretion and major diarrhoea.

Lactose-fermenting Enterobacteriaceae

- *E. coli*
- *Klebsiella*
- *Enterobacter*

Capsulated organisms

- *Strep. pneumoniae*
- *Haemophilus*
- *Klebsiella*
- *Pseudomonas*
- *Neisseria meningitidis*
- *Cryptococcus* (which exists only in the yeast form)

Diseases of animal origin (zoonotic)

- Brucellosis (from milk)
- Leptospirosis (rodent urine)
- Anthrax (inhalation of spores from animal carcasses)
- Bovine tuberculosis
- Food poisoning (with *Salmonella* and *Campylobacter*)

Diseases transmitted by insect bites

- Yellow fever
- Malaria
- Dengue fever
- Typhus

Types of vaccines

Live vaccines	Killed vaccines	Toxoids (modified bacterial toxins)	Vaccines from subunit of organism
Polio (Sabin)	Polio (Salk)	Diphtheria	Hepatitis B virus
Mumps	Hepatitis A virus	Tetanus	*N. meningitidis*
Measles	Rabies		*Strep. pneumoniae*
Rubella	Cholera		Pertussis
Yellow fever			Influenza
Varicella-zoster			

Hepatitis B, D, and E virus infections

- Chronic HBV infection is defined by HBsAg production beyond 6 months of onset of infection, persistent serum HBsAg, and no production of antibodies to HBsAg.
- Antibodies to HBcAg are present following HBV infection, whether fully resolved (95%) or persistent as chronic infection (5%). HBcAg is *not* seen in patients who have had hepatitis B vaccine.
- Hepatitis D virus (or delta virus) is a defective blood-borne RNA virus, the smallest known human virus. It needs HBV infection to replicate.
- HEV is transmitted via the oro-faecal route like HAV but it is dangerous in pregnancy with a mortality rate of approximately 20%.

Interferons (IFN)

- These are cytokines produced by immune cells (WBC produce α-IFN; fibroblasts produce β-IFN; and macrophages, natural killer, and other cells produce γ-IFN) in response to viruses, parasites, and tumour cells.

- They inhibit viral replication within host cells by:
  1. inhibiting viral protein synthesis
  2. inhibiting viral protein kinases
  3. activating RNA endonucleases, which digest viral RNA.
- IFN activates NK cells and macrophages, increases antigen presentation to lymphocytes, and induces host cells' resistance to viral infection.

Fungi and antifungal agents

- Ergosterol is a major component of fungal cell membranes with identical function to cholesterol in animal cells. It is also found in the cell membranes of trypanosomes, hence the efficacy of some antifungal agents against sleeping sickness. Ergosterol provides a good target for antifungal drugs since it is absent in animal/human cell membranes and will therefore not produce unwanted side effects in host cells.
- Amphotericin B binds to ergosterol and creates a polar pore in fungal membranes, allowing ions (mostly K^+ and H^+) and other molecules to leak out, leading to cell death. The azole group of antifungal agents including miconazole and clotrimazole inhibits the synthesis of ergosterol.

CHAPTER 9

Pharmacology

General principles

Drugs are chemicals that, when introduced into the body, selectively interfere with its functions. They may not have tissue specificity and may therefore give rise to unwanted side effects. The actions of a drug are determined by its chemical properties and how these interact with bodily processes. For example:

- Highly ionized drugs are not readily absorbed from the gut and do not readily enter the CNS.
- Once in the body, drugs may distribute widely in body water or have a much more restricted distribution, giving rise to the concept of the *volume of distribution* (see below), which is large if they are widely distributed or strongly bound to some molecular site in the body.
- Some drugs are readily metabolized by the liver into inactive compounds and a few are converted to more active compounds. Metabolism generally increases their water

solubility and the rate at which they are excreted by the kidneys. The processes of metabolism and excretion determine how long a drug remains in the body, which in turn determines how often it needs to be administered to maintain an effective therapeutic concentration. Some very fat-soluble drugs can remain in body fat for very long periods.

- Not all drugs are excreted via the urine. Some, such as general anaesthetics, are largely (although not exclusively) excreted by the lungs and pass out in the expired air. Others may appear in breast milk, semen, saliva, or sweat, pass out in faeces, or cross the placenta to reach the fetus. Also, variations can occur due to age (for example with children or the aged) or due to genetic constitution. The latter can cause serious problems on some occasions and genotyping may be required.

Route of administration

- Patients may not comply with drugs that require non-oral routes of administration.
- Orally-administered drugs may be absorbed at different points in the gastrointestinal tract. The rate of absorption depends on numerous factors; for example, on whether food has been taken or the level of gut motility, which in turn can be influenced by drugs or physiological state.
- Glyceryl trinitrate is fat-soluble and well absorbed if placed under the tongue; if it passes to the intestine it is transported by the venous portal system and extensively metabolized by the liver.
- In general, drugs that are extensively ionized do not readily pass across epithelia such as that of the gut. Thus, weak bases (e.g. chloroquine, propranolol) and weak acids (e.g. penicillins, aspirin) that may be ionized at the pH of the stomach or intestinal contents are absorbed in their unionized form, provided they are sufficiently

fat-soluble for this to occur. As the unionized form achieves equilibrium across the epithelium, the total concentration of the drug on the two sides of the epithelium may become very unequal, as the degree of ionic dissociation will depend on the pH of the respective body compartments (i.e. 'ion trapping' may occur).

- Aminoglycosides, e.g. streptomycin, are not very fat-soluble in the unionized form and are even less able to pass epithelia in their ionized form, so they are poorly absorbed from the gut. Poor gut absorption is also true for amphotericin B, which can be used to treat fungal infection of the gut with minimal systemic absorption (important since nephrotoxicity may be a problem).
- Sometimes slower, more prolonged intestinal absorption is desired and encapsulated slow-release preparations are used. Particle size may influence gut absorption (digoxin). Corticosteroids and oestrogenic and progestogenic

steroids (e.g. oral contraceptives) are satisfactorily absorbed, but testosterone (except as the undecanoate) is not because of first-pass metabolism by the liver, and so depot preparations or injections are the rule.

- Anabolic steroids, which are alkyl-substituted testosterone analogues, are, however, well absorbed orally. Rectal administration is used when other routes are not possible or difficult (vomiting, collapsed veins, unconscious, convulsions).
- Drugs administered intravenously reach the bloodstream quickest but this may not be reflected in rapid or significant access to the CNS, the eye, or the interior of abscesses. Also, intravenous administration of some drugs may cause unwanted effects on the heart unless given by slow infusion.
- Intramuscular injection results generally in a slow absorption into the bloodstream, which may be sufficiently rapid for some purposes but some drugs may be painful, irritant, or unsuitable for administration by this means.

The rate of absorption depends very much on the blood supply and whether injection was actually into muscle or into surrounding fat. Where rapid absorption is not required, such as with depot preparations, then subcutaneous injection may be satisfactory.

- Rapid access to the central nervous system may be obtained by intrathecal injection.
- Inhalation of aerosols may be the most suitable route of therapy for respiratory disease and has even been successful as a method of administering insulin, a peptide that is destroyed if given orally.
- Absorption across epithelia is generally accelerated if they are inflamed due to the increased blood supply and to a less effective epithelial barrier.
- Skin patches can provide a suitable method of absorption where the drug is very fat-soluble (e.g. nicotine skin patches) and fat-soluble insecticides may be absorbed through the skin leading to long-term toxicity.
- Occasionally, drugs may be enclosed in liposomes.

Distribution of drugs within the body

The volume of distribution (VoD) is a measure of the extent of distribution of a drug in body water. It is obtained by dividing the dose given by the plasma concentration. So, if the drug is confined to the bloodstream then the VoD will equal the plasma volume (about 50 ml/kg). If the drug escapes from the bloodstream into the extracellular fluid then the VoD will increase (to about 200 ml/kg). Entry into intracellular water will further increase the VoD (to >550 ml/kg). If the drug is bound to some component of the body, or sequestered in fat, then its VoD will accordingly increase to a value greater than the total body water. Conversely, if it is strongly bound to components of the blood then it can be used to measure blood volume. In pregnancy the total body water increases by around 8 litres.

In the simple case, drug concentration in the plasma may decline at a rate directly proportional to the concentration and so exhibit first-order kinetics. The time taken for the

concentration to decline to half is called the half life. Many drugs, because they are absorbed into various compartments of the body at different rates, fail to obey these simple kinetics. However, the approximation can be useful. In the case of alcohol, phenytoin, and aspirin there is an upper limit at which the drugs can be eliminated, which is easily exceeded so that in practice they exhibit saturation or zero-order kinetics. This means that when the dose is increased, the time for complete elimination of the drug is increased more than when first-order kinetics occurs. If a drug is given either by infusion, or at regular intervals at the same dosage, then the concentration in the plasma or at its site of action will rise until the rate of elimination is equal to the rate of administration. In the case of drugs that have approximately first-order kinetics this will take three or four half lives. For this reason, loading doses are sometimes given to achieve the final steady-state (therapeutic) level more quickly.

Metabolism

- The majority of drugs are metabolized in the liver, where the microsomal P450 enzyme system plays a major role. Polar water-soluble drugs tend to be excreted by the kidney and more lipid-soluble ones are able to pass across the cell membrane of the hepatocytes and access microsomal P450 enzymes.
- Two main types of metabolism of the drug occur in the liver: simple oxidation to create hydroxyl and other groups (phase 1); and conjugation of these with various

sulphate, acetyl, methyl, glycyl, and glucuronyl groups (phase 2). These molecular modifications generally increase water solubility and therefore facilitate renal excretion. They also generally reduce the pharmacological effects of the drug, although this is not always the case.

- Some benzodiazepines are metabolized into active compounds that can persist to exert longer-term effects (e.g. diazepam into nordazepam). Sulindac is a prodrug that is virtually pharmacologically inactive until metabolized.

Renal excretion

- The metabolites of drugs are generally more water-soluble than the parent drug and are more readily excreted by the kidney. Filtration at the glomerulus, transport through the epithelium of the kidney tubules, and diffusion are the three mechanisms involved.

- Compounds are carried in the glomerular filtrate into the tubular fluid or may attach to exchange mechanisms in the renal tubule and be transported into the tubular lumen. In the former case the portion of the drug (or metabolite) bound to plasma proteins does not affect filtration as water and drug are filtered together, whereas in the latter case, as drug (or metabolite) binds to the exchanger and is removed, then more dissociates from its bound state to become available to the exchanger.

- Where diffusion of lipid-soluble compounds across the tubular epithelium is important, because of the 'ion trapping', weak acids (e.g. aspirin) are better excreted into alkaline urine and weak bases (e.g. propranolol) are better excreted into acid urine (in both cases the lipid-soluble form equilibrates across the tubule epithelium between blood and tubule luminal fluid, but in the latter case dissociation into the ionized form is greater).

- Drug clearance is a concept defined as the equivalent volume of plasma containing the drug completely cleared of the drug per unit time. Because a compound may be actively pumped into the lumen of the renal tubules, the clearance of some compounds can approach that of renal blood flow (e.g. para-aminohippuric acid).

- The rate at which compounds are moved from the plasma into the urine is usually proportional to the plasma concentration, so overall clearance is usually independent of plasma concentration. Renal clearance is important because it dictates the rate at which a drug needs to be administered to maintain a steady plasma concentration.

Receptors and their mechanisms

Communication between cells within the body is often by means of chemical messengers, with the exception of electrical connections between certain syncytial tissues such as the heart and most smooth muscle organs/tissues. Thus, the endocrine glands control or affect their target cells, tissues, and glands by means of hormones released into the bloodstream. Nerves affect other nerves (in the central nervous system) and muscles and glands (peripherally) by means of neurotransmitters. A large number of cells release local hormones, many of which are as yet unknown. Communication by means of chemical messengers shows a number of features:

- The chemical messenger needs to be produced and stored, either ready for release or as a precursor, such that synthetic and storage mechanisms are the norm. There needs to be a trigger for release, and a release mechanism. Finally, the target cells must have mechanisms to detect the released chemical messenger; this is done by means of receptors to which the messenger substance binds and which are then activated.

- Many drugs exert their effects by combining with receptors normally utilized by endogenous compounds. However, drugs may also combine with endogenous molecules in the body that do not act as receptors for endogenous compounds; for example, they may bind to enzymes such as angiotensin-converting enzyme, or to membrane transporters that have no known endogenous ligands. Some receptors have secondary allosteric sites at which drug binding may occur, modulating the primary function of the receptor exerted through its primary binding site.

- Receptors come in a variety of forms, which vary depending on the chemical properties of the messenger, the speed of response required, and other factors. If the transmitter or hormone is ionized at the pH of the extracellular fluid, then rather little if any of it will be able to enter the cell, and so its receptors need to be on the surface of the cell. In this case the target cell must have mechanisms to express the genes for the receptor and mechanisms responsible for transporting it, or a precursor, to the surface of the cell and inserting it in the membrane. Also, mechanisms are needed to regulate the number or density of the receptors on the cell surface in relation to the amount of transmitter or hormone that reaches the cell over time. These involve various mechanisms for internalization and possibly re-utilization of the receptors.

- A large number of different types of receptor are linked by GTP-binding proteins (G-proteins) to effector mechanisms (ion channels or enzymes) in the cell. In other cases, such as the insulin receptor, binding of insulin to the receptor initiates a cascade of reactions involving receptor dimerization and autophosphorylation, followed by an amplifying cascade of further phosphorylation reactions. In still other cases, when fast reactions are required, the receptor may form part of an ion channel that has a low probability of existing in the open state unless the chemical messenger is bound to it. Other types of receptors also exist.

- Where messengers are lipid-soluble, as in the case of steroids, then they can readily cross the cell membrane and enter the nucleus of the cell. Here specialized receptors exist, which recognize and bind the steroid. This causes the receptor to bind to particular parts of the DNA, acting as a promoter of transcription, and causing up- or down-regulation of various genes.

- Receptors for drugs may also be enzymes; for example, enalapril binds to and inhibits angiotensin-converting enzyme (ACE), which converts angiotensin I to angiotensin II. Diuretics combine with ion transporters in the kidney tubules; frusemide inhibits the $Na^+/K^+/2Cl^-$ symporter in the ascending limb of the loop of Henle. Protease-activated receptors, of which the thrombin receptor is an example, cleave a portion of the receptor and the residue then activates itself to produce the response.

Pharmacology of sex steroids

Oestrogens exert a wide range of reproductive and metabolic effects in the body, including the development of secondary sexual characteristics of puberty, growth, menstrual cycle, and a crucial negative feedback effect on the hypothalamic-hypophyseal complex, which inhibits FSH production. Oestrogens are used therapeutically in cases of delayed puberty or hypogonadal syndromes, although other hormones may be preferred such as GnRH analogues. A number of analogues are used, particularly as constituents of contraceptive pills and patches. Apart from their use in males to suppress androgen-dependent tumours, oestrogens are commonly used in post-menopausal women for replacement therapy. The natural oestrogens, oestradiol, oestrone, and oestriol, are preferred over synthetic analogues because of their advantageous spectrum of actions. Tibolone, which has oestrogenic, progestogenic, and androgenic activity, is also used. Continuous use of oestrogen may cause excessive endometrial hyperplasia; therefore, a progestogen is given in combination, which converts the endometrium into its secretory phase and suppresses oestrogen receptor expression in this tissue, thus reducing the risk of hyperplasia or cancer of the endometrium.

- In post-menopausal women, dryness and atrophy of the vaginal epithelium, hot flushes, and osteoporosis may be a problem. Hormone replacement therapy (HRT) can help these conditions. However, HRT has been linked with increased risks of breast and endometrial cancer, and with thromboembolism and stroke.
- Receptors for oestrogens are of two types, alpha and beta. In addition, in different tissues activation of the same receptor by the same ligand may produce different effects. This gives rise to the concept of selective oestrogen receptor modulators, of which tamoxifen and raloxifene are examples.
- Tamoxifen has agonist activity in brain, bone, liver, and endometrium but antagonist activity in breast tissues; hence its use in cancers of the breast. Raloxifene is used for osteoporosis but also causes hypertriglyceridaemia and thromboembolism and promotes breast cancer.
- Clomifene is a pure oestrogen antagonist used to inhibit the inhibitory action of oestrogen on FSH secretion, which results in a surge of FSH promoting ovulation in non-ovulating women.
- Aromatase inhibitors such as anastrozole are also used in breast cancer.

The menstrual cycle

Cyclical changes in oestrogens and progesterone control the menstrual cycle and ovulation, and influence conception and implantation. Analogues of these hormones suppress ovulation and are used successfully as contraceptives. These are marketed in different formulations:

- The low-dose combined preparations of ethinylestradiol with norethisterone, desogestrol, or gestodene, or standard-dose combined preparations containing slightly more ethinylestradiol (or mestranol) with these three progestogens or with levonorgestrel, norgestimate, or drospirenone. In addition there are patches in which ethinylestradiol is combined with norelgestromin.
- The progestogen-only pills, injections, and implants.
- Emergency contraception within 72 hours of intercourse is achieved with levonorgestrel. After 72 hours efficacy declines but if pregnancy ensues the fetus is unharmed.

These preparations work by inhibiting the release of gonadotropin-releasing hormone (GnRH) and FSH in the early part of the cycle when FSH normally rises and causes a batch of follicles to develop. Normally, as the level of oestrogen produced by the follicles rises to a critical point, the negative feedback to the hypothalamico-hypophyseal complex switches to a positive feedback and LH (along with more FSH) is produced, causing ovulation normally of the single largest follicle. This resultant corpus luteum starts to produce progesterone, which inhibits further ovulation.

- The combination of oestrogen and progestogen, or progestogen alone (although slightly less effective), activates the negative feedback on the hypothalamico-hypophyseal complex and follicles do not develop and ovulation does not occur.

- Progestogen-only preparations are considered to exert a major component of their effect through creating a thick, viscid cervical mucus through which sperm are unable to penetrate easily.
- Combined contraceptives in general reduce dysmenorrhoea, menorrhagia, premenstrual tension, fibroids, benign breast disease, ovarian cysts, and ovarian and endometrial cancer. They do not significantly alter lipoprotein profile but triglycerides increase.
- During pregnancy the incidence of venous thromboembolic disease is about 60 per 100 000 women, whereas with low-dose pill it is about 15 per 100 000, and it is about 25 per 100 000 with combined contraceptives containing desogestrel and gestodene.

- Drugs that induce liver enzymes or antibiotics affecting the gut flora, so reducing the enterohepatic re-absorption of ethinylestradiol, may impair the effectiveness of the pill.
- Heavy smokers or women with diabetes mellitus or hypertension (both exacerbated by oestrogens) are better maintained on progestogen-only pill, which is also suitable for lactation (does not reduce milk flow), proximity to recent birth (not thrombogenic), older women, and after surgery.
- The incidence of breast and cervical cancer is slightly increased on low-dose combined preparations but this increased risk disappears 10 years after ceasing medication.

Drugs in pregnancy

Termination of pregnancy

- For therapeutic termination of pregnancy, initial treatment with mifepristone, a progesterone antagonist, opposes progesterone support of the pregnancy and sensitizes the uterus to prostaglandin action. Misoprostol (oral or vaginal) or gemeprost (vaginal) PGE$_1$ analogues, or rarely dinoprostone (PGE$_2$), can then be given.
- For induction of labour, dinoprostone is recommended prior to artificial rupture of membranes; after rupture of membranes dinoprostone or oxytocin may be used (although sequential use of both is recommended clinically). Misoprostol or dinoprostone are given vaginally, whilst oxytocin is given by slow IV injection. Oxytocin should not be given for 6 hours after intravaginal prostaglandins.
- For premature labour, atosiban (an oxytocin-receptor antagonist) or nifedipine (a calcium channel antagonist) may be used. Oxytocin increases intracellular Ca^{2+} release from the sarcoplasmic reticulum by modulating cAMP systems. The oxytocin antagonist atosiban inhibits this process by specifically antagonizing the oxytocin receptor. Calcium channels control the influx of Ca^{2+} into the cell during action potential to effect the cycling of actin and myosin. Blockade of these channels reduces the influx of extracellular calcium into the myometrial cell leading to relaxation. However, calcium channel blockers including the vascular selective nifedipine and its relatives may also exert a negative inotropic and chronotropic effect on the cardiac cell leading to profound cardiodepression.
- Beta-agonists such as isoxsuprine, salbutamol, ritodrine, or terbutaline also cause uterine relaxation by increasing intracellular uptake of Ca^{2+} into the sarcoplasmic reticulum. They are, however, associated with marked cardiovascular side effects including left ventricular failure and fluid overload and are no longer recommended as first-line tocolytic agents.
- Postpartum haemorrhage: ergometrine with oxytocin is recommended. If these are not effective, prostaglandins carboprost or misoprostol are the next line.

- Patent ductus arteriosus: the prostaglandin antagonist indometacin is used to accelerate closure after birth. Alprostadil (PGE$_1$) can be used to maintain patency when this is required.

Teratogenesis, pregnancy, and lactation

Drugs and alcohol are best avoided in pregnancy and may pass to suckling infants during lactation. Treatment of women of child-bearing age always runs the risk that they are pregnant and the fetus is particularly susceptible to drug-induced malformations in the first trimester. However, the test is always whether the benefit to the mother outweighs the possible harm to the unborn child. The increase in the incidence of malformations with some drugs, although real, is small.

- Drugs known to cause or that have been implicated in fetal malformations include:
  - cytotoxic anti-cancer drugs
  - anti-epileptic agents
  - some antirheumatic drugs
  - many antibiotics
  - oral hypoglycaemic agents
  - some antihypertensives
  - tranquillizers.
- High doses of vitamin A have been implicated and isotretinoin (for acne) should only be used in males, or in females if they apply strict contraception for 1 month before and for 2 years after administration as it is very persistent in body fat.
- Treatment of pregnant women should only be carried out when absolutely necessary and with the lowest possible drug dose.
- Most cytotoxic anti-cancer drugs inhibit rapid cell growth and so are likely to be detrimental to fetal growth. Methotrexate and other anti-folate drugs may cause cleft palate and other abnormalities of development. Thalidomide

has returned as an anti-cancer agent and must be avoided in pregnancy.

- The potential teratogenic effects of phenytoin, phenobarbitone, carbamazepine, valproate, and trimethadione are well documented. The use of two or more anti-epileptic drugs simultaneously is liable to exacerbate teratogenicity and should be avoided. The lowest possible dose of anti-epileptic drug along with folic acid supplementation should be used. Several anti-epileptics induce liver enzymes and CYP3A4 induction especially increases the incidence of contraceptive failure, so barrier methods should be used. Hypoprothrombinaemia may also occur necessitating vitamin K injection.

- Aspirin and other cyclo-oxygenase (COX) inhibitors are potentially teratogenic in pregnancy and care should be exercised with newer COX2 inhibitors. Leflunomide has reported teratogenicity. Prolonged use of high-dose aspirin or other non-steroidal anti-inflammatory drugs (NSAIDs) during pregnancy is associated with reduced birth weight and may cause closure of the ductus arteriosus *in utero*, lead to prolonged pregnancy, and increase the risk of postpartum haemorrhage. Low-dose intermittent aspirin use is probably without effect.

- Many antibiotics have detrimental effects on the fetus. Metronidazole has not been shown to be teratogenic. Streptomycin, gentamycin, and kanamycin may cause deafness in the fetus and susceptibility to deafness is increased in the case of certain genetic mutations.

- The antiviral agent ribavirin is contraindicated in pregnancy and ciprofloxacin is not recommended.

- In malaria prophylaxis or treatment, proguanil (with folate) should be postponed until pregnancy is over. Quinine is safe. Breast-feeding infants should receive separate therapy as amounts in breast milk are unreliable.

- Tetracyclines may damage tooth growth in children under the age of 8, and may lodge in bone and should be avoided in pregnancy.

- In tuberculosis avoid streptomycin during pregnancy and use isoniazid/rifampicin/pyrazinamide combination.

- Benzodiazepines should be avoided if at all possible in early pregnancy and regular use in pregnancy should be avoided. They also pass into the breast milk and may depress the infant.

- Small and occasional amounts of alcohol is permissible but daily intake of 1–2 units/day is associated with a two-fold increase in the risk of second trimester miscarriage. Higher usage may trigger fetal alcohol syndrome and growth restriction.

- Statins are not recommended for use in pregnancy.

- Many antihypertensives can be used, although methyl dopa is frequently used as first-line. Hydralazine is used for acute blood pressure control in severe pre-eclampsia/eclampsia.

- Warfarin is teratogenic and may also cause intracranial bleeding. Heparin is preferred during pregnancy but has been associated with maternal osteoporosis and thrombocytopenia. It should be discontinued before labour and delivery, especially if regional analgesia is contemplated.

- Nausea and vomiting in pregnancy may be treated with promethazine or a phenothiazine. Dexamethasone can be used to prevent respiratory distress syndrome in infants at risk of premature delivery but fluorinated analogues are teratogenic, so lowest dose of natural steroids should be used.

- Hyperthyroidism may be treated with carbimazole. Carbimazole crosses the placenta, so the minimum effective dose should be used. Propylthiouracil is preferred during lactation as it has a lesser tendency to enter the breast milk.

- Antidepressants may be used in pregnancy. Some withdrawal symptoms in the newborn are described with selective serotonin reuptake inhibitors (SSRIs) paroxetine and fluoxetine. Tricyclic antidepressants have been reported to cause tachycardia and muscle spasms in the newborn, whilst lithium is associated with a low incidence of malformations. Abuse of cocaine increases the risk of premature labour and placental abruption.

Pharmacology of blood coagulation

The coagulation cascade

Coagulation involves a complicated interplay of numerous plasma and endothelial factors, and platelets. A simplified scheme is shown in Figure 9.1. Conspicuous are a number of positive feedback and autocatalytic pathways, which amplify an initial signal involving endothelial damage, release of tissue factors such as von Willebrand's factor, and platelet activation. Following initiation and amplification, consolidation of the thrombus occurs, increasing the mechanical strength of the thrombus and normally effecting haemostasis.

In normal individuals mechanisms exist to limit the extent of thrombus formation. Where these are deficient, disseminated coagulation may occur.

Thrombus formation can be considered to involve four stages: initiation, amplification, consolidation, and limitation of spread. The endothelial cells have a number of mechanisms that normally inhibit thrombus formation. These include a covering of heparan sulphate, a co-factor for antithrombin III, and the secretion of prostacyclin (PGI_2), which inhibits platelet attachment. However, they contain von Willebrand's factor and thromboxane A2 (TXA_2), which when released promotes attachment of platelets.

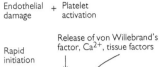

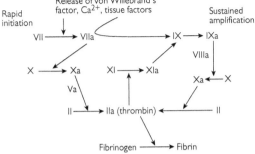

Figure 9.1 The coagulation cascade.

When there is damage/removal of the endothelium, the underlying connective tissue fibres are exposed, to which these attach.

Platelets play a crucial role in thrombus formation, and deficiency states (thrombocytopenia) result in thrombocytopenic purpura, where multiple petechia of haemorrhage occur in the skin and internal organs. Platelets contain a variety of clotting factors: ADP, TXA_2, 5HT, and platelet-derived growth factor (PDGF). The release of ADP from a few platelets triggers further platelet activation (positive feedback, autocatalysis) and release of calcium, an important co-factor in thrombus formation. TXA_2 release promotes platelet adhesion. Activation of platelets causes them to express glycoprotein receptors IIb and IIIa, which bind fibrinogen. Exposure of acidic phospholipids on their surface promotes fibrin formation from fibrinogen and links adjacent platelets.

The **endothelium** has a number of mechanisms that inhibit thrombus formation and, should it occur in response to localized damage, limit the extent to which the thrombus spreads.

1. The glycoproteins (heparan sulphate, heparin, and dermatan), which cover the endothelial surface and bind to antithrombin III and thrombomodulin.

2. As a result, the power of antithrombin III to inhibit thrombin is increased substantially, while the substrate specificity of thrombomodulin is altered from fibrinogen to Protein C, a circulating proenzyme that is activated.

3. Activated Protein C inactivates activated factors VIII and V (VIIIa and Va), so inhibiting thrombin formation. Protein S is required for this reaction. Congenital lack of Protein C (a hereditary thrombophilia) leads to a fatal postnatal thrombosis.

4. The endothelium also produces the potent anticoagulation prostaglandin I_2 (PGI_2; also known as prostacyclin) and also NO, which acts to inhibit vasoconstriction and also coagulation.

5. The endothelium synthesizes plasminogen activator inhibitor. Plasminogen activator diffuses into a thrombus where it converts plasminogen to plasmin; this degrades fibrin and other clotting factors resulting in clot dissolution. When the endothelium is damaged or lost then these anticoagulation influences are reversed.

Emphasis is placed on measurements of the ability of the blood to clot as estimated by the INR (international normalized ratio), which is calculated by reference to the time taken (the prothrombin time) for blood from normal individuals to clot. The normal value is 1.0 and as INR increases above this level, the risk of clotting decreases and that of bleeding and bleeding-related events increases. In most of the conditions mentioned, INR values above 2.5 or 3.0 are desired and are achieved by the use of anticoagulants. In pregnancy and during oestrogen administration there is hypercoagulability.

In disorders of clotting, largely caused by genetic deficiencies of clotting factors or platelets, treatment is aimed at replacing the deficient factor or accelerating clotting by drugs. Newborns are routinely given vitamin K as they may be deficient in this substance. Vitamin K is important in maintaining activity of factors II, VII, IX, and X and Proteins C and S, as it is a necessary co-factor for the carboxylation of residues in these proteins, without which they are inactive in the coagulation cascade.

Anticoagulant drugs

Anticoagulants

Indications for use

- Venous thrombosis
- Pulmonary embolism
- Atrial fibrillation, where there is a danger of coronary or cerebral embolism
- Unstable angina
- Prosthetic valve replacement
- During the use of extracorporeal circulation

Anticoagulants generally interfere with the liver's production of coagulation factors or the actions of these factors in the coagulation cascade (Figure 9.2). The 'coumarins' class of anticoagulants exert their effect on coagulation by inhibiting the recycling of vitamin K oxide. Vitamin K is an essential co-factor for a carboxylase enzyme that catalyses the γ-carboxylation of glutamic acid residues on vitamin K-dependent proteins, which include the coagulation factors II (prothrombin), VII, IX, and X, and the anticoagulation proteins, proteins C, S, and Z. Vitamin K is necessary for the synthesis and also the activation of these proteins. Vitamin K is absorbed from the intestine with the aid of bile salts and there is very little storage. It undergoes a cycle of oxidation and reduction that allows its reuse and is active only in the reduced form, and the reduction process takes several days (Figure 9.2).

- Vitamin K (usually K_1) is reduced to vitamin KH_2 by a reductase.
- Oxidation of vitamin KH_2 provides the energy to drive the carboxylation reaction, leading to formation of γ-carboxyglutamic acid residues and vitamin K oxide.

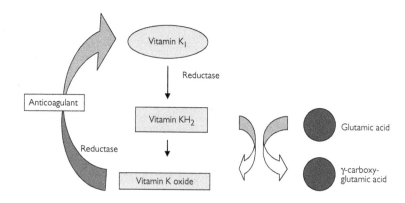

Figure 9.2 Vitamin K cycle.

- Vitamin K oxide is reduced by another reductase back to vitamin K, ready to re-enter the cycle. Anticoagulants such as warfarin block the reduction of vitamin K oxide to vitamin K.

Warfarin

- Warfarin is an analogue of vitamin K, which competitively inhibits its reduction by competing for the active site of the reductase enzyme that reduces vitamin K oxide back to vitamin K.
- Because of the slow production of the reduced form, Proteins C and S may be inhibited before other factors initially. As a result of the loss of these activated proteins, which normally inhibit coagulation by inactivating factors VIIIa and Va, an anomalous reduction in INR and increase in intravascular coagulation may result.
- Heparin may be given before warfarin to prevent these effects. An INR between 2 and 4 is desirable where patients are predisposed to thrombosis or its consequences.
- Although warfarin is rapidly absorbed and peak plasma concentrations are achieved within an hour, the effects on clotting take 12 hours to develop and last 4–5 days.
- Warfarin is teratogenic during the first trimester of pregnancy and is also contraindicated in later pregnancy because of the danger of fetal intracranial haemorrhage. It passes into the breast milk in small amounts and may theoretically cause increased bleeding tendencies in the infant. Administration of vitamin K reduces this risk.
- Necrosis of breast or buttock caused by intravascular thrombosis of small vessels due to inhibition of Protein C

and, with overdose, haemorrhage may occur. Other oral anticoagulants are phenindione and acenocoumarol.

Heparin

Standard or unfractionated heparin consists of a variety of molecules of different length, and low-molecular weight heparins (LMWHs) are generally preferred. Fondaparinux is a synthetic LMWH.

- Heparin activates antithrombin III produced by the endothelium, which inhibits the action of thrombin (factor IIa) and factors IXa, Xa, Xia, and XII.
- Heparin is administered intravenously or subcutaneously and has a half life of about 1 hour. Usually it is given by infusion after a bolus loading and APTT monitored.
- LMWHs have a longer half life and zero-order elimination so their effects are more predictable.
- Heparins are large molecules and do not cross the placenta; however, they should be discontinued before delivery.
- The main side effect is haemorrhage, which can be treated by ceasing administration and, if necessary, administration of protamine, which is less good at reversing the actions of LMWHs.
- Heparin-induced thrombocytopenia may occur due to the development of antibodies after 4–5 days administration, and osteoporosis with much longer periods of treatment.
- Other anticoagulants that inhibit the action of thrombin include hirudin derivatives and danaparoid (heparan, dermatan, and chondroitin sulphates).

Antibiotics and antimicrobial agents

Antimicrobials fall into four classes in which synthesis of essential parts of the infective organism is inhibited: cell wall synthesis, protein synthesis, membrane synthesis, and nucleic acid synthesis.

Inhibitors of cell wall synthesis

- As the bacterial cell wall is unique to bacteria, agents acting in this way generally have good therapeutic ratios, and are the safest antimicrobials to use in pregnancy.

This group includes the penicillins and their derivatives and the cephalosporins. Vancomycin, bacitracin, and cycloserine also fall into this group.

- The narrow spectrum benzylpenicillin is very rapidly excreted as it is transported into the renal tubule. Its half life is therefore very short and large doses need to be given at frequent intervals to maintain effective therapeutic plasma concentrations. Probenecid blocks the renal transport mechanism and prolongs the action of benzylpenicillin. Others in this group are procaine penicillin, which is given intramuscularly once a day, and phenoxymethylpenicillin.

- The β-lactam ring of benzylpenicillin can be broken by bacteria that possess the enzyme β-lactamase. Modification of this structure has created antibiotics such as flucloxacillin with a resistance to β-lactamase action but reduced activity against *Neisseria*, pneumococci, and β-haemolytic *Streptococcus*. Broader spectrum activity has been obtained in the case of ampicillin and amoxicillin. In co-amoxiclav, amoxicillin is combined with clavulinic acid, which binds to β-lactamase, thus reducing its action against the β-lactam ring and increasing the effectiveness of amoxicillin.

- Penicillins may cause convulsions if given intrathecally but are otherwise relatively free of side effects, with the important exception of allergic or, rarely, anaphylactic reactions due to penicillin metabolites combining with proteins in the body and the resulting complex acting to elicit hypersensitivity reactions. IgE antibodies can be detected in hypersensitive patients.

- Methicillin-resistant *Staphylococcus aureus* (MRSA) infection may be difficult to treat and sensitivity needs to be determined. Tetracyclines, clindamycin, and a glycopeptide such as vancomycin are possible depending on sensitivity, but specialist advice is generally needed.

- First, second, and third generation cephalosporins are also β-lactam antibiotics, which by manipulation of the β-lactam ring have resistance to β-lactamase and various improved spectra of activities against Gram-negative and Gram-positive bacteria. They may show hypersensitivity, which may cross-react with penicillin hypersensitivity. Prolonged use or high doses may result in thrombocytopenia and other organ damage.

Hypertension and cardiovascular pharmacology

Pathophysiology of hypertension

The relationship between flow, pressure, and resistance in a system can be represented by the Poiseuille's equation:

$$Q = P_1 - P_2 / R$$

where: Q = flow; $(P_1 - P_2)$ = pressure gradient, the net force that is pushing the fluid through the system; and R = resistance of vessel between P_1 and P_2.

Applying the Poiseuille's equation to the entire cardiovascular system gives the following:

$$CO = MAP/SVR \text{ or } BP = CO \times SVR$$

where: CO = cardiac output; MAP = mean arterial pressure; and SVR = systemic vascular resistance.

There are four key alterations in homeostasis that characterize increased blood pressure in humans. They involve the dysregulation of salt and water retention (therefore blood volume), vascular tone, and cardiac output:

1. Increased sympathetic tone
2. Decreased vagal tone to the heart
3. Increased renin-angiotensin system activity
4. Sodium and water retention

Treatment of hypertension

The aim of treatment of hypertension will thus include a reduction in sympathetic tone, blood volume, and vascular tone and will aim to deal with the compensatory effects elicited by these interventions (Table 9.1).

Table 9.1 Treatment of hypertension

Blood pressure determinant	Pathophysiologic factors in hypertension	Potential agents
Cardiac output—heart rate	Reduced vagal tone	β-blockers Calcium channel blockers
Cardiac output—contractile force	Increased sympathetic tone	β-blockers
Systemic vascular resistance	Increased sympathetic tone	Sympathoplegics Calcium channel blockers Direct-acting vasodilators
Blood volume	Increased renin-angiotensin activity	Diuretics ACE inhibitors Angiotensin II antagonists

Antihypertensive agents

(a) Centrally acting α_2-adrenoceptor agonists (e.g. methyldopa, clonidine)

- Stimulation of α_2-receptors in the brainstem exerts an inhibitory effect on sympathetic tone and outflow leading to a reduction in peripheral vascular tone.
- This is mediated through blockade of presynaptic release of noradrenaline and acetylcholine.
- Methyldopa and clonidine act through this mechanism. Other α_2-adrenoceptor effects include contraction of vessels in the skin and mucous membranes. This effect, however, is activated by circulating noradrenaline, in contrast to the α_1 effect exerted through noradrenaline released at the nerve terminals.
- Methyldopa is a prodrug, which is metabolized to its active metabolite α-methyl noradrenaline. It is α-methyl noradrenaline that preferentially activates central α_2-receptors, thereby reducing sympathetic outflow and vasomotor tone. The delay in the onset of action of methyldopa observed clinically is in part due to the time required to convert methyldopa to its active metabolite.
- The resultant reduction in peripheral vascular resistance lowers systemic blood pressure. There are no significant compensatory effects because it has no effect on α_1-receptors. There are, however, central side effects including sedation, drowsiness, dizziness, and reduced libido because of its primary site of action.
- Other side effects include oedema and positive Coombs test. Clonidine is associated with severe rebound hypertension if discontinued abruptly and is rarely used in clinical practice. It also causes drowsiness and dry mouth.

(b) β-blockers (labetalol and other '-olols')

- The cardiovascular effects of α- and β-adrenoceptor responses may be summarized as follows:
  - α_1 response—vasoconstriction, increase in mean arterial pressure (MAP)
  - β_1 response—increased heart rate, stroke volume, cardiac output, contractility, and blood pressure because β_1 receptors are expressed mostly in the heart
  - β_2 response—reduced peripheral vascular resistance mainly in the skeletal muscle.
- Labetalol is a non-selective β-blocker and it also exhibits additional α-blocking action.
- It exerts its antihypertensive effect mainly through blockade of the β_1-receptors expressed in the heart. It reduces myocardial contractility, heart rate, cardiac output, myocardial oxygen demand, and blood pressure. It is not associated with orthostatic hypotension but there may be atrioventricular block and congestive cardiac failure.
- A selection of cardio-selective β_1-blockers are available including acebutolol, metoprolol, bisoprolol, and atenolol.
- The action of labetalol on the heart prevents reflex tachycardia following a drop in blood pressure.

- It opposes renin release through blockade of β_2 effect in the juxtaglomerular apparatus; thus there is no sodium and water retention.
- For some as yet inexplicable reason, white and younger patients respond better to β-blockers compared to black and older patients respectively.
- β_2-receptors are expressed in the bronchioles, pancreas, and peripheral skeletal muscle vasculature. For this reason labetalol should be avoided in asthmatics, diabetics, and in people with peripheral vascular disease where β-receptor blockade may lead to bronchospasm, hypoglycaemia, or ischemic limb respectively.
- Fetal effects include growth dysregulation with prolonged use. There may be neonatal hypoglycaemia and therapy should be discontinued gradually. Central effects include depression, fatigue, and sexual dysfunction.

(c) Calcium channel blockers (nifedipine and other '-dipines')

- The voltage-dependent long latency type (L-type) calcium channels are present in the nodal tissues (SA and AV) of the cardiac cells. These channels control the influx of calcium into the cell during action potential to effect the cycling of actin and myosin leading to contraction.
- Blockade of these channels reduces the influx of extracellular calcium into the intracellular compartment and as such exerts negative inotropic and chronotropic effects on the cardiac cell. Thus, calcium channel blockers may cause profound cardiodepression.
- These slow-response cells are also present in the vascular smooth muscles where their blockade leads to vasodilatation.
- Nifedipine is the prototype of a class of vascular selective calcium channel antagonists known as the 'dihydropyridines'. Nifedipine causes a marked vasodilatation in the hypertensive patient. This elicits a compensatory reflex tachycardia, which may be sufficiently severe to induce cardiac arrhythmias, myocardial infarction, and/or sudden death. This is particularly important in patients with underlying cardiac impairment.
- The coronary arteries are perfused during the diastolic phase of the cardiac cycle. Therefore, during tachycardia the time available for the perfusion of the coronaries may be significantly reduced, with deleterious effects on the myocardium.
- The side effects of nifedipine include gastrointestinal distress, constipation, headaches, gingival overgrowth with prolonged use, and proteinuria.
- Unlike the β-blockers, nifedipine is a very good antihypertensive for black and elderly people.

(d) Direct-acting vasodilators (hydralazine)

- Hydralazine exerts vasodilatory effects by acting directly on the vasculature. It increases the release of endothelial-derived relaxation factor (EDRF), which was subsequently shown to be nitric oxide, a potent vasodilator.

- Nitric oxide causes a direct ateriolar dilatation and reduces peripheral vascular resistance in a variety of vascular beds, including renal, coronary, and cerebral.
- The potent vasodilatation of cerebral vessels leads to headaches, whilst dilatation of other vascular beds elicits flushing and compensatory tachycardia, sweating, and fluid retention.
- Hydralazine is metabolized by N-acetyltransferase, so it may accumulate in people with systemic lupus erythematosus and in slow acetylators.
- Hydralazine can be administered orally for the management of moderate to severe hypertension, but its main role in obstetrics is as a rapidly acting antihypertensive for severe hypertension and pre-eclampsia.
- Other direct-acting vasodilators include nitroprusside, minoxidil, and diazoxide, although these are rarely if ever used in obstetric practice.
- In general these agents do not interfere with the sympathetic tone, innervation of the vasculature, or responses to such innervation.

(e) The renin-angiotensin-aldosterone system

- This system is responsible for the long-term control of blood pressure and is therefore the target of major classes of antihypertensive agents (Figure 9.3).
- *Renin* is a circulating enzyme produced in the kidney by the *juxtaglomerular apparatus* (JGA) cells (modified smooth muscle cells that surround the afferent arterioles). The JGA cell is designed to monitor the pressure of blood coming into afferent arterioles.
- *Renin* is not a hormone. There are no known receptors in target tissues. It digests *angiotensinogen* (produced in the liver) into a pro-hormone, *angiotensin-I* (AT-I).
- AT-I is converted into its active form, AT-II, by *angiotensin-converting enzyme* (ACE), a peptidase produced by the endothelial cells of the pulmonary capillaries.
- AT-II exerts its physiologic effects via AT-I receptors on two major targets relevant to blood pressure homeostasis, namely the *zona glomerulosa* of the adrenal cortex (where it stimulates the release of *aldosterone*) and the blood vessels (where it causes vasoconstriction and elevation of blood pressure).
- Aldosterone stimulates the Na^+-K^+ pump, mainly in the basement membrane of the collecting ducts of the kidney, to increase the re-absorption of Na^+ and with it water. It also promotes the secretion and excretion of K^+ and H^+ by the collecting ducts.
- Aldosterone also replicates these same effects in the distal colon.
- Blockade of AT-II production by pharmacological inhibition of ACE leads to a reduction in aldosterone output and vascular tone.
- Furthermore, the vasodilator peptide *bradykinin* is a substrate for ACE and the inhibition of ACE leads to the accumulation of bradykinin, nitric oxide-mediated vasodilatation, and reduction in peripheral vascular resistance. This added BP lowering action is not exploited by angiotensin receptor antagonists such as losartan.
- The accumulation of bradykinin following the use of ACE inhibitors (ACEI) is believed to be responsible for the dry cough observed in a third of patients on ACE inhibitors, and also angioedema, which is found more commonly in black patients compared to their Caucasian counterparts.
- Other side effects include hypotension, hypovolaemia, hyperkalaemia, and acute renal failure.
- These agents are associated with fetal hypotension, renal failure, and renal and skull malformations, and are therefore contraindicated in pregnancy.

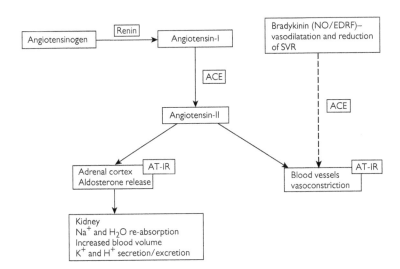

Figure 9.3 The renin-angiotensin-aldosterone system (RAAS).

Neuropharmacology

Antipsychotics (aka neuroleptics and major tranquillizers)

This is a large group of drugs used to treat schizophrenia and other psychoses.

Pathophysiology

Schizophrenia is thought to be due to an overactivity of dopaminergic pathways innervating the limbic system and frontal cortex. There is good evidence of a strong genetic component, but no genes of major effect have been identified. There is also good evidence that schizophrenia may result from a problem of neurodevelopment *in utero*, with a long latent period.

Antipsychotics are divided into two major groups: typical (or classical) and atypical.

Typical antipsychotics (e.g. chlorpromazine, haloperidol)

These are older drugs (pre-1980) and are effective against positive symptoms of schizophrenia such as hallucinations and delusions, but not against negative symptoms such as flattened affect and social withdrawal. The beneficial effect is related to blockade of dopamine (DA) receptors, particularly D_2 receptors.

Adverse effects

- Movement disorders (termed extrapyramidal side effects, EPSEs), which include parkinsonism (classical features of Parkinson's disease, although the bradykinesia is often most marked), dystonia (abnormal postures and sustained muscle contractions), and akinesia (motor restlessness). These usually occur early in treatment (weeks or months). Tardive dyskinesias are late onset (usually after years of treatment) and include abnormal repetitive movements (lip smacking, tongue protruding, choreiform limbs). These may become irreversible.
- Increased prolactin secretion (hyperprolactinaemia), which can lead to hypogonadism and gynaecomastia in males, breast engorgement, inappropriate lactation, and amenorrhoea in females.
- EPSE and increased prolactin are both mediated by DA receptor blockade.
- Blockade of other neurotransmitter receptors results in adverse effects. Blockade of α_1NA receptors results in orthostatic hypotension (marked with chlorpromazine); blockade of histamine H_1 receptors results in sedation; blockade of muscarinic acetylcholine receptors results in atropine-like effects including dry mouth and constipation (both marked with chlorpromazine and thioridazine); sulpiride and haloperidol produce less of these adverse effects than chlorpromazine and thioridazine.

Atypical antipsychotics (e.g. risperidone, olanzepine)

These are newer drugs and are effective against positive and negative symptoms. They produce fewer EPSEs (particularly dystonias and tardive dyskinesia) and less elevation of prolactin than typical antipsychotics. Other atypical antipsychotic agents include clozapine (see below) amisulpiride, quetiapine, and zotepine.

Adverse effects

- Weight gain is very common, and marked with olanzepine.
- Hyperglycaemia (leading to a higher than expected incidence of type 2 diabetes) and increased cholesterol and triglycerides. Olanzepine has the highest incidence; risperidone the lowest.
- Increase in QT interval (shared by some typical antipsychotics).
- Increased incidence of stroke and myocardial infarction.

Clozapine

- The first atypical antipsychotic. Causes leucopenia and (rarely) fatal agranulocytosis (not shared by other atypicals). Blood monitoring is mandatory. Licensed for treatment-resistant schizophrenia (patients unresponsive or intolerant to other antipsychotics). Adverse effects include sedation, hypotension, hypersalivation, and seizures at high doses. High incidence of weight gain and type 2 diabetes. Fatal myocarditis and cardiomyopathy have been reported.
- The mechanism of atypical antipsychotics is not clear; all block D_2 receptors, but generally block 5-HT$_2$ receptors with higher affinity than D_2.

Aripiperazole

- Termed a 'dopamine stabilizer' (to distinguish it from typicals or atypicals).
- Claimed to offer the advantages of atypicals (low incidence of EPSE, little effect on prolactin, effective against positive and negative symptoms) without their disadvantages (no weight gain, no effect on QT interval).
- Adverse effects include somnolence, orthostatic hypotension, and increased risk of seizures.
- Novel pharmacology—partial agonist at D_2 and 5-HT$_{1A}$ receptors, antagonist at 5-HT$_{2A}$ receptors.

Antipsychotics are routinely administered orally, in single or divided doses. Long-acting depot injections are often used as maintenance therapy, particularly when compliance with oral medication is unreliable. Depots are oily preparations, administered by deep intramuscular injections at intervals of 1–4 weeks. Several typical antipsychotics are available as depots, e.g. haloperidol, fluphenazine, and flupentixol. Risperidone is the only atypical antipsychotic available as a depot.

NICE guidelines recommend that newly diagnosed patients are given a trial of oral atypical antipsychotics. They also recommend that patients treated with typical antipsychotics who fail to respond or suffer severe adverse effects should be considered for oral atypical antipsychotics.

Antipsychotics and pregnancy

- Limited evidence suggests that exposure to low-potency typical antipsychotics in pregnancy is associated with a small additional risk of congenital malformations. Even less is known about atypical antipsychotics, although manufacturers recommend that they are avoided.
- Antipsychotics can produce respiratory depression, extrapyramidal movements, and difficulty with oral feeding in newborn infants medicated in the womb, although these adverse effects usually resolve within days.
- Antipsychotics are excreted in breast milk. Manufacturers recommend avoidance of these drugs during breast-feeding, although there is limited evidence of toxicity or impaired development.

Antidepressants

Pathophysiology of mood disorders

- Depression is thought to be related to an under-activity of monoamine neurotransmitters, particularly serotonin and noradrenaline, and mania to be due to their over-activity. There is strong evidence of a genetic component to bipolar affective disorder, although no gene of major effect has been identified. There is less evidence of a genetic component for unipolar depression.
- The major groups of antidepressant drugs are: selective serotonin reuptake inhibitors (SSRIs), tricyclic antidepressants (TCAs), and monoamine oxidase inhibitors (MAOIs).

Selective serotonin reuptake inhibitors (SSRIs)

- These include fluoxetine, paroxetine, citalopram, escitalopram, fluvoxamine, and sertraline.
- They are selective inhibitors of 5HT reuptake, and thus increase the synaptic concentration of 5HT. They have little or no effect on the uptake of other monoamines and minimal direct interaction with neurotransmitter receptors. They have fewer cardiovascular effects and are safer in overdose than other antidepressants.
- Adverse effects include nausea, GI discomfort, reduced appetite, decreased libido and anorgasmia, agitation, anxiety, and nervousness (early in treatment), movement disorders, particularly orofacial dystonia, and lower seizure threshold.

Tricyclic antidepressants (TCAs)

- These include imipramine, amitriptyline, desimipramine, nortriptyline, dothepin, doxepin, lofepramine, clomipramine, and trimipramine.

- They inhibit the reuptake of serotonin and noradrenaline and thus increase the synaptic concentration of these neurotransmitters.
- Adverse effects: Atropine-like effects, e.g. dry mouth and constipation, due to marked but variable blockade of muscarinic acetylcholine receptors. Cardiovascular effects, e.g. tachycardia, arrhythmias, and orthostatic hypotension, due to blockade of noradrenaline (NA) reuptake, α-NA receptors, and K^+ channels. Lower seizure threshold. Some TCAs are sedative, e.g. amitriptyline. TCAs are toxic in overdose and are often used in attempted suicide. There are no specific antidotes.

SSRIs and TCAs have not been found to have serious effects on the fetus, but SSRIs have been associated with decreased gestational age (1 week) and birth weight (175 g). There are reports of neonatal withdrawal symptoms after use of SSRIs and TCAs during late pregnancy. There are no serious adverse effects in children whose mothers were taking SSRIs or TCAs during breast feeding.

Monoamine oxidase inhibitors (MAOIs)

- These include phenelzine and tranylcypromine.
- They inhibit the enzyme monoamine oxidase (MAO) and thus increase the concentration of monoamine neurotransmitters. The enzyme is present in nerve terminals but is also present in the liver and the GI tract. Inhibition is irreversible (and thus the effects are long-lasting) and affects both isoforms of MAO.
- Adverse effects: 'Cheese effect'—hypertensive crises following ingestion of foods rich in tyramine. Tyramine (an indirect-acting sympathomimetic) is normally metabolized by MAO in the GI tract but following MAOI treatment it is absorbed and causes a release of NA from nerve terminals, causing vasoconstriction and tachycardia. Dietary restrictions are necessary to avoid tyramine-rich foods such as fermented milk products, certain beers and wines, meat extracts, and yeast products. Other sympathomimetics, e.g. ephedrine and phenylephrine, also need to be avoided. Atropine-like adverse effects occur, but are less of a problem than with TCAs. Hypotension is common and is the opposite of what one might expect (with increased stores of NA).
- Moclobemide is a reversible inhibitor of the MAO_A subtype. The 'cheese effect' is much reduced and dietary restriction is not necessary.

Venlafaxine

This is an inhibitor of 5HT and NA reuptake (serotonin-noradrenaline reuptake inhibitor or SNRI) but lacks the direct receptor interaction seen with TCAs. At low doses venlafaxine inhibits only 5HT reuptake and is therefore similar to SSRIs and has the same adverse effects. At higher doses NA reuptake is inhibited and additional adverse effects emerge, e.g. nausea, agitation, insomnia, and hypertension. Duloxetine is also an SNRI.

Mood stabilizers

- These drugs are used in the treatment and prophylaxis of mania, bipolar affective disorder, recurrent depression, and the mood changes associated with schizophrenia.

- Lithium carbonate has been the major mood stabilizer in the UK for over 40 years. The therapeutic range of plasma concentration is narrow: 1–1.5 meq/l. Below 1 meq/l there is no psychotropic effect, whilst above 1.5 meq/l toxic effects begin to develop. The half life of lithium is long and it takes about 2 weeks to reach steady-state concentration. Therefore, regular monitoring of plasma concentrations is necessary, particularly early in treatment and following change in dosage.

- The mechanism of action of lithium is unclear, partly because lithium has so many effects and it has proved difficult to establish which are most critical. Two of the most important actions of lithium are inhibition of cyclic AMP production and reduction in receptor-stimulated phosphatidylinositol turnover.

- Adverse effects of lithium include fatigue, diuresis, weight gain, tremor, and a metallic taste in the mouth. Long-term lithium is associated with hypothyroidism, so regular thyroid function tests are recommended. Lithium toxicity is associated with a number of neurological effects including nystagmus, ataxia, coma, and convulsions. Lithium toxicity can be precipitated by renal impairment, diuretics, low sodium diet, and dehydration.

- Carbamazepine, valproate, and lamotrigine (all introduced and still used in the treatment of epilepsy) have recently gained in popularity as first-choice mood stabilizers in preference to lithium, because of better side effect and safety profiles.

Hypnotics and anxiolytics

Anxiolytics are drugs that reduce the symptoms of anxiety. Hypnotics are drugs used to treat insomnia. There is a degree of overlap between these classes of drugs, as most anxiolytics will produce some degree of sedation and hypnosis. There are, however, some sedatives/hypnotics that lack specific anxiolytic properties.

Benzodiazepines (e.g. diazepam, temazepam, and other '-azepams')

- This is a large group of drugs with similar chemical structures and similar pharmacological properties. They are anxiolytic, hypnotic, anticonvulsant, and muscle relaxant and fall broadly into two groups—short-acting and long-acting. Short-acting (e.g. temazepam and oxazepam) have short half lives and are metabolized to inactive glucuronides. Long-acting (e.g. diazepam and nitrazepam) have long half lives or give rise to active metabolites with long half lives.

- Benzodiazepines produce their pharmacological actions by interacting with specific binding sites on a receptor

for γ-aminobutyric acid (GABA) termed the GABA-A receptor, and potentiating the inhibition action of GABA. The benzodiazepine binding sites are distinct from the sites at which GABA binds and are termed modulatory sites.

- Flumazenil is a selective benzodiazepine antagonist. It binds competitively to the same site as benzodiazepines and reverses their pharmacological action. It is used to treat benzodiazepine overdose.

- Careful choice of dose can produce anxiolytic effects without marked daytime sedation. As hypnotics, benzodiazepines reduce the time taken to get to sleep and increase total sleep time. The hypnotic effects of benzodiazepines are also used preoperatively, to facilitate endoscopy, in fracture realignment, and in dental work. Anterograde amnesia following IV administration is a beneficial feature when undertaking such procedures.

- Benzodiazepines are not routinely used for the long-term management of most forms of epilepsy because they are too sedative. They are the drug of choice for termination of status epilepticus. Diazepam or clonazepam (IV) are often used.

- Adverse effects are largely restricted to the CNS. There can be impairment of intellectual and motor performance, coordination, and reaction time, hence the need to advise patients not to drive or operate potentially dangerous machinery. Benzodiazepines normally have a calming effect but paradoxical hostility is sometimes seen, particularly in the elderly.

- Benzodiazepines are CNS depressants and their effects are additive with other CNS depressants, particularly alcohol. An overdose of benzodiazepines taken alone is rarely fatal, but the same dose combined with alcohol can be fatal.

- A major problem with benzodiazepines is the development of tolerance and dependence. High dependence potential seems to be related to high potency and short half life, e.g. triazolam has far greater dependence potential than temazepam. The Commission on Human Medicines (CHM) recommend that benzodiazepines are limited to 2–4 weeks of treatment for anxiety and are used only for the short-term treatment of insomnia when it is severe and disabling.

The ZEDs (e.g. zopiclone, zolpidem, and zalepon)

- These are non-benzodiazepine hypnotics licensed for the short-term treatment of insomnia. They have largely replaced benzodiazepines in the treatment of insomnia.

- They have short half lives and no active metabolites.

- Although chemically distinct from benzodiazepines, the Zeds bind to the same binding sites. However, whereas benzodiazepines bind equally well to α_1, α_3, and α_4 subunits of the GABA-A receptor, the Zeds bind selectively to the α_1 subunit. This explains why the Zeds lack the anticonvulsant and muscle relaxant properties seen with benzodiazepines.

- Tolerance and dependence are not fully established; dependence has been reported in small numbers of patients.

Buspirone

- This is anxioselective. It is less sedative than benzodiazepines and not anticonvulsant or muscle relaxant.
- It has slower onset of action than benzodiazepines (2 weeks). There is no potentiation with alcohol.
- It acts as a partial agonist at 5-HT_{1A} receptors.

Selective serotonin reuptake inhibitors (SSRIs)—see under 'Antidepressants'

As well as their role as antidepressants, SSRIs are licensed for the treatment of a range of anxiety disorders, including generalized anxiety disorder, panic disorder, social anxiety disorder, and post-traumatic stress disorder. Recommended doses are somewhat higher than those used to treat depression. SSRIs are also licensed for the treatment of severe premenstrual tension and premenstrual dysphoric disorder.

β-Adrenoceptor blockers (e.g. propranolol)

These are used to treat the physical symptoms of anxiety, such as sweating, tremor, and tachycardia.

Opioid analgesics (e.g. morphine)

These are a large group of drugs used primarily for their pain-relieving properties. Some are naturally occurring in the seed pods of the poppy, *Papaver somniferum* (e.g. morphine, codeine), others are semi-synthetic (e.g. diamorphine), but most are synthetic (e.g. pethidine, fentanyl, methadone).

Effects and adverse effects of morphine

- Opioid analgesics are used to treat moderate to severe pain, but are less useful in neuropathic pain. Opiates also reduce the affective component of pain. Patients report that they are aware of the pain but less troubled by it.
- Analgesia is mediated at various levels of the central nervous system. At the spinal cord, opioids act presynaptically in the dorsal horn to inhibit the release of excitatory neurotransmitters from the primary afferent neurons carrying the nociceptive stimuli from the periphery. They also act at higher brain centres, particularly the periaqueductal grey matter, the nucleus raphe magnus, and the nucleus reticularis paragigantocellularis, to prevent ascending nociceptive impulses reaching the cortex.
- Morphine produces a powerful feeling of contentment and wellbeing. Codeine does not produce euphoria and nalorphine produces dysphoria.
- Morphine and other opiates cause respiratory depression. This is mediated by a decrease in the sensitivity of the respiratory centre to pCO_2. This is the most troublesome and dangerous unwanted effect of opiates because it occurs within the analgesic dose range. Death from acute opiate poisoning is due to respiratory depression.
- Morphine suppresses the cough reflex, i.e. it is antitussive. This property does not correlate with analgesia or respiratory depression. Codeine is antitussive at sub-analgesic doses and is often used in cough medicines. Pholcodine is a modified opiate that has strong antitussive effects but little or no analgesia.
- Morphine increases tone and reduces motility in the GI tract. Peristaltic contractions are reduced, resulting in slower passage of material and increased re-absorption

of water, leading to constipation. This effect is used to treat diarrhoea. Loperamide, which is unable to cross the blood-brain barrier and so does not cause analgesia or respiratory depression, is widely used to treat diarrhoea.

- Morphine can cause nausea and vomiting on first administration, due to an action on the chemoreceptor trigger zone in the medulla. This effect is usually transient and disappears on repeat administration.
- Morphine causes pin-point pupils. This is centrally mediated and is an important diagnostic aid in opiate overdose.
- Morphine (but not other opiates) releases histamine from mast cells. This can result in itching, urticaria, hypotension, and bronchoconstriction.
- Tolerance occurs when a drug is administered repeatedly and the dose has to be increased to maintain the desired effect. Tolerance may occur with most opiate effects including analgesia and respiratory depression, but not with miosis or constipation.
- Dependence is where adaptive changes have taken place in response to repeated administration of drugs and are most clearly seen as a withdrawal syndrome when the drug is withheld or its pharmacological action blocked. Opiate withdrawal comprises physical and psychological effects. Physical effects include abdominal cramps, diarrhoea, shivering, yawning, goose bumps, anxiety, and convulsions. Psychological effects are manifest as intense craving. Physical effects typically start within 12 hours, peak between 24–72 hours, and may last up to 14 days. Psychological effects typically last much longer, sometimes years.

Opioid antagonists

Naloxone and naltrexone are opioid antagonists. They bind with high affinity at all opioid receptors (although they are less potent at δ receptors) and reverse the effects of opioid agonists, but have no effects of their own. They are used to reverse respiratory depression in opioid overdose. They precipitate withdrawal symptoms in opioid-dependent individuals. Naloxone has a short half life, so repeat injections may be necessary. Naltrexone has a longer duration of action.

Kinetic aspects

- Morphine undergoes considerable first pass metabolism. It is therefore markedly less potent when taken orally than when injected. Intravenous or intramuscular morphine is commonly used to treat severe acute pain. Oral preparations are useful in chronic pain.
- Morphine is metabolized by conjugation with glucuronic acid. Glucuronides invariably lack pharmacological activity, but unusually morphine-6-glucuronide is more active as an analgesic than morphine itself.

Other opioids

- Diamorphine (heroin): Produces a faster, more intense euphoria than morphine because of its greater lipid solubility. Metabolized in the body to morphine, therefore produces the same effects. Shorter duration of action.
- Codeine: About one-fifth the potency of morphine. Little or no euphoria and rarely addictive. Used mainly as oral analgesic, antitussive, and to treat diarrhoea.
- Pethidine: More sedative and has a more rapid onset and a shorter duration of action than morphine. Pethidine is preferred to morphine for analgesia during labour because the metabolism of morphine, but not pethidine, is dependent upon conjugation reactions that are deficient in the newborn.
- Methadone has a longer duration of action than morphine. It binds to a variety of proteins in various tissues and its slow release from these binding sites, when administration is stopped, leads to a milder abstinence syndrome than with morphine. Regular oral doses of methadone are used as a replacement strategy to wean addicts from morphine or heroin.
- Fentanyl is 80 times more potent than morphine but with a much shorter duration of action. It is widely used in patient-controlled analgesia, where a short duration of action is an advantage.

Mechanism of action

- Opioids produce their effects by acting as agonists at a family of G-protein receptors, termed opiate receptors. They mimic the effects of a family of endogenous peptide neurotransmitters, comprising enkephalins, endorphins, and dynorphins.
- There are three major classes of opioid receptors, termed μ (mu), δ (delta), and κ (kappa) receptors. Mu receptors are responsible for the spinal analgesic effects and the respiratory depression and euphoria. Endorphins and enkephalins are the endogenous neurotransmitters at these receptors. Delta receptors are responsible for the supraspinal analgesia. Enkephalins and endorphins are the endogenous neurotransmitters at these receptors. Kappa receptors contribute to analgesia at the spinal level. Dynorphins and endorphins are the endogenous neurotransmitters at these receptors. Some analgesics, e.g. pentazocine, are relatively κ selective.
- At the molecular level opioid receptors are linked to inhibition of adenylate cyclase. They also mediate opening of potassium channels (causing hyperpolarization) and prevent the opening of calcium channels (inhibiting transmitter release).

Anaesthetics

Local anaesthetics (LAs)

- LAs reversibly block the conduction of action potentials in nerve fibres. They are used clinically to produce loss of sensation when applied locally or regionally. Small-diameter nerve fibres are more readily blocked than large-diameter fibres, thus pain sensation is more readily blocked than other sensory modalities or motor nerves. In practice, block of pain sensation is usually accompanied by other sensory loss and local paralysis.
- LAs consist of an aromatic ring linked to a basic side-chain by an ester or amide bond. Those containing ester bonds (e.g. procaine, amethocaine) are metabolized by non-specific esterases and are shorter-acting than those LAs containing amide bonds (e.g. lidocaine, bupivacaine).
- Most LAs are weak bases and so are mainly (but not completely) ionized at physiological pH.

Mechanism of action

LAs block the generation and propagation of action potentials by blocking the Na+ channels responsible for the upstroke of the action potential. Many drugs exhibit 'use-dependent' block, i.e. the more channels that are active, the greater the block produced, because the LA can enter the channel more easily when the channel is open.

Routes of administration

- Surface anaesthesia, e.g. lidocaine: LA applied directly to mucous membranes (e.g. pharynx/larynx to aid intubation/endoscopy).
- Infiltration anaesthesia (most LAs): LA injected directly into the tissue (e.g. wound stitching, episiotomy).
- Intravenous regional anaesthesia, e.g. lidocaine, prilocaine: LA injected intravenously with a pressure cuff to restrict flow (e.g. for limb surgery).

- Nerve block anaesthesia (most LAs): LA injected close to nerve trunk (e.g. mandibular nerve for dentistry, brachial plexus for shoulder and arm procedures, sural nerve for ankle or foot procedures).
- Spinal anaesthesia, e.g. lidocaine: LA injected into the subarachnoid space of the spine (e.g. for caesarean section or other abdominal surgery).
- Epidural block, e.g. lidocaine, bupivacaine: LA injected into the epidural space to block nerve roots (e.g. in obstetrics).

Adverse effects of LAs

- LAs are administered in such a way as to minimize their spread. The most dangerous adverse effects result when significant concentrations reach the systemic circulation, either by absorption from the injection site or accidental injection directly into a blood vessel. Vasoconstrictors, such as adrenaline or felypressin, are sometimes added to LAs to restrict absorption into the systemic circulation.
- Fall in blood pressure due to a combination of myocardial depression and vasodilatation.
- CNS effects range from light-headedness, restlessness, and tremor, sometimes progressing to respiratory depression or convulsions.
- Urinary retention is common with spinal and epidural administration.
- Prilocaine and benzocaine can induce methaemoglobinaemia and should not be used in obstetric procedures or in neonates.

General anaesthetics

There are two main types: intravenous and inhalational.

Intravenous anaesthetics, e.g. thiopentone, propofol

- These are fast-acting, producing unconsciousness in seconds. They are used to induce anaesthesia, which is then often maintained with inhalational agents.
- Thiopentone is a barbiturate. It is very lipid-soluble and thus enters the brain quickly, producing rapid and smooth anaesthesia. Given alone, anaesthesia is of short duration (approximately 5 minutes), because as soon as the blood level begins to fall, thiopentone leaves the brain and is redistributed to other tissues. It is metabolized slowly and

therefore has a long after-effect (sedation can persist for 24 h). It has no analgesic effect and the margin between anaesthetic dose and dose causing cardiovascular and respiratory depression is narrow.

- Propofol produces rapid anaesthesia and, because it is rapidly metabolized, recovery is also rapid and with little hangover. It can produce marked bradycardia, which can be minimized with an antimuscarinic agent. It can be administered by infusion as the sole anaesthetic agent. Caution is needed when used in day surgery because of reports of delayed convulsions.
- Etomidate is similar to thiopentone, but is metabolized rapidly and thus produces less after effect. There is less hypotension than with thiopentone or propofol. It causes involuntary movements during induction. Not recommended for maintenance of anaesthesia because of the risk of adrenal suppression.

Inhalation anaesthetics, e.g. enflurane, isoflurane

- These are volatile liquids administered via calibrated vaporizers using air, oxygen, or gas mixtures as the carrier gas. Can be used for induction and maintenance, or for maintenance following induction with an intravenous agent.
- Blood: gas partition determines the rate of induction and recovery. Low blood: gas partition gives faster induction and recovery. Oil: gas partition is used as measure of fat solubility. The higher the ratio, the lower the minimum alveolar concentration (MAC) needed to maintain anaesthesia, but recovery may be delayed by accumulation of agent in fat (see Table 9.2).
- Halothane provides smooth induction and is non-irritant, but it is not analgesic. It causes a fall in BP. Associated with severe hepatotoxicity (particularly with repeated exposure).
- Isoflurane lowers BP and depresses respiration. Produces muscle relaxation and the effects of muscle relaxants are potentiated. Possibility of hepatotoxicity.
- Desflurane gives fast induction and recovery, so is popular for day surgery. May cause respiratory tract irritation, so not recommended for induction. Hepatotoxicity possible but very rare.
- Servoflurane is similar to desflurane but is more potent and is non-irritant, so can be used for induction.

Table 9.2 Characteristics of commonly used inhalational agents

Drug	Blood: gas partition	Induction recovery	Oil: gas partition	MAC (%)
Halothane	2.4	Medium	220	0.8
Isoflurane	1.4	Medium	91	1.2
Desflurane	0.4	Fast	23	6.0
Servoflurane	0.6	Fast	53	2.0

- All inhalational anaesthetics can induce malignant hyperthermia (muscle rigidity, tachycardia, hyperthermia, hypermetabolic state) in susceptible individuals.

Nitrous oxide

Nitrous oxide is a gas widely used in anaesthesia. It has low potency and is thus not suitable as a sole anaesthetic agent. It is, however, used (as a 70% mixture with oxygen) as a carrier gas for volatile anaesthetics, allowing them to be used in lower concentrations. It has fast onset (because of its low blood: gas partition) and is a good analgesic in sub-anaesthetic concentrations. A 50% mixture of nitrous oxide and oxygen is used to provide analgesia during childbirth.

Prolonged or repeated exposure to nitrous oxide can result in depression of bone marrow function.

Mechanism of action

The mechanism of action of this mixture of gases is ill understood despite their use for 150 years. However, the action seems to be dependent on the physicochemical properties of these rather inert molecules. Lipid solubility is certainly an important determinant of anaesthetic potency. More recent theories have focused on enhancing inhibitory neurotransmission or inhibiting excitatory neurotransmission by an action on receptors or ion channels. At the cellular level the effects are mainly at the level of synaptic transmission, rather than impulse conduction.

Drug dependence

Drug abuse is the non-medical use of a substance.

Dependence is defined in terms of substance use leading to clinically significant impairment or distress as manifest by three of the following:

1. Tolerance (either increased amounts of substance or diminished effects with the same amount).
2. Withdrawal (a characteristic syndrome on removal of the drug).
3. Escalating dosage.
4. Desire or attempts to reduce substance use.
5. Significant time spent on activities to obtain, use, or recover from the substance.
6. Social, recreational, or occupational activities given up because of substance use.
7. Continued use despite knowledge of physical or psychological problems caused by the substance.

Some drugs that are abused have limited dependence liability, e.g. psychotomimetics such as LSD and ecstasy.

Ethanol

- 3–5% of adult population dependent; 20–30% are 'problem drinkers'.
- Two distinct types:
  1. Type 1—consistent intake, slow onset of problem, low novelty-seeking, and high harm avoidance.
  2. Type 2—high intermittent consumption (bingeing), young, impulsive, often antisocial, high novelty-seeking, and low harm avoidance.
- Ethanol is a CNS depressant. Acute effects of talkativeness, increased confidence, and euphoria are due to disinhibition. Effects on CNS of chronic abuse include neurological degeneration and peripheral neuropathy.
- Chronic use damages the liver, progressing from fatty liver through to cirrhosis and to liver failure.

- There is a well characterized withdrawal syndrome in dependent individuals. In the early phase tremor, nausea, and sweating are apparent, which may develop to seizures. Over several days a confusional state with agitation, aggression, and sometimes hallucinations develops (delirium tremens or DTs). Benzodiazepines are used to alleviate the withdrawal syndrome.
- Excessive ethanol consumption in pregnancy can give rise to the 'fetal alcohol syndrome' (impaired fetal development, small size, abnormal facial development and other physical abnormalities, and mental retardation). Alcohol-related neurodevelopmental disorder (ARND) involves less impairment but is more common.
- Pharmacological approaches to treatment include naltreone (an opioid antagonist) and acamprosate (an antagonist at NMDA receptors—a type of receptor for excitatory amino acid neurotransmitters). Disulfiram is used as an aversion therapy in compliant individuals. Disulfiram is an inhibitor of acetaldehyde dehydrogenase (catalyses the conversion of acetaldehyde to acetate). Alone it has no effect. When ethanol is consumed, acetaldehyde concentration builds up causing flushing, tachycardia, and hyperventilation. The reaction is very unpleasant, but harmless.

Nicotine

- Nicotine is the major pharmacological constituent of tobacco, although smoked tobacco also contains carcinogenic tars and carbon monoxide. Nicotine is an agonist at nicotinic acetylcholine receptors causing neuronal excitation. Behaviourally subjects report arousal and increased alertness, with reduced anxiety and tension. Peripheral effects include tachycardia, increased BP, and increased GI motility.
- Nicotine is highly addictive. Tolerance develops to the peripheral effects, but much less so to the central effects, although desensitization of central receptors occurs.

- A well characterized withdrawal syndrome in a dependent individual includes irritability, aggressiveness, insomnia, and abdominal cramps.
- Cigarette smoking is the biggest avoidable health risk, with markedly increased risks of cancer of the lung and upper respiratory tract (largely from the tars). Increased risks of coronary heart disease, peripheral vascular disease, and chronic bronchitis are associated with long-term cigarette smoking.
- Smoking while pregnant reduces fetal growth and increases perinatal mortality. Premature delivery and spontaneous abortion are also significantly more likely in women who smoke. The carbon monoxide in cigarette smoke may contribute to these effects.
- Pharmacological strategies to help individuals give up smoking include maintenance therapy—replacing nicotine from smoking by safer methods of administration (patches, chewing gum). Bupropion is a different strategy, although the mechanism is not clear.

Opioids

- Opioids are abused for the euphoria they produce when injected or smoked. The euphoria is intense but short-lived. Heroin and morphine are the drugs most often abused. Tolerance develops quickly but the mechanism is unclear.
- A well characterized withdrawal syndrome in dependent individuals resembles influenza, with fever and sweating. Pupillary dilatation, diarrhoea, and yawning are also seen. The withdrawal syndrome can be precipitated in dependent individuals by μ-receptor antagonists and can be alleviated by μ-receptor agonists. The physical withdrawal syndrome lasts a few days, but psychological dependence can persist for months.
- Pharmacological strategies to treat opioid dependence consist of replacement oral therapy with a long-acting μ-receptor agonist, e.g. methadone, or a partial agonist, e.g. buprenorphine.

Psychostimulants

Amphetamine

- Amphetamine and related compounds, such as dextro-amphetamine (dexamphetamine) and methamphetamine, produce marked central effects (euphoria, anorexia, wakefulness, increased performance at repetitive tasks) and peripheral effects (increased BP and heart rate). The central effects last a few hours and are followed by a period of lethargy and depressed mood. They are effective orally but more rapidly absorbed from tthe nasal mucosa, so are often 'snorted'.
- Tolerance develops to the anorexia, but more slowly to the other effects. Withdrawal syndrome is much less clear than with ethanol or opiates. Binge use over a period of several days is not uncommon.

- Amphetamine and related compounds cause the release of monoamines, especially dopamine and noradrenaline, from nerve terminals.
- Repeated use of amphetamine can produce a schizophrenia-like psychosis with hallucinations and paranoid thoughts. This toxic state results in amphetamine being classified as both a CNS stimulant and a psychotomimetic.

Ecstasy

Ecstasy is an amphetamine-related compound that produces feelings more of empathy and benevolence than euphoria. It is referred to as an 'entactogen' or 'empathogen'. Peripheral effects include: increased HR and pulse, pupil dilation, jaw clenching, and teeth grinding. Adverse effects include hyperthermia and hyponatraemia (from drinking too much water). Effects of ecstasy are dependent on the release of 5-HT (serotonin). Use has been claimed to be toxic to 5-HT neurons.

Cocaine

- Produces effects similar to amphetamine but with shorter duration. Psychotomimetic effects are rare. Hydrochloride salt is snorted or used intravenously. The free base form of cocaine (crack) can be smoked, giving an effect as rapid as intravenous doses.
- Cocaine blocks the reuptake of dopamine and noradrenaline.
- The withdrawal syndrome is much less clear than for thanol or opiates. Escalated use and binging is not uncommon.
- Acute toxicity can include cardiac dysrhythmias, thrombosis, and cardiac failure. Cocaine can have marked effects on brain development *in utero*, with small brain size and neurological abnormalities. Limb malformations and sudden infant death also increase in cocaine-exposed babies.

Psychotomimetics

Produce distortions of perception, particularly visual disturbances. Can produce a persistent psychotic state. No physical withdrawal syndrome.

- LSD (lysergic acid diethylamide) is synthetic and very potent. Sometimes produces menacing or paranoid delusions ('bad trips') with 'flashbacks' occurring for months. Acts as an agonist/partial agonist at 5-HT receptors.
- Mescaline (derived from a Mexican cactus) and psilocybin (the active constituent of magic mushrooms) produce similar effects to LSD but are much less potent.
- Phencyclidine is a hallucinogenic but can also produce stimulant behaviours, like amphetamine. It is an antagonist at a subtype of excitatory amino acid receptor (called NMDA receptors).

Cannabinoids

- These are the active ingredients of the hemp plant, *Cannabis sativa*. Δ9-tetrahydrocannibinol (THC) is the major active substance. Effects include a feeling of relaxation and wellbeing and enhanced sensory awareness. Peripheral effects include tachycardia and vasodilation (particularly bloodshot eyes). Potential medicinal effects include bronchodilation, analgesia, antiemetic, antispasmodic, and lower intraocular pressure.

- Rapid absorption occurs when smoked, with much slower absorption when taken orally. It remains in the body for days.

- There are adverse effects on short-term memory and reaction times. There are concerns that cannabis may precipitate psychotic episodes, particularly in the young.
- Specific receptors for cannabis exist in the brain and periphery. Anandamide (an amide derivative of arachidonic acid) is an endogenous compound at cannabinoid receptors.

ADDITIONAL FACTS AND REVISION MATERIAL

Blood pressure regulation

- The carotid and aortic baroreceptor systems control acute changes in blood pressure via neural (and therefore instant) reflexes modulated by the vasomotor centre in the brainstem.
- The renin-angiotensin system, on the other hand, controls blood pressure in the long term. It is mediated via hormonal mechanisms and therefore takes time to exert its effect.

- ACE inhibitors reduce glomerular efferent resistance and slow down the progression of nephropathy in diabetics.
- ACTH may stimulate the release of aldosterone, but this is only an early and transient effect. ACTH is not considered a significant regulator of aldosterone release.
- The juxtaglomerular apparatus is innervated by sympathetic neurons via β_2 receptors.

CHAPTER 10

Epidemiology and Statistics

Epidemiology

Epidemiology is the study of factors that affect the health and disease of populations, and constitutes the main methodology of public health research. In clinical medicine, the doctor evaluates the patient, undertakes tests, makes a diagnosis of disease, and treats that individual patient. Epidemiology, on the other hand, regards disease as something that is distributed in the larger population and uses numbers and the relationships between the numbers (e.g. rates) to describe disease in the population.

Definitions

- The crude rate of a disease is: $\dfrac{\text{number of diseased people}}{\text{total population}}$.

  It is unrefined compared to specific rate, which is the rate in a specific subset of the population (e.g. age group, sex, or ethnic group). Rates are usually given per 100 000 of the population.

- The incidence of a disease is:

  $$\dfrac{\text{number of new cases of disease}}{\text{number of people at risk of getting disease}} .$$

  Note that the denominator may exclude certain subsets of the population to be valid; for example, to calculate the incidence of prostate cancer in a given population, all the women in that population and all the men under 40 should be excluded from the denominator. With some infectious diseases recovery means conferment of lifelong immunity such that the individual is no longer at risk of catching that disease; such individuals are also removed from the denominator. Incidence is usually applied to acute conditions such as influenza and food poisoning. The incidence of a disease may be reduced by the introduction of a new effective vaccine, but is unaltered by a new effective treatment or improved survival from the disease.

- The prevalence is all cases of a given disease per (say) 100 000 people in the population. It is commonly used to describe chronic conditions such as diabetes mellitus and hypertension. The prevalence of a disease may be reduced by the introduction of a new effective vaccine

or treatment, and increased by improved survival from the disease.

Characteristics of screening tests

Screening tests are imperfect and their limitations make it impossible for us to conclude that an abnormal test definitively signifies the presence of disease, or that a normal test means the absence of disease. The accuracy of a test is rated by applying the complex and counterintuitive principles of sensitivity and specificity, which may be translated into the more useful 'positive and negative predictive values' by taking into account the prevalence of a particular disease in the population being tested.

- Sensitivity—the ability of the test to detect every case of the disease, calculated as the probability of a positive test in

  the presence of disease or $\dfrac{\text{true positive}}{\text{true positive} + \text{false negative}}$.

  Sensitivity = 'positive in disease (PID)'. A test with a perfect sensitivity will detect all the diseased individuals, and it doesn't matter about the number of healthy people it also labels as diseased!

- Specificity—the ability of the test to exclude healthy, non-diseased individuals; that is 'negative in health (NIH)'. It is the probability of a negative test in the absence

  of disease: $\dfrac{\text{true negative}}{\text{true negative} + \text{false positive}}$. A test with a

  perfect specificity will classify all healthy individuals as negative even though it will almost certainly label some diseased people as healthy. That doesn't matter; specificity is about the healthy!

- Positive predictive value (PPV)—the probability of having the disease if the test is positive, or

  $\dfrac{\text{true positive}}{\text{true positive} + \text{false positive}}$. It is concerned with only

  the diseased people and is more clinically useful than sensitivity.

- Negative predictive value (NPV)—the probability of being disease-free if the test is negative, or

$$\frac{\text{true negative}}{\text{true negative} + \text{false negative}}$$. A NPV of 90% means

that you have a 90% chance of being normal if you have a normal test.

- Accuracy of a test—the probability that the results of the test will accurately predict the presence or absence of disease, i.e.

$$\frac{\text{true positive} + \text{true negative}}{\text{true positive} + \text{true negative} + \text{false positive} + \text{false negative}}.$$

- Generally, the more sensitive a test is for a particular disease, the higher its false-positive rate, lowering its specificity. Equally, a test with a higher specificity will usually sacrifice sensitivity by increasing its false-negative rate. This makes a highly sensitive test ideal for screening, whilst highly specific tests are best for confirmation of disease.

- Screening tests are concerned with diseases that are already present in the population; therefore they do not give information on the incidence of disease. Sensitivity and specificity are properties of the test and are not influenced by the incidence or prevalence of the disease in the population.

- An increase in the prevalence of a disease will, however, increase the PPV and reduce the NPV of a test.

Types of bias

In everyday language the term 'bias' describes a tendency towards a particular perspective, which interferes with the ability to be impartial or objective. In statistics there are several types of bias:

- Selection (or sampling) bias—there is a problem with the process of selection such that the sample is not representative of the population; for example, selecting from members of a gym to measure the prevalence of hypertension in the wider population.

- Measurement bias—the process of data gathering distorts the information, e.g. asking respondents leading questions in a questionnaire or making people obviously aware that they are being observed, which might change their behaviour.

- Confounding bias—there is a characteristic or something else associated with the factor being studied (confounder) and it cannot not be separated out whether the findings are due to the factor being studied or due to this other factor (the confounder).

- Recall bias—when subjects fail to accurately recall events.

- Experimenter expectancy bias—when the investigator's expectation is inadvertently communicated and alters the parameter being estimated.

- Late look bias—when information is collected so late that the most severe cases are less likely to be uncovered because they have died.

Types of study design

Study designs can be divided into two basic types, namely observational and experimental designs. In observational studies, the investigator is simply observing and recording what is happening or has happened; there is no treatment or intervention involved. In an experimental design there is an intervention, treatment, advice, or procedure involved and the investigator seeks to record the effect of this intervention on the outcome of interest.

Observational studies

1. Case report—this describes a single clinical subject, N = 1.
2. Case series—this describes the characteristics of a group of clinical subjects, N > 1: what they have in common; whether these subjects are different from non-diseased people; i.e. there is comparison.
3. Cross-sectional study—addresses the questions of how widespread a disease is and what risk factors are shared by sufferers. A cross-sectional study may provide prevalence but not incidence data, or causality. The results of cross-sectional studies are usually analysed using Chi square.
4. Case control study—a sample of diseased individuals is compared with disease-free people by examining them retrospectively for the presence or absence of some hypothesized risk factors. This type of study can provide some insight into causality, but not incidence or prevalence. The results of case control studies are usually presented as odds ratio (OR).
5. Cohort study—samples of disease-free individuals with a given risk factor and those without the risk factor are followed forward over time for the appearance or not of a disease. Because of its temporal sequence it can indicate causality and incidence but not prevalence. The results of cohort studies are usually presented as relative risks (RR) and absolute risks (AR).

Experimental study designs

1. Randomized controlled trial (RCT)—the participants are randomly allocated to the study and control groups, reducing the chance of bias.
2. Double-blind RCT—the blinding of the investigator removes his/her expectations in addition to random allocation of the participants.
3. Crossover study (trial)—a longitudinal study in which subjects receive a sequence of different treatments or exposures; it allows participants to receive treatment at some stage of the study and not be disadvantaged by exposure to placebo only, for example.

Descriptive statistics

Descriptive statistics provides us with a way of describing datasets so that we do not have to deal with individual data. Two key characteristics of the data allow us to achieve this, namely a measure of central tendency and a measure of spread or variation.

Measures of central tendency

1. Mean—average
2. Median—the midpoint, the 50th centile
3. Mode—the most frequent value

In a unimodal, perfectly symmetrical normal distribution, the mean, median, and mode are the same value (Figure 10.1).

Skewed curves

The distribution of a variable is said to be skewed if it is not symmetrical around the mean or median. The distribution has a positive skew if the tail of high values is longer than the tail of low values, and a negative skew if the reverse is true. It is easier to simply remember that in a positively skewed

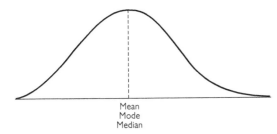

Figure 10.1 The mean, median, and mode are the same value in a unimodal normal distribution curve.

curve the tail of the curve points towards the positive direction, whereas the tail of a negatively skewed curve points in the negative direction (Figure 10.2).

Of the measures of central tendency, the mean is the most sensitive to extreme values, followed by the median, and the least sensitive is the mode. Therefore, in a skewed distribution, the mean gets dragged furthermost towards the tail of the skew, followed by the median, and lastly the mode, in that order from the tail of the curve towards the hump. A helpful pneumonic is to line them up in alphabetical order from the tail to the hump (Figure 10.2). In a skewed distribution (e.g. income), the median is a better representation of the central value than the mean.

Measures of spread or variation

- Range—the smallest interval that contains all the data, calculated by subtracting the smallest observation from the largest. It is not a good measure of spread because it uses only the two extreme measurements—the highest and the lowest values. Extreme values are most likely to shift and if measured repeatedly regress to the mean. The range provides an indication of statistical dispersion.
- Sample variance—calculated by subtracting the sample mean from each individual observation, squaring this difference, adding these differences for all observations, and dividing this total by the number of observations minus 1. Therefore, the further an observation is away from the mean, the larger its contribution to the variance, and datasets that show a large spread around the mean will have large sample variance, compared to datasets with a smaller spread.
- Standard deviation—a measure of the dispersion of a dataset, calculated as the root-mean-square deviation of its values from the mean. It is a measure of how much

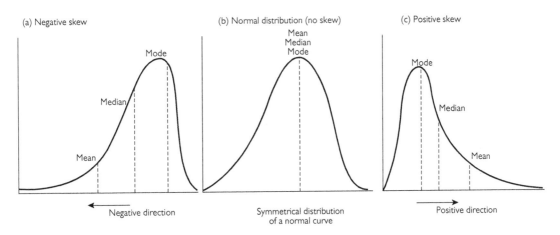

Figure 10.2 Normal and skewed distributions.

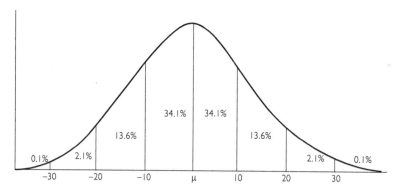

Figure 10.3 Percentage of cases that fall within ±1, ±2, and ±3 standard deviations (σ) around the mean (μ) in a normal distribution curve. These percentages are constant and are 68%, 95.5%, and 99.7% respectively.

variation there is from the 'average', or how far away the data points are from the mean. A low standard deviation indicates that the data points tend to be close to the mean, whereas a high standard deviation indicates that the data are spread out over a wide range of values.

- Interquartile range (IQR)—the difference between the third quartile and the first quartile of the data. It is a consistent estimate of the standard deviation if the population is normally distributed.

Inferential statistics

Whereas descriptive statistics simply describe what is going on in our data, inferential statistics make inferences from our data to the general population. Inferential statistics is the process by which we extend the findings from our sample to reach conclusions about the general population, and make judgements of the probability that an observed difference between groups is dependable, or might have happened by chance in the study. The exact mean (or value) of interest in the population (i.e. the true reality) is unknown but we are certain to a degree that it is somewhere around the mean (or value) obtained from the study sample. This range of possibilities is the confidence interval.

Calculating the confidence interval (CI) of the mean

$$CI = \mu \pm z \left(\frac{\sigma}{\sqrt{N}} \right)$$

where μ = mean, z = standard score, and σ = standard deviation.

z—score—is a score taken from a particular distribution with clearly known properties, by convention mean μ = 0 and standard deviation σ = 1 (that is, the measurements are in standard deviation units, therefore if z = −2 then the score is 2 standard deviations below the μ).

Standard error of the mean (SEM)

This is an indication of how well the mean of a sample estimates the mean of a population. It is measured by the standard deviation of the means of randomly drawn samples of the same size as the sample in question:

$$SEM = \frac{sd}{\sqrt{N-1}}$$

95% CI = ±2 (approximated from 1.96)

99% CI = ±2.5 (approximated from 2.58)

The most important number in the interpretation of the CI is 1.0. Unless the CI excludes 1.0, there is no difference between the groups. If the CI includes 1.0, then the difference between the groups is not significant (see Table 10.1).

Hypothesis testing

In statistics we cannot prove anything, we can only disprove things. Therefore, if you want to demonstrate that a drug works, you have to disprove the proposition that it does not work. In other words, you must prove that the proposition

Table 10.1 Examples of confidence interval values and their interpretation

Relative risk (RR)	Confidence interval (CI)	Interpretation
1.68	(1.19 – 2.32)	Significant increase in risk
1.46	(0.75 – 3.24)	Not significant, risk the same
0.71	(0.56 – 0.91)	Significant decrease in risk

that it does not work is false—a completely counterintuitive double negative approach but that is how it works! The opposite proposition of what you want is the null hypothesis (H_0) and this should be defined and stated at the outset of a study.

The p-value and type 1 (α) and 2 (β) errors

The p-value informs decision making in statistics. It is the probability of obtaining a test statistic at least as extreme as the one that was actually observed, assuming that the null hypothesis is true. It is conventionally set at 0.05 (or 5%) and if achieved in a study, the H_0 is rejected leaving us with the proposition that the opposite is true, that the drug works, for example. However, the fact that the drug worked in the study does not mean that it would work in the wider population, in which case we have made a type 1 or α error—that is, we rejected H_0 when we shouldn't have, and concluded that the drug works when it doesn't. We never know for sure whether we made a type 1 error or not; the p-value simply tells us the probability that we did, for example p = 0.01 means that there is a 1% chance that we are wrong in rejecting H_0. Furthermore, we reject H_0 or fail to reject H_0; we never accept H_0. It is similar to a jury verdict—the accused is either guilty or not guilty; the jury does not find the accused innocent. The p-value is limited in several ways, in that it does not tell us the chance that an individual patient will benefit, or the proportion of patients that will benefit, or the magnitude of such benefit for a given patient.

We make a type 2 (or β) error if we fail to reject H_0 when we should have; in other words, we conclude that the drug does not work when in actual fact it does. Clinically this is not as bad as type 1 error because people may be denied a drug that might have helped them, whereas with a type 1 error people may be taking a drug that does not help. The relationship between the power of a study and type 2 error is expressed in the equation $\beta = 1 - power$. Power is directly related to the sample size; therefore one way of reducing a type 2 error is by increasing the sample size.

Meta-analysis

This is a mathematical synthesis of the results of different studies conducted in different populations, by different investigators and at different times, to obtain a single p-value that summarizes all the studies. Put differently, it is a mathematical tool for literature review and overcomes the problems of clinicians reading the same literature and coming to subjectively different conclusions.

Correlation coefficient (r)

Correlation coefficient applies only to a linear relationship, not any other relationship, and therefore a correlation of 0 (r = 0) does not mean that there is no relationship but that there is no linear relationship. The sign simply indicates the direction of the correlation rather than the magnitude, therefore r = –0.68 is greater than r = +0.50.

Steps for drug approval (stages of clinical trials)

- Phase 1 trial—the drug is tested in a small number of healthy volunteers to test for safety.
- Phase 2 trial—establishing efficacy, dosage, and protocol for administration.
- Phase 3 trial—evaluation for efficacy and the occurrence of side effects.

Data analysis and statistical testing

The type of statistical test used for data analysis depends on the type of data generated in the study represented as scales.

Types of scales in statistics

- Nominal (or categorical) scale—for example, different groups or gender; Chi square is used for analysis if all data are nominal.
- Ordinal scale (or rank order data)—some sequence or order but without a clear value between the ranks, e.g. gold, silver, or bronze medals; hotel star system.
- Interval level data—exact and measureable differences between data points, e.g. heights, weights, or temperatures. Correlation is used if all data are interval; for combined interval and nominal data Student t-test is used.
- Ratio—this is interval data plus a true zero point below which one cannot go, e.g. temperatures measured in Kelvin scale.

CHAPTER 11

Medical Physics

Ultrasound

Ultrasound waves are longitudinal compression waves with frequencies >20 kHz. The frequency range used for medical imaging is normally between 2 MHz and 15 MHz. In obstetrics and gynaecology this is usually 2 MHz and 6 MHz for abdominal ultrasound and 7 MHz–9 MHz for transvaginal ultrasound scan. Ultrasound is the most common imaging modality in obstetrics and gynaecology.

- There are various ways that an ultrasound wave can interact with tissues, namely:
  - reflection
  - refraction
  - diffraction
  - absorption
  - scatter.
- Reflection occurs when a wave front travelling through a medium reaches an interface with another medium causing the wave front to return into the medium from which it originated (Figure 11.1). The angle at which the wave front reaches the surface equals the angle at which it will be reflected. The strength of reflection from an object, i.e. what proportion of the original wave front will be reflected, depends on the difference between the acoustic properties of the two media, known as acoustic impedance.
- Refraction occurs when a wave front travelling through a medium reaches an interface with another medium and then passes through it (Figure 11.1). If the two media have different acoustic impedance then the speed at which the wave front travels in each medium will be different. This causes a change in the direction of the wave front as it passes from one medium to another (Figure 11.1).
- Diffraction occurs when a wave encounters an obstacle that has a diameter comparable to its wavelength. This phenomenon manifests itself in the apparent bending of waves around small obstacles and the spreading out of the waves as they pass through small openings (Figure 11.2). There is a resultant change in the direction of travel of the wave. Higher-frequency waves, with a short wavelength, are rarely diffracted.

- Scatter is the combination of irregular reflection, refraction, and diffraction of a wave front in multiple directions.
- Absorption is the direct conversion of sound energy into heat as it travels though a medium.
- The above principles, combined with the acoustic properties of bone and air, limit the ability of ultrasound to image through these two media.

Generation of ultrasound wave

Ultrasound imaging uses the pulse echo principle. This is where a pulse of known speed is emitted and the time taken for the reflected echo to return is measured, assuming that the speed of sound in all tissues is 1540 ms⁻¹. An ultrasound probe consists of two elements, a transducer and a receiver. The transducer is made from materials that exhibit piezoelectric behaviour such as quartz and ceramic. When an electrical current is applied across these materials they deform mechanically with resultant changes in their thickness. Conversely, piezoelectric materials generate an electric charge when mechanically deformed. Rapid application of voltage changes across piezoelectric material is used to induce mechanical deformation, displacement of the surrounding air, and ultrasound waves. The signals picked up from the receiver are used to produce an image by converting

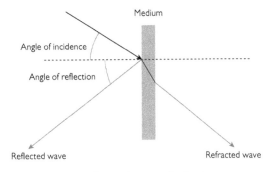

Figure 11.1 Wave front reflection and refraction.

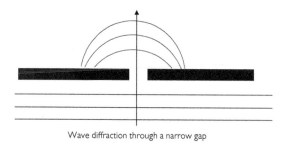

Wave diffraction through a narrow gap

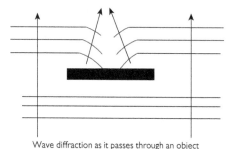

Wave diffraction as it passes through an object

Figure 11.2 Wave diffraction.
Reproduced from Arisudhan Anantharachagan, Ippokratis Sarris, Austin Ugwumadu, *Revision notes for the MRCOG Part 1*, 2011, Figure 12.2, page 350, with permission from Oxford University Press.

mechanical deformation into voltage changes. Modern probes contain an array of transmitters and receivers making it possible to construct a grey-scale two-dimensional image on a screen.

- Resolution is the ability to distinguish two adjacent points from each other. Most ultrasound machines can achieve a maximum resolution of 0.3–1 mm (depending on the frequency and axis in question).
- Frame rate is the frequency at which an imaging device produces unique consecutive images (frames) and is expressed in frames per second. There is a trade-off between resolution of an image and frame rate, since the higher the resolution, the longer it takes for the ultrasound probe to generate an image, limiting the maximum achievable frame rate. This becomes relevant when imaging fast-moving objects like the fetal heart.
- Acoustic intensity is a measure of the energy flux over a certain time period (or sound power) through a unit area. The SI unit is watts per square metre (W/m2).
- Although ultrasound is considered to be a relatively safe imaging modality, it can still produce biological effects in three ways:
  - cavitation
  - micro-streaming
  - heating.

- Cavitation is the production, growth, oscillation, and decay of small gas bubbles under the influence of an ultrasound wave, and micro-streaming is the formation of small, local fluid circulations. These effects can occur intracellularly or extracellularly.

Three-dimensional (3D) ultrasound imaging consists of a sweep of multiple two-dimensional scans in parallel and then reconstruction of a third Z-plane, creating a volume box containing three-dimensional voxels instead of two-dimensional pixels. The addition of time as a fourth dimension gives rise to real-time 3D scanning, or 4D scanning.

Doppler ultrasonography

The Doppler effect is based on the principle that reflected or scattered ultrasound waves from a moving interface will undergo a frequency shift, called a Doppler shift. This is the change in frequency of a wave as observed by an observer moving relative to the source of the wave. The Doppler shift frequency is the difference between the transmitted and received frequencies.

The Doppler effect is used in medicine to detect and measure blood flow (red blood cells act as the reflectors). The shift frequency depends on the frequency of the insonating wave, the velocity of the moving blood, and the angle between the sound beam and the direction of movement of the blood.

- There are three types of Doppler techniques in ultrasound machines:
  - pulse
  - power
  - colour.
- Pulse Doppler allows a sampling gate to be positioned over a vessel visualized on the grey-scale image. The amplitude of the signal is approximately proportional to the number of moving red blood cells. Pulse Doppler provides information on direction and velocity of blood flow along with flow characteristics. Therefore, it is angle dependent with flow perpendicular to the transducer being difficult to detect.
- Power Doppler is also known as energy or amplitude Doppler. It allows detection of a larger range of Doppler shifts and thus better visualization of small vessels. However, this occurs at the expense of information on direction and velocity. The advantages of power Doppler include the following: it is not angle dependent; it has a higher sensitivity to detect low flow or small blood vessels; and it has better penetration.
- Colour Doppler provides an estimate of the mean velocity of flow within a vessel by colour-coding the information. The flow direction is assigned red colour for flow towards the transducer and blue colour for flow away from it. Unlike power Doppler, colour Doppler provides information on flow and velocity of blood. However, it has poor temporal resolution and is angle dependent.

Radiation

Ionizing radiation

Radiation can be broadly divided into ionizing and non-ionizing radiation.

Ionization is the process of converting an atom or molecule into an ion by adding or removing charged particles. A positively charged ion is produced when an atom or molecule releases an electron, whilst a negatively charged ion is produced when an atom receives an electron. Radioactive decay is the process by which an unstable atomic nucleus spontaneously loses energy by emitting ionizing particles and radiation. It is impossible to predict when a given atom will decay (i.e. it is a stochastic process). The SI units of radioactive decay activity are the becquerel (Bq), defined as one decay per second, and the curie (Ci), with 1 Ci = 3.7×10^{10} Bq. The half life is the time taken for the activity of a given amount of a radioactive substance to decay to half of its initial value.

- Ionizing radiation produced by radioactive decay includes:
  - alpha (α) radiation
  - beta (β) radiation
  - gamma (γ) radiation.
- Alpha particles are emitted from the nucleus of an atom and consist of two neutrons and two protons. They are heavily ionizing with a high mass and high energy but low depth of penetration. They can act as a power source for cardiac pacemakers.
- Beta particles are divided into beta minus ($\beta-$) and beta plus ($\beta+$) particles. A $\beta-$ particle is an electron that arises from $\beta-$ decay of a neutron, whilst a $\beta+$ particle is a high-energy positron (same mass as an electron but with a positive charge) arising from $\beta+$ decay of a neutron.
- Gamma rays are high-frequency (>1019 Hz) electromagnetic waves. They can be produced by radioactive decay, fusion, or fission. Gamma rays are used for sterilization of medical equipment, gamma knife surgery, and gamma-emitting radioisotopes in nuclear medicine (e.g. technetium-99m). Shielding from gamma rays requires a large amount of mass (e.g. lead), whilst for alpha particles a single sheet of paper would suffice.
- X-rays are a form of electromagnetic radiation with a wavelength in the range of 10 to 0.01 nm. They differ from gamma rays only in their origin, since electrons emit them. A measure of an X-ray's ionizing ability is the roentgen. One roentgen represents the amount of radiation required to create one electrostatic unit of charge of each polarity in one cubic centimetre of dry air. The gray (Gy) and the rad are measures of the absorbed dose of ionizing radiation. One Gy is defined as the amount of radiation required to deposit one joule of energy in one kilogram of matter. One rad is equal to 1 Gy. A measure

of the biological effect of radiation on human tissue, called the equivalent dose, is measured in sievert (Sv) units or a roentgen equivalent man (rem). One Sv = 100 rem. As an illustration, the ionizing radiation threshold dose for fetal malformation is 100–200 mGy and the ionizing radiation dose for permanent sterility is 3500–6000 mGy in men and 2500–6000 mGy in women. For comparison, the absorbed dose of ionizing radiation from an abdominal X-ray is 4.2 mGy and for a chest X-ray is <0.01 mGy.

- Ionizing radiation can be used for the management of both malignant and non-malignant conditions in the form of radiation therapy. Radiation causes DNA damage by direct or indirect ionization of the atoms that make up the DNA chain. Oxygen is a potent radiosensitizer and therefore tumour cells in hypoxic environments are more resistant to radiation damage. This is common for solid tumours that can outgrow their blood supply and thus be in a low-oxygen environment. In order to allow normal cells time to recover between treatments, the method of fractionation is employed when administering radiation therapy. This also helps with treatment response, since tumour cells that are in a radio-resistant phase of the cell cycle during the radiation exposure are allowed to cycle into a more sensitive phase for the next dose. Furthermore, fractionation allows time for re-oxygenation of hypoxic tumour cells between treatments, thus increasing their sensitivity to the subsequent dose. Sometimes drugs can be administered that are radiosensitizing, such as cisplatin.
- Ionizing radiation is also used in the field of nuclear medicine, where radioactive isotopes may be administered internally. These radionuclides are atoms with an unstable nucleus and their radioactive decay emits ionizing radiation, which is then captured by a gamma camera. This is useful both for imaging (e.g. positron emission tomography) and for treatment (e.g. ingestion of iodine-131 (I^{131}) for hyperthyroidism). Compared to other forms of imaging that predominantly show tissue anatomy, nuclear medicine imaging may reveal the physiological function of a tissue or an organ system.

Non-ionizing radiation

Non-ionizing radiation refers to any type of electromagnetic radiation that does not carry enough energy per quantum to ionize atoms or molecules. This includes magnetic resonance imaging (MRI) and light amplification by stimulated emission of radiation (LASER).

Magnetic resonance imaging (MRI)

MRI relies on the fact that spinning nuclei produce or absorb radio waves. The frequency of these radio waves depends on the magnetic field that they are in, and their energy state. Within the MRI machine a radio frequency (RF) transmitter is turned on briefly to produce an electromagnetic field. These align atomic nuclei within the body tissues, causing them to produce a rotating electromagnetic field. Different RF fields will align different nuclei, but the one most commonly chosen is that for hydrogen (i.e. a single proton) since that is the most common nucleus in the body. After the field is turned off, the nuclei revert to their original state and the difference in energy between the two states is released as a photon, which is detected by the MRI machine. During application of the RF fields, nuclei gain energy. Once the field is turned off, this energy is dissipated to the surrounding lattice and the nuclei revert to their original energy state. The time taken for this is called the spin-lattice relaxation time (T_1). Fluids have a long T_1, whilst structured tissues have a short T_1. In T_1-weighted MRI images, the output is set so that fluid-containing tissues are dark whilst fat-containing tissues are bright. Once the RF fields are off, the nuclei cease to be aligned and there is an increased lack of synchronization. This is described by the spin-spin relaxation time (T_2). In T_2-weighted images, water and fluid-containing tissues are bright whilst fat-containing tissues are dark. Tesla (T) is the SI unit for magnetic field. Most magnets in medical MRI equipment produce a magnetic field of 0.5 to 3 T.

Light amplification by stimulated emission of radiation (LASER)

LASER is a type of electromagnetic radiation. An electron can transit to other energy levels by absorbing or releasing energy accordingly. Transition from a lower to a higher energy level requires absorption of photons, whilst transition from a higher to a lower energy level requires photons to be released. During this transition, the energy of the photon absorbed or released governs the wavelength of the light that is absorbed or emitted. In laser devices, the transitions of the electrons are purposefully stimulated by other photons, causing a specific stimulated photon emission from the excited atoms. The resultant beam is monochromatic and through a series of mirrors and lenses it is also perfectly parallel and highly focused. Therefore, energy is concentrated in a very small area causing very high local temperatures. Thus, in brief, a laser device comprises of an optical resonator and a gain medium. Lasers can be of any state including gas, liquid, solid, plasma, and semiconductor.

A laser beam can cause thermal destruction of tissues. This effect depends on the laser's wavelength, its power, the time duration of the application, and the tissue properties. Laser thermal injury can lead to coagulation, which is produced by desiccation, blanching, and a shrinking of the tissues through denaturation of proteins and collagen. This effect can be used for haemostatic purposes. If the settings are altered, then volatilization can occur. At temperatures above 100°C various tissue constituents disappear as smoke. A cutting effect is obtained when the volatilization zone is narrow with coagulation necrosis occurring at the edges of this zone. Apart from thermal effects, a laser beam can also cause mechanical effects as a result of cavitation and explosive vaporization.

Electrosurgery

Electrosurgery is the application of high-frequency electric current (100 kHz–5 MHz) to tissue to incise/excise, coagulate, desiccate, or fulgurate. It uses alternating current (AC) to directly heat the tissues. In tissues, electric conduction is due to interstitial fluid.

Electrodes can be monopolar with a high-power unit (400 W) generating a high-frequency current, bipolar with a low-power unit (50 W), or tripolar. There are four electrosurgical modalities. Cutting occurs when a high power density is applied to vaporize the water content of the tissue. Coagulation uses waveforms with lower average power to achieve haemostasis. Desiccation occurs when the electrode touches the tissue but the amount of generated heat is lower than that required for cutting. The tissue surface and some of the tissue more deep to the probe dries out and forms a dry patch of dead tissue. When the electrode is held away from the tissue, the air gap between the electrode and the tissue becomes ionized. Consequently, an electric arc is discharged and superficial tissue burning occurs. This is referred to as fulgaration.

Electrocautery is the process of destroying tissue using heat conduction. It uses direct current (DC) to produce heat, leading to cauterization.

Index

191